Progress in Drug Research

Vol. 57

Edited by Ernst Jucker, Basel

Authors
Pushkar N. Kaul and Balawant S. Joshi
E. Domingo, A. Mas, E. Yuste, N. Pariente,
S. Sierra, M. Gutiérrez-Rivas and
L. Menéndez-Arias
Doreen Ma
Chaman Lal Kaul and Poduri Ramarao
Jay A. Glasel

Springer Basel AG

Editor

Dr. E. Jucker
Steinweg 28
CH-4107 Ettingen
Switzerland
e-mail: jucker.pdr@bluewin.ch

Visit our PDR homepage: http://www.birkhauser.ch/books/biosc/pdr

ISBN 978-3-0348-9512-5 ISBN 978-3-0348-8308-5 (eBook)
DOI 10.1007/978-3-0348-8308-5

Originally published by Birkhäuser Verlag 2001
Softcover reprint of the hardcover 2001

Member of the BertelsmannSpringer Publishing Group
Printed on acid-free paper produced from chlorine-free pulp. TCF ∞
Cover design and layout: Gröflin Graphic Design, Basel

ISBN 3-7643-6266-9
9 8 7 6 5 4 3 2 1

Contents

Alternative medicine: Herbal drugs and their critical appraisal – Part II 1
By Pushkar N. Kaul and Balawant S. Joshi

Virus population dynamics, fitness variations and the control of viral disease: an update 77
By Esteban Domingo, Antonio Mas, Eloisa Yuste, Nonia Pariente, Saleta Sierra, Mónica Gutiérrez-Rivas and Luis Menéndez-Arias

Applications of yeast in drug discovery 117
By Doreen Ma

Sympathetic nervous system and experimental diabetes: role of adrenal medullary hormones 163
By Chaman Lal Kaul and Poduri Ramarao

From outer to inner space: Traveling along a scientific career from astrochemistry to drug research 181
By Jay A. Glasel

Index Vol. 57 247

Index of titles, Vol. 1–57 253

Author and paper index, Vol. 1–57 269

Foreword by the Editor

This 57th volume of the series *Progress in Drug Research* presents five extensive reviews which all highlight latest insights and discoveries in drug research and application. The first article is devoted to herbal drugs and summarizes the existing chemical, pharmacological, toxicological and clinical data of the three of them, namely Kava-kava, garlic and ginger. These natural products have been, and still are, widely used all over the world and the available data indicate their usefulness on the one hand and the need for further extensive evaluation on the other. The following article provides an overview of the viral quasispecies and emphasises the resistance of human immunodeficiency virus and some human DNA viruses to antiviral agents. This review is of particular interest in view of the rapid growth of drug resistance which is becoming one of the major problems of human health and therapy of many life threatening diseases. The yeast *Saccharomyces cerevisiae* is probably the best-studied eukaryotic organism, and its experimental tractability, combined with the remarkable conservation of gene function throughout evolution, makes yeast an ideal model genetic organism. Identification of antifungal targets suitable for drug development is crucial for elucidation of mechanisms of action of antifungal agents. In the fourth article, the role of the sympathetic nervous system in experimental diabetes is described and the ability of various drugs and pharmacological agents to produce hyperglycemia in experimental animals for screening new chemical entities and differentiating the modes of action of these agents is emphasised. Of great interest is the last article by Jay Glasel since it describes an unusual career of a research scientist whose activities embraced physical chemistry, biophysical chemistry, molecular pharmacology, immunology, biochemistry, molecular biology and biology, leading, finally, to the present occupation: interaction of drugs with gene expression.

All of these reviews contain extensive bibliographies, thus enabling the interested reader to have easy access to the original literature. The various indices facilitate the use of these monographs and also help to use PDR as an encyclopedic source of information in the complex and fast-growing field of drug research.

The series *Progress in Drug Research* was founded in 1958/59. In the 42 years of its existence, drug research has undergone drastic changes, but the original purpose of these monographs remained unchanged: dissemination of information on actual trends, discussion of crucial points and creation of new prospects for future drug design. The Editor is anxious to maintain the high standard of PDR and is grateful to the authors for their willingness to undertake the hard work of writing comprehensive review articles for the benefit of all involved with drug research. It is their high qualification and experience on which the success of these monographs is based.

In ending this foreword, I would like to thank the authors for their contributions, the members of the Board of Advisors for their help and advice and the reviewers for improving these monographs. Last but not least, I am greatly indebted to Birkhäuser Publishers and in particular to Daniela Brunner, a biologist, for her critical attitude and active help with scientific and also technical aspects of individual articles. Ruedi Jappert, Bernd Luchner, Eduard Mazenauer and Gregor Messmer have contributed their vast experience and intimate technical knowledge. My sincere thanks are also due for their personal engagement and for the rewarding, harmonious cooperation.

My very special thanks go to Mr. Hans-Peter Thür, Birkhäuser Publishing's CEO. For the decades of our cooperation, Mr. Thür gave PDR and its Editor his full support and he never ceased to give this series impulses which go far beyond his function as CEO. It is due to Mr. Thür's encouragement that I continue with great enthusiasm with the editorship of PDR.

Basel, September 2001 Dr. E. Jucker

Progress in Drug Research, Vol. 57 (E. Jucker, Ed.)

Alternative medicine: Herbal drugs and their critical appraisal – Part II

By Pushkar N. Kaul[1] and Balawant S. Joshi[2]

[1]Clark Atlanta University
223 J. P. Brawley Street, SW
Atlanta, GA 30314, USA
<pkaul@cau.edu>

[2]230 Ashbrook Dr.
Athens, GA 30605-3954, USA
<bsjoshi@prodigy.net>

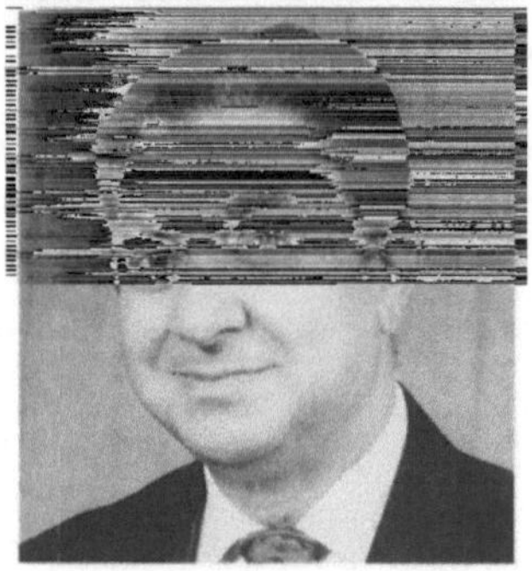

Pushkar N. Kaul

Pushkar N. Kaul was born in Kashmir, India. He earned his B.Sc. and M.Sc. degrees in pharmaceutical sciences from Banaras University, his Doctorate from the University of California Medical Center at San Francisco, and I.E.M. from Graduate Schools of Education and Business Administration of Harvard University.
Having received over a dozen awards for academic and research excellence, Professor Kaul's research contributions include his pioneering work in the field of preclinical drug discovery from marine natural products, clinical pharmacology of psychotropic drugs, and drug metabolism.

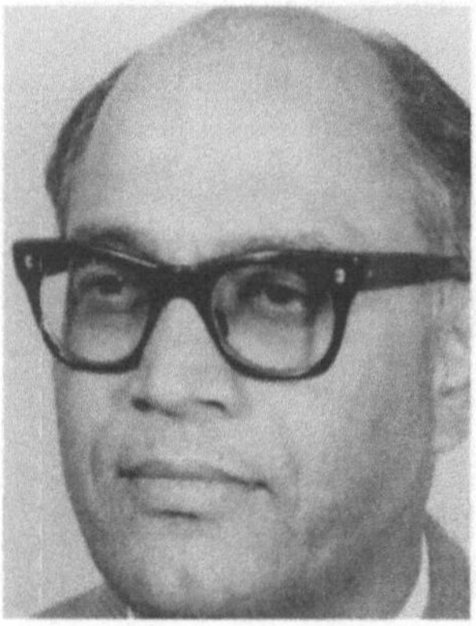

Balawant S. Joshi

was born in Jamkhandi (Karnataka State), India. He received his B.Sc. and Ph.D. (Tech) degrees from the University Department of Chemical Technology, Bombay. For further studies he went to King's College, Cambridge (UK), where he obtained Ph.D. and Sc.D. degrees in chemistry. Dr. Joshi worked as a scientist in the National Chemical Laboratory, Poona, and served as head of the Natural Products Chemistry group at the CIBA Research Centre, Bombay. For the past 18 years he has been a research scientist at the Institute for Natural Products Research, University of Georgia. He has used proton, carbon-13 NMR and mass-spectral techniques in the structure determination of many novel alkaloids, di- and triterpenoids, and oxygen heterocyclics. He has published over 200 research papers on natural products and synthesis.

Summary

The availability of herbal products as "over-the-counter" drugs and their increasing usage in the US and Canada have caused concern at the US FDA, since these products are not currently monitored for their safety, efficacy and quality. Reliable information on these aspects of the products is not available. Most of the clinical trials carried out to date have been lacking in scientific design, data collection and interpretation, and systematic toxicological evaluation. A critical review of the existing data on three of the widely used herbs and their products is presented. Of the three herbs, garlic and ginger, through both experimental and clinical data, as well as their liberal consumption by man over millennia, appear to be very safe for therapeutic use. However, further and large-scale, well-designed clinical investigations are needed to establish their efficacy before they can enter the mainstream drug market of North America. It is hoped that this review will equip the physicians and interested biomedical scientists with a comprehensive summary of the total information available to date on the herbs described.

Contents

1	Introduction	4
2	Kava-kava	5
2.1	Chemistry	6
2.1.1	Yangonins	7
2.1.2	Methysticins	8
2.1.3	Kavains	10
2.1.4	Chalcones and flavanones	13
2.1.5	Conjugated dieneketones	14
2.1.6	Kava alkaloids	14
2.2	Analysis and quality control	16
2.3	Pharmacology	17
2.4	Mechanisms of action	19
2.5	Clinical studies	22
2.6	Adverse reactions	23
3	Garlic	24
3.1	Chemistry	25
3.1.1	Alliin and alk(en)ylcysteine sulfoxides	26
3.1.2	γ-Glutamyl peptides	27
3.1.3	Dipeptides	29
3.1.4	Allicin and other thiosulfinates	29
3.1.5	Ajoenes and vinyldithiins	29
3.1.6	Organosulfides	30
3.1.7	Organoselenium compounds	30
3.1.8	Miscellaneous compounds	31
3.2	Analysis and quality control	33
3.3	Pharmacology	34
3.3.1	Cardiovascular effects	35
3.3.2	Anticancer potential	36
3.3.3	Immunomodulation	37
3.3.4	Enzyme inhibition	37
3.3.5	Other activities	38
3.4	Clinical studies	39
3.4.1	Drug-drug interactions	42
4	Ginger	43
4.1	Chemistry	44
4.1.1	Essential oils	44
4.1.2	Gingerols	48
4.1.3	Gingerdiones	49
4.1.4	Gingediols	49
4.1.5	Gingesulfonic acid	51
4.1.6	Shogaols	51

4.1.7	Diarylheptanoids	52
4.1.8	Miscellaneous compounds	55
4.2	Analysis and quality control	57
4.3	Pharmacology	57
4.3.1	Gastrointestinal activity	58
4.3.2	Anti-inflammatory activity	58
4.3.3	Anticancer activity	59
4.3.4	Other activities	60
4.3.5	Mechanisms of action	61
4.4	Toxicity	62
4.5	Clinical studies	63
	References	65

Key words

Herbal, kava, garlic, ginger, kavalactones, yangonins, methysticins, kavains, chalcones, flavanones, alkaloids, allicin, alliin, thiosulfinates, organosulfur- organoselenium compounds, gingerols, shogaols, gingediones, diarylheptanoids, analysis and quality control, pharmacology, clinical studies, antidepressant, anxiolytic, antioxidants, hyperlipidemia, hypercholesteremia, anticancer, anti-emetic, enzyme inhibition, clinical trials, drug-drug interactions

Glossary of abbreviations

^{1}HNMR, ^{13}CNMR, proton and carbon-13 nuclear magnetic resonance; IR, infra-red; TLC, thin-layer chromatography; HPLC, high-pressure liquid chromatography; ORD, optical rotatory dispersion; GC, gas chromatography; MS, mass spectrometry; FAB, fast bombardment; ACE, angiotensin converting enzyme; ATP, adenosinetriphosphate; DNA, deoxyribonucleic acid; 5-HT, serotonin; GABA, γ-aminobutyric acid; NE, norepinephrine; DA, dopamine; NMDA, N-methyl-D-aspartate; CYP, cytochrome P_{450}; PAF, platelet activating factor; FDA, Federal Food and Drug Administration; NCCAM, National Center for Complementary and Alternative Medicine; NIH, The National Institutes of Health; BP, British pharmacopaeia; COX, cyclooxygenase; LOX, 5-lipoxygenase; PGE-2, prostaglandin E2; LT-B4, leukotriene B4.

1 Introduction

The use of herbs to alleviate pain and pestilence is as old as mankind itself, but it has now been dubbed as one of the alternative therapies in the allopathic system of medicine. Our previous review summarized a critical assessment of various alternative therapeutic modalities [1a]. A literature survey of the chemistry, pharmacology, clinical studies and toxicology of four of the most commonly used herbs, along with their limitations as well as their potential in allopathic medicine, was published more recently [1b].

The allopathic community in the United States (US) is being confronted with the dilemma of public and political pressures to endorse the use of herbal medicine on one hand, and the lack of quality control and valid clinical assessment data on the other. The US Congress recently converted the relatively small Office of Alternative Medicine, created in 1995, into the National Center for Complementary and Alternative Medicine (NCCAM) under the umbrella of the National Institutes of Health (NIH). The NCCAM is charged with the clinical evaluation of all types of alternative therapies, including herbal medicine, through currently acceptable, well-controlled studies. It is particularly encouraging that the NCCAM has lately been receiving appreciable funding to carry out its mission.

This review summarizes the known chemical, pharmacological and clinical characterizations of three herbs, namely kava, garlic and ginger.

2 Kava-kava

Piper methysticum Forster (meaning intoxicating pepper, family Piperaceae, common names Kava-kava, awa, hereafter referred to as kava) is a perennial shrub resembling bamboo. The plant is endemic to Polynesia, including the Sandwich or Hawaiian Islands, and to other South Sea Islands where it plays an important cultural role. Kava rhizome extract has been traditionally used as a beverage and is claimed in folk medicine to have many beneficial health effects, including soothing of nerves and inducing relaxation and sleep. Fermented liquor made from the upper portion of the rhizomes, known as "kava" or "yaqona", is used in feasts and rituals as an intoxicating drink [1].

In 1616 the Dutch explorers Jacob Le Maire and William Schouten observed the ritualistic consumption of the kava plant by natives of the French Hoorn Islands. Wallis and Futuna, later travelers in the Pacific region, provided a wealth of detail on this highly valued and widely used pepper plant [2]. Captain James Cook, who observed the use of kava in his world voyage of 1768–1771, thought that its effects resembled those of opium [3]. Lewis Lewin, a pioneer pharmacologist in the field of mind-altering drugs, referred to it as a narcotic sedative but noted that these effects followed a period of quiet euphoria. Currently, kava is considered a psychoactive and a muscle-relaxing anxiolytic agent similar to the synthetic benzodiazepines, e.g., Valium [4]. Kava promotes relaxation and sociability, but its effects are very different from those of either alcohol or synthetic tranquilizers. It is claimed that kava does not give a hangover or cause dependency or addiction. Kava has been found valuable in the treatment of neuralgic pain in the facial trigeminal nerve, tooth-, ear- and ocular-aches, and reflex neuralgia. It has also been claimed to be beneficial in treating anorexia, gonorrhoea, vaginitis, leucorrhoea, nocturnal incontinence and ailments of the urino-genital tract. Other claims refer to its local anaesthetic, aphrodisiac, diuretic, anti-rheumatic and bronchodilatory effects [5].

In the 1950s and 1960s, two teams of German scientists, headed by H.J. Meyer in Freiburg and R. Hänsel in Berlin, found that the various activities of the kava plant were due to some 15 different kavapyrones or kavalactones. German Commission E, the group responsible for evaluating the safety and efficacy of herbal medicine, reviewed the data on kava and in 1990 approved its use for conditions such as nervous anxiety, stress and restlessness. In Europe, it is frequently marketed as an anxiolytic [6].

2.1 Chemistry

Chemical analysis of the kava roots shows that the fresh material on average contains 80% water. The dried root consists of ~ 43% starch, 20% fibers, 12% water, 3.2% carbohydrates, 3.6% proteins, 3.2% minerals and 15% kavalactones. The lactone content varies between 3 to 20% of the dry roots, depending on the age of the plant. Kava resin containing the biologically active lactones can be extracted with organic solvents. The constituents of the resin fall into the general categories of arylethylene-pyrones, chalcones, flavanones and conjugated dieneketones and alkaloids [7].

It appears that most of the biological activity is present in the water-insoluble nonpolar kavalactones extracted by organic solvents. The chemical investigations of kava resin in the past 100 years have been laborious and controversial, especially while identifying the pharmacologically active constituents. In 1857, Cuznet, a pharmacist in the French navy, isolated a crystalline substance "kavahine" [8] while at about the same time Gobley isolated a compound named "methysticin" [9]. Both these compounds appeared to be impure but the major component was identical with methysticin. Borsche et al. [10–21] isolated kavain, methysticin, dihydrokavain and dihydromethysticin. Table 1 gives a list of the isolated kavalactones and their physical properties.

2.1.1 Yangonins

The fully unsaturated 4-methoxy-α-pyrone yangonin (**1**) was isolated by Riedel in 1904 and its name was given by Lewin [22]. By treatment with alcoholic alkali, yangonin gave yangonic acid (**10**) which on heating afforded yangonol (**11**). Although Borsche interpreted correctly the structures of many of the compounds of kava resin, he failed to assign the correct structure for yangonin [10]. Based on degradation and synthetic studies, he proposed a γ-pyrone structure 12 [8, 13]. The correct structure (**1**) for yangonin was assigned by Chmielewska et al. [23] based on UV and IR spectral studies. Bu'Lock and Smith [24] reported an unambiguous synthesis of **1** by the condensation of *p*-methoxybenzaldehyde and 4-methoxy-6-methyl-α-pyrone in the presence of magnesium methoxide. 11-Methoxyyangonin (**2**) was isolated from *P. methysticum* and 11-methoxy-12-noryangonon (**6**) was isolated from a Piper species of New Guinea. Hänsel et al. [25] confirmed structures **2** and **6** by synthesis. 12-Noryangonin (12-*O*-demethylyangonin, 4'-hydroxy-5,6-dehydrokavain) was isolated from the whole plant *Anaphalis adanta* DC.

Structure **3** was assigned with a *trans*-configuration of the side-chain double bond based on ^{1}H NMR and mass spectral evidence and its conversion to the methyl ether yangonin (**1**) [26]. The isolation of yangonin from the kava roots and assignments of the ^{1}H NMR spectra have been reported [27, 28] while Harris et al. [29] accomplished its synthesis. Paulino et al. [30] carried out both the isolation and synthesis of **1**. Its X-ray crystal structure was determined by Engel et al. [31]. Yangonin and 5,6,7,8-tetrahydroyangonin (**9**) were extracted by supercritical-fluid extraction of kava roots with CO_2 containing 15% EtOH at 60 °C and 250 atm. for 1 h, 350 atm. for 1 h and 450 atm. for 1 h, and identified by GC-70eV EIMS. Tetrahydroyangonin (**9**) and the 11-methoxyl derivative (**9A**) have been isolated from *Aniba gigantifolia* [33]. A reversed-phase HPLC method has been developed for the isolation of yangonin and 12-demethoxyyangonin [34]. The identification of the lactones **1**,

Table 1.
Naturally occurring lactones from kava

Name	Color	mp	$[\alpha]_D$	λmax mμ
Yangonin	Greenish-yellow (blue fluor.)	153–154°		217, 260, 357
11-Methoxyyangonin	Yellow	162–164°		
11-Methoxy-12-noryangonin		268° (dec.)		
7,8-Dihydroyangonin				
5,6,7,8-Tetrahydroyangonin				
5,6-Dihydroyangonin				
10-Methoxyyangonin				
11-Hydroxyyangonin				
Methysticin	White	139–140°	+95°	206, 226, 260, 305
7,8-Dihydromethysticin	White	117–118°	+20.7°	233, 287
-"- Racemic	White	110–111°		
10-Methoxymethysticin				
5,6-Dehydromethysticin	Yellow	233–234°		221, 250, 364
Kavain	White	105–106°	+105°	244, 281, 291
-,,- Racemic		146–147°		
7,8-Dihydrokavain(Marindinin)	White	56–58°	+ 30°	235, 343
-,,- Racemic		73–74°		
5,6-Dehydrokavain	Greeenish	138–140°		208, 230, 255, 343
7,8-Dihydro-11-hydroxy-12-methoxykavain				230, 280
5,6-Dehydro-12-hydroxy-11-methoxykavain				
5-Hydroxykavain				
7,8-Dihydro-11,12-dimethoxykavain				205, 232, 275
7,8-Dihydro-5-hydroxykavain				228, 270

2, 11-hydroxyyangonin (**4**), 10-methoxyyangonin (**5**), 7,8-dihydroyangonin (**7**), 5,6-dihydroyangonin (**8**) and (**9**) from kava extracts has also been accomplished by electrospray HPLC-MS [35].

2.1.2 Methysticins

The first substance to be isolated from kava was methysticin (also known as kavatin, kavahin, kanakin). Pomeranz [36] undertook the chemical investigation after the original isolation by Cuznet [8] and proposed structure **17**,

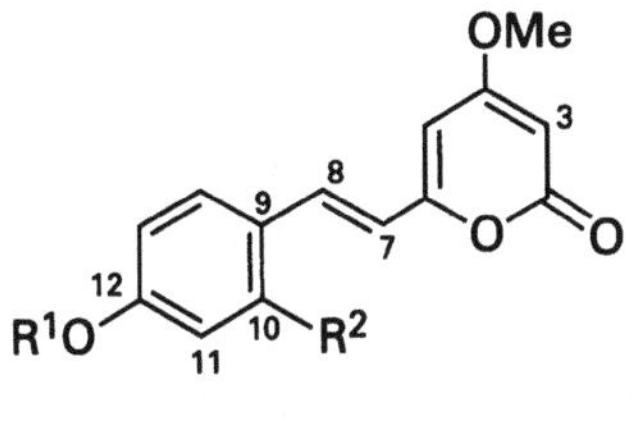

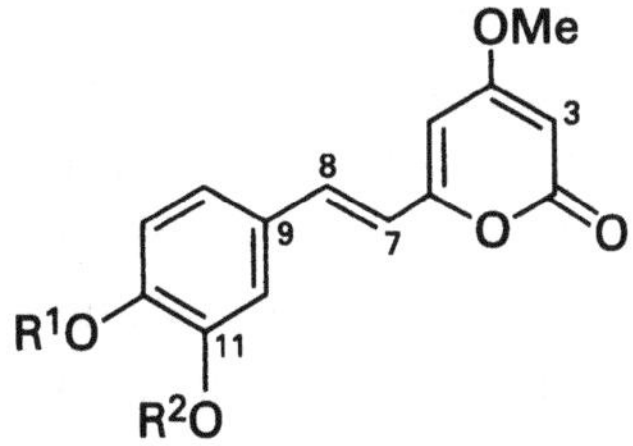

Yangonin (**1**) R^1 = Me, R^2 = H
12-Noryangonin (**3**) R^1, R^2 = H
10-Methoxyyangonin (**5**) R^1 = Me, R^2 = OMe

11-Methoxyyangonin (**2**) R^1, R^2 = Me
11-Hydroxyyangonin (**4**) R^1 = Me, R = H
11-Methoxy-12-noryangonin (**6**) R^1 = H, R^2 = Me

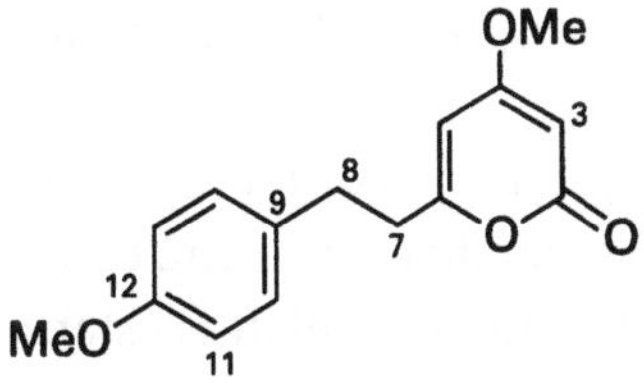

7,8-Dihydroxyangonin (**7**)

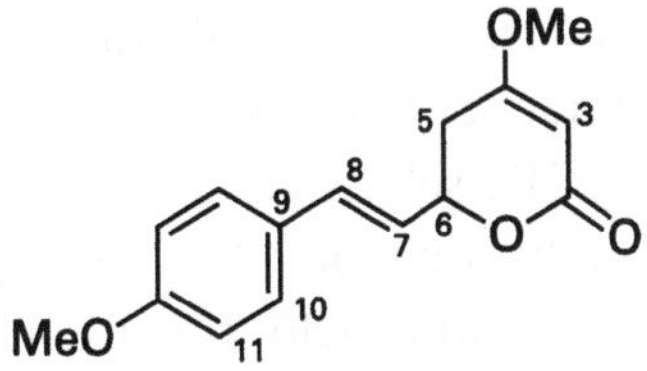

5,6-Dihydroxyyangonin (**8**)

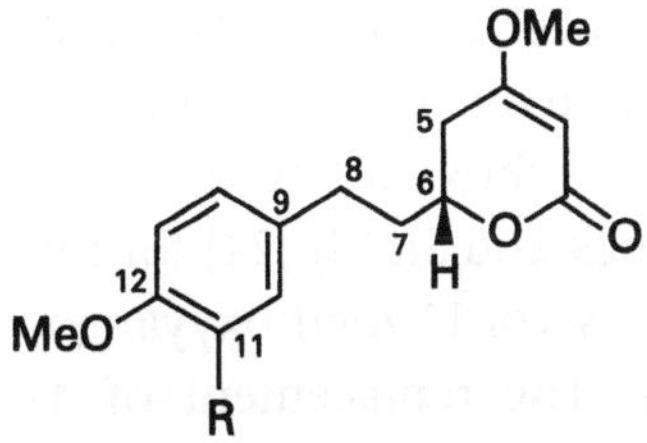

5,6,7,8-Tetrahydroyangonin (**9**) R = H
11-Methoxy-5,6,7,8-tetrahydroyangonin (**9A**) R = OMe

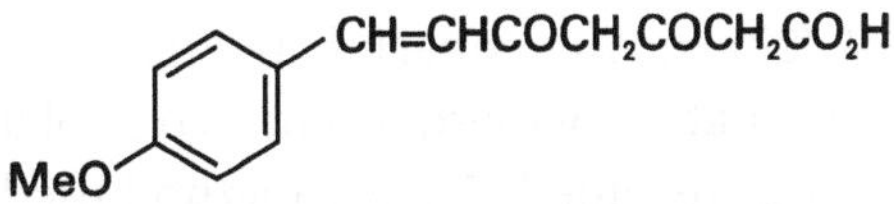

Yangonic acid (**10**)

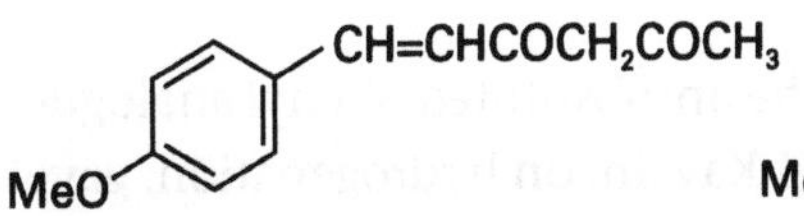

Yangonol (**11**)

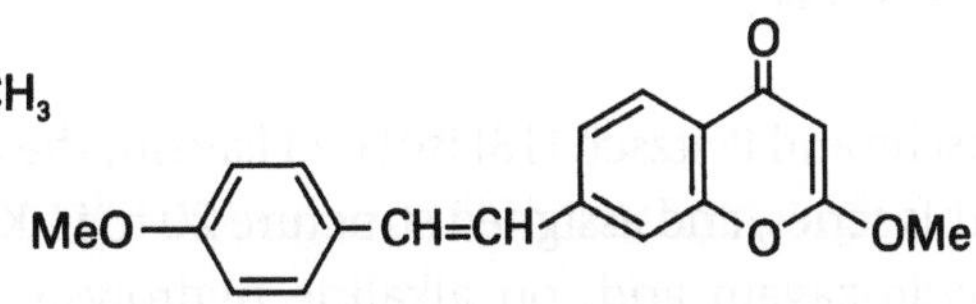

Borsche's structure of yangonin (**12**)

based on degradation studies; Murayama and Shinozaki [37], however, revised it and assigned structure **18**. Winzheimer in 1906 [38] isolated the ethylenic dihydroanalogue dihydromethysticin. The correct structures for methysticin, (5-hydroxy-3-methoxy-7-[3,4-methylenedioxyphenyl]-2,6-heptadienoic-acid-α-lactone) (**13**) and 7,8-dihydromethysticin (also called ψ-methysticin) (**14**) were given by Borsche et al. [15, 16] from an interpretation of the degradation products of earlier workers and a synthesis of methystic acid (**19**), which is an alkaline hydrolysis product of methysticin. Dihydromethysticin (**14**) was also isolated from *Aniba grandiflora* [33]. The fully conjugated analogue 5,6-dehydromethysticin **16** has been observed as a component of kava [39] and it has been synthesized [25]. 5,6-Dehydromethysticin (**16**) has been identified in the electrospray HPLC-MS of the chloroform extract of kava [35].

Snatzke and Hänsel assigned the absolute configurations of methysticin and dihydromethysticin based on a study of the circular dichroism and comparison with parasorbic acid, the absolute configuration of which is established [40]. Thus **13** and **14** have the (6*R*) and (6*S*) configurations respectively, according to the Cahn, Ingold, Prelog convention of assignments [41].

Klohs et al. [42, 43] reported the isolation and synthesis of *dl*-dihydromethysticin. These compounds were also isolated from *Aniba gigantifolia* [33]. The proton NMR spectra of methysticins have been determined by Beak et al. [27] and Achenbach [44]. Engel et al. [45] carried out an X-ray structure determination of methysticins. The isolation of 10-methoxymethysticin (**15**) has been recorded [7]. The method used by Bu'Lock and Smith [24] for the synthesis of yangonin was employed for the synthesis of 11-methoxyyangonin (**2**) and 5,6-dehydromethysticin (**16**) [46]. The replacement of 4-methoxyl of methysticin with an ethoxyl group (ethysticin) appears to give a pharmacologically active derivative that has been tested clinically [47].

2.1.3 Kavains

Borsche and Peitzsch [18] isolated kavain, the unsubstituted phenyl analogue of this series, and assigned structure **20** to it. Kavain, on hydrogenation, gave dihydrokavain and, on alkaline hydrolysis, kavaic acid. Dutta et al. [28] described the isolation, mass and ^{1}H NMR spectra of **20**. Hänsel et al. [48] also reported the isolation and syntheses of kavain and its derivatives. Kimura et

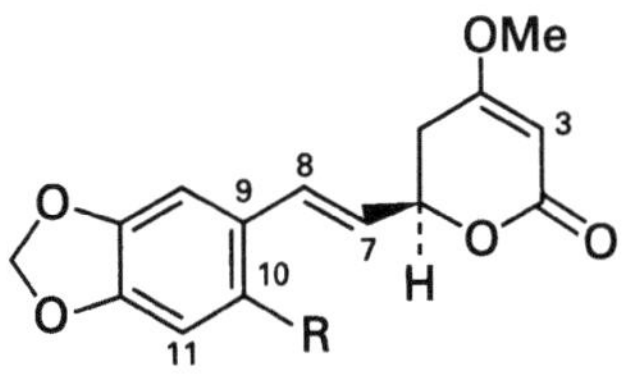

Methysticin (**13**) R = H
10-Methoxymethysticin (**15**) R = OMe

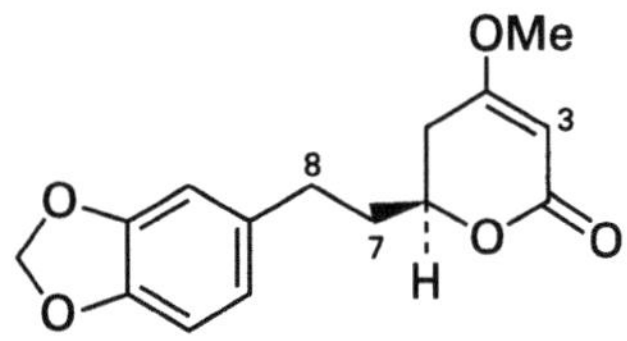

7,8-Dihydromethysticin (**14**)

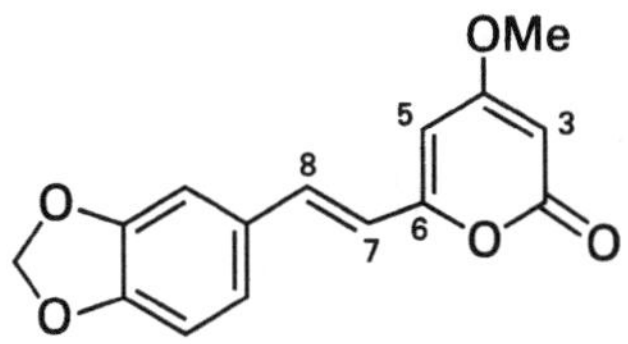

5,6-Dehydromethysticin (**16**)

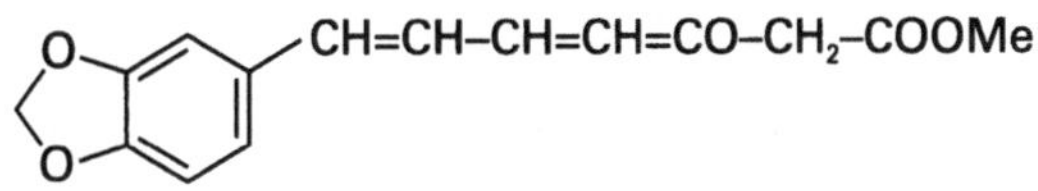

Pomeranz's structure of methysticin (**17**)

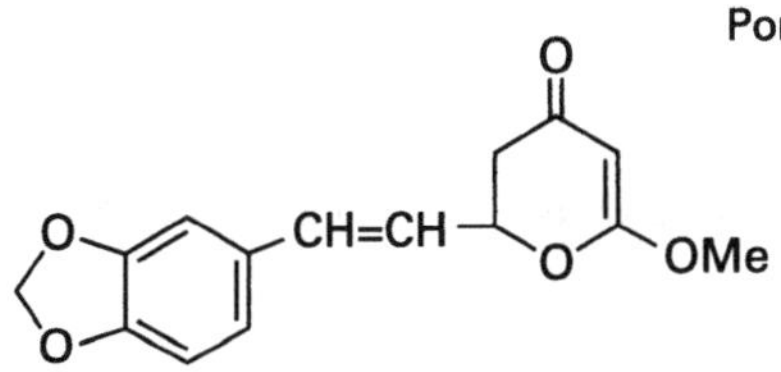

Murayama's structure of methysticin (**18**)

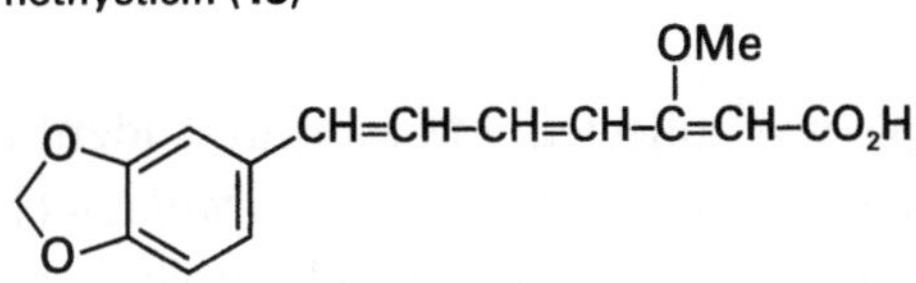

Methystic acid (**19**)

al. [49] and Reffstrup et al. [50] recorded the ^{1}H NMR spectra while Achenbach et al. [51] and Møller et al. [52] described the mass spectra of kavains. Izawa et al. [53], Israili et al. [54] and Castellino [55] carried out the synthesis of kavains. Van Veen [56] isolated a crystalline compound, $C_{14}H_{16}O_{3,}$, and named it marindinin, after the Marindanim people of Irian Jaya where the

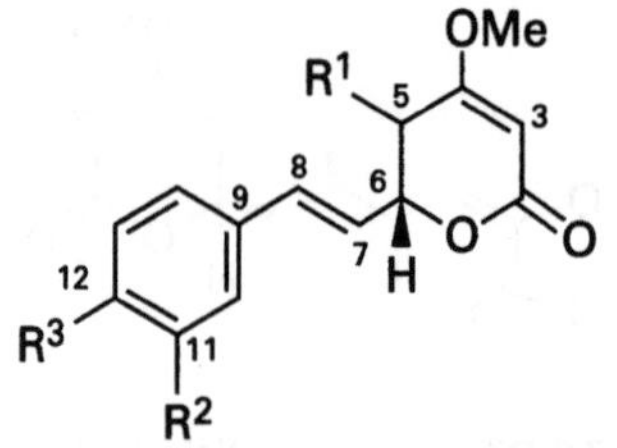

Kavain (**20**) $R^1, R^2, R^3 = H$
5-Hydroxykavain (**25**) $R^1 = OH$
$R^2, R^3 = H$

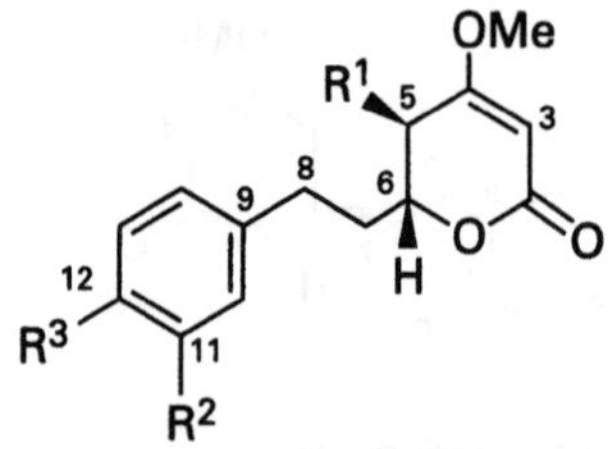

7,8-Dihydrokavain (**21**) $R^1, R^2, R^3 = H$
7,8-Dihydro-11-hydroxy-12-methoxykavain (**23**) $R^1 = H, R^2 = OH, R^3 = OMe$
7,8-Dihydro-11, 12-dimethoxykavain (**26**) $R^1 = H, R^2, R^3 = OMe$
7,8-Dihydro-5-hydroxykavain (**27**) $R^1 = \beta\text{-}OH, R^2, R^3 = H$

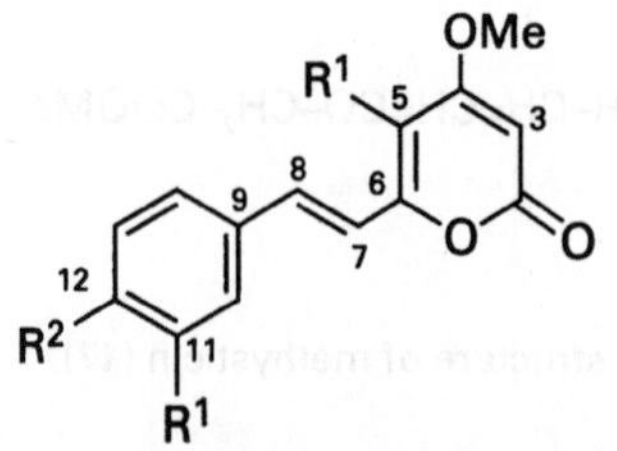

5,6-Dehydrokavain (**22**) $R^1, R^2 = H$
5,6-Dehydro-12-hydroxy-11-methoxykavain (**24**)
$R^1 = OMe,\ R^2 = OH$

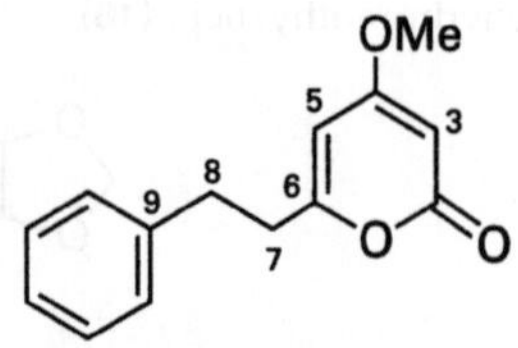

5,6-Dehydro-7,8-dihydrokavain (**28**)

kava sample was collected. Marindinin is identical with 7,8-dihydrokavain (**21**) and it is also isolated from *Aniba gigantifolia* [33]. The dihydro derivative and the dehydro analogue, 5,6-dehydrokavain (12-desmethoxyyangonin) (**22**), are both identically comparable with the methysticin derivatives **14** and **16** described earlier. Kavain (**20**), 5,6-dehydrokavain (**22**), and 7,8-dihydrokavain (**21**) have been isolated by supercritical-fluid extraction of kavalactones [32]. 5,6-Dehydrokavain (**22**) was synthesized by Macierewicz and later by Hänsel et al. [25]. It was actually synthesized prior to its isolation from kava resin. 5,6-Dehydro-7, 8-dihydrokavain (**28**) and 5,6-dehydrokavain (**22**) were identified in the aqueous extracts of *Alpinia zerumbot* based on their UV, ^1H, ^{13}C NMR and hydrolysis data [57]. The absolute configurations of kavain

(**20**) and dihydrokavain (**21**) were established as (6*R*) and (6*S*), respectively, based on CD measurement [39]. Achenbach [58] also determined the absolute stereochemistry of the kavains. The X-ray crystal structure of kavains has been determined [59, 60]. The lactones **20** and **28** were identified in a number of archaeological artifacts using selected ion-monitoring techniques in conjunction with GC-EIMS [61].

7,8-Dihydro-5-hydroxykavain (**27**) was isolated from kava [62] and its structure was established by the selenium dioxide oxidation of kavain and Pd/C reduction of one of the epimers [63]. The α-pyrones 7,8-dihydro-11-hydroxy-12-methoxykavain (**23**), 7,8-dihydro-5-β-hydroxykavain (**27**), and 7,8-dihydro-11, 12-dimethoxykavain (**26**) were isolated by preparative column HPLC, and **20**, **21**, **22**, 5,6-dehydro-12-hydroxy-11-methoxykavain (**24**) and 5-hydroxykavain (**25**) were identified by electrospray HPLC-MS of kava root [39]. Two additional syntheses of (+)-dihydrokavain-5-ol (**27**) have recently been reported [64, 65]. The lactone **27** was also identified by CI-GC-MS of kava from Vanuatu [66].

2.1.4 Chalcones and flavanones

Two pigment materials, flavokavain A and flavokavain B, were isolated from the kava rhizome by chromatography in 0.04% and 0.004% yield, respectively [67]. Based on syntheses, they were shown to be 6-hydroxy-2,4,4'-trimethoxychalcone (**29**) and 6-hydroxy-2',4'-dimethoxychalcone (**30**), respectively [68].

These chalcones are relatively devoid of any major biological activity and are believed to be responsible for the skin discoloration of people with chronic exposure to kava extracts. Flavokavain C was isolated from the benzene extract of kava and assigned structure (**31**) based on IR, UV and MS spectral data [28]. Two other chalcones from a New Guinea Piper species are reported as pinostrobinchalcone (**32**) and alpinetinchalcone (**33**) [69].

Some flavanones related to the chalcones have been isolated from a New Guinea Piper species, but these might be artifacts formed during the isolation procedure by cyclization. Dihydrotectochrysin (**34**) is the cyclization product of pinostrobinchalcone (**32**), and alpinetin (**35**) is related to alpinetinchalcone (**33**). A third flavanone, dihydrooroxylin A (**36**), has been obtained, but no corresponding chalcone has as yet been isolated [69].

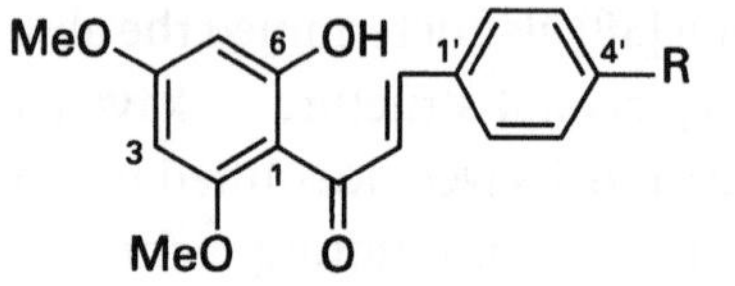

Flavokavain A (**29**) R = OMe
Flavokavain B (**30**) R = H
Flavokavain C (**31**) R = OH

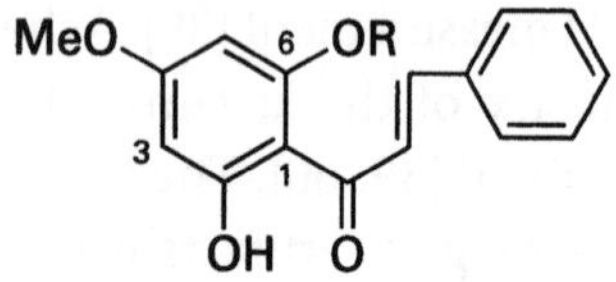

Pinostrobinchalcone (**32**) R = H
Alpinetinchalcone (**33**) R = Me

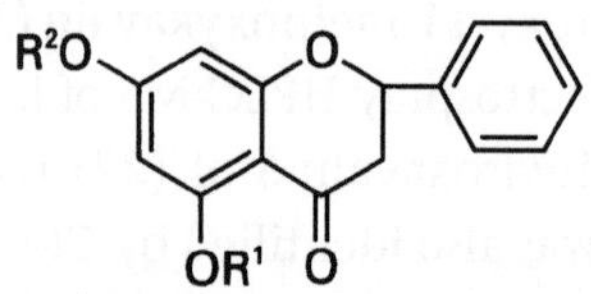

Dihydrotechtochrysin (**34**) R^1 = H, R^2 = Me
Alpinetin (**35**) R^1 = Me, R^2 = H

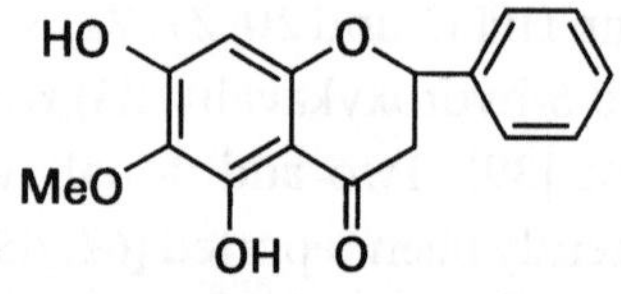

Dihydrooroxylin A (**36**)

2.1.5 Conjugated dieneketones

Two conjugated diene ketones, cinnamylidineacetone (37) and 3,4-methylenedioxy-cinnamylidineacetone (38) have been obtained from kava. That these are not artifacts resulting from hydrolysis and decarboxylation of kavain and methysticin, respectively, has been confirmed by appropriate experiments [70]. Bornylcinnamate has been found in both the kava resin and its steam distillate.

2.1.6 Kava alkaloids

The fact that α-pyrones, which are nitrogen-free compounds, can give an alkaloid-positive reaction to Dragendorff's reagent, misled the earlier studies to infer the presence of alkaloids in the kava resin [71]. However, the resin contains some unstable alkaloids that are adsorbed on the Al_2O_3 column.

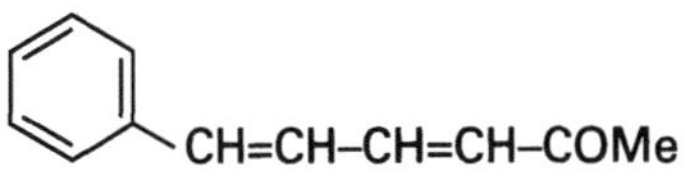

Cinnamylidineacetone (**37**)

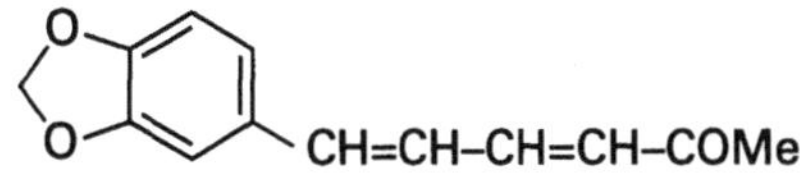

3,4-Methylenedioxycinnamylidineacetone (**38**)

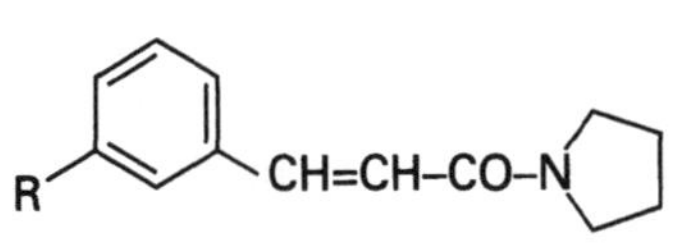

N-Cinnamoylpyrrolidine R = H (**39**)
N-(*m*-Methoxycinnamoyl)pyrrolidine R = OMe (**40**)

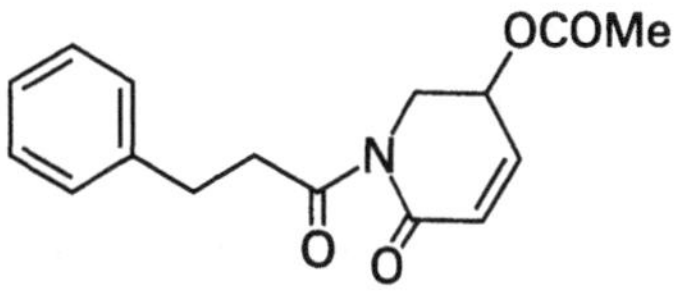

Pipermethystine (**41**)

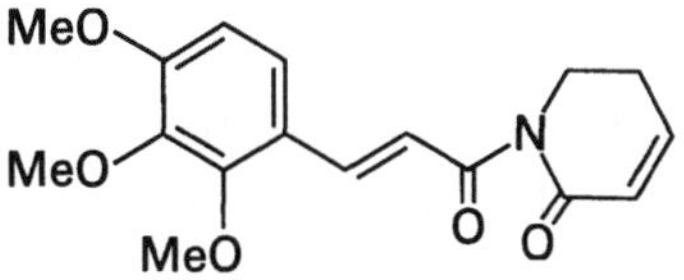

Piplartine (**42**)

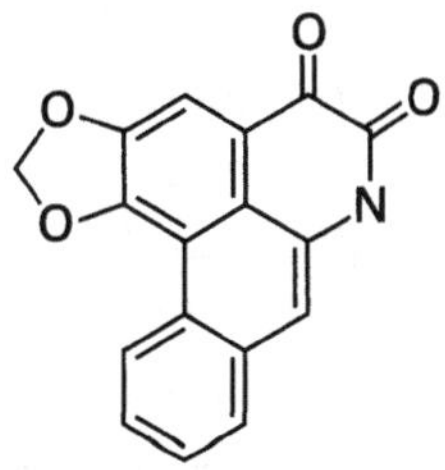

Cepharadione A (**43**)

Achenbach and Karl isolated two pyrrolidine alkaloids by MeOH extraction of the roots, and identified them as *N*-cinnamoylpyrrolidine (**39**) and *N*-(*m*-methoxycinnamoyl)pyrrolidine (**40**) based on IR, mass and proton NMR spectroscopy. The double bond in both alkaloids was shown to have a *trans*-configuration [72]. 1-Cinnamoylpyrrolidine (**39**) has been detected in the mass spectrum of kava resin from Fiji and Vanuatu [66]. Smith [73] isolated the alkaloid pipermethystine from the leaves by chromatographic purification on SiO_2. Pipermethystine was shown to have structure **41** by ^{1}H NMR, ^{13}C NMR and MS data and by chemical degradation studies. Structure **41** closely resembles that of piplartine (**42**) [74]. A minor alkaloid, cepharadione

A (**43**), has been isolated and its structure determined by ^{13}C NMR studies [75–77]. This alkaloid occurs in kava as well as in other piper species [78–80].

2.2 Analysis and quality control

Kavalactones have been investigated by several analytical techniques, including chromatography, GC and HPLC [81]. The determination of the relative amounts of the various compounds present in the intact plant is difficult, as different separation procedures lead to different analyses. Young et al. [82, 85] have separated the various fractions and assayed the isolates by column chromatography, since GC might lead to artifacts not present in the plant. A separation into major and minor components has been made as follows: kavain, dihydrokavain and methysticin (1% or more); flavokavain A, pinostrobinchalcone, dihydrotectochrysin, alpinetinchalcone, alpinetin, dihydrooroxylin A, flavokavain B (0.1–1%) [42, 68, 69, 82].

Gas chromatographic analysis was first used for the qualitative analysis of kava [83], and later in 1986 for the identification of the α-lactones **1**, **13**, **20** and **21** and their derivatives [84]. The concentration of the major constituents of six samples from Hawaii was estimated by TLC and spectrophotometry [85]. Similar methods were employed for the estimation of yangonin (**1**), methysticin (**13**) and kavain (**20**) [86]. Gas chromatography and HPLC have been used in more recent studies [87]. The leaves, stem and roots of two samples of kava from Fiji have been analyzed for the composition of kavalactones **1**, **9**, **14**, **20–22** and pipermethystine (**41**) by GC [88]. Six kavalactones (**1**, **13**, **14** and **20–22**) were separated and estimated quantitatively by preparative HPLC on a Dynamax-60A SiO_2. Column [34]. Supercritical fluid extraction of kava roots with CO_2 yielded kavalactones **1**, **9**, **13**, **14**, **20** and **22** [32]. A reversed-phase HPLC method has been developed for the quantitative determination of the kavalactones [89]. By HPLC separation on a ChiraSpher® NT column, enantioselective determination was carried out of the chiral kava pyrones **13**, **14**, **20**, **21** and the achiral compounds **1** and **22** [90]. Ganzera and Khan [91] compared the GC and HPLC methods of analysis for the determination of the kavalactones. Specific interactions between a tetramethylrhodamine-labeled kavain and human cortical neurons were found for the first time using fluorescence spectroscopy [92].

2.3 Pharmacology

Kava has enjoyed a long history of both social and clinical use in Polynesian culture and among the Aboriginal people of Arnhem Land in the Northern Territory of Australia. The latter, however, appear to consume socially much larger quantities at a steady tempo, which may amount to 37 g of kava powder containing 3800 mg of kavalactones in two-thirds of a liter per hour [93]. Clinically, kava has been used in these cultures for a variety of disorders, some based on real effects and others on mere hearsay. The past two decades of investigations on kavalactones, which are claimed to be the active principles of the herb, have revealed anticonvulsive, analgesic, anxiolytic and centrally acting muscle-relaxant activities.

Duffield et al. [94] tested the aqueous (lactone-free) and nonpolar (lactone-rich) extracts of kava on the conditioned avoidance response in rats in a shelf-jump apparatus and on the amphetamine-induced hypermotility in mice. Both the extracts reduced the hypermotility. However, the aqueous extract in i.p. doses of 30 to 500 mg/kg had no effect on the conditioned avoidance response in rats. The lactone-rich nonpolar extract at 125 mg/kg dose, on the other hand, reduced this response by 18%. Higher doses produced only a slight increase in this activity, but did induce sedation and ataxia. The effect of the nonpolar extract was relatively small compared to the usual doses of the anti-psychotic drugs chlorpromazine and haloperidol. In other studies, the aqueous extract was found to produce a loss of spontaneous activity in mice without loss of muscle tone, slight analgesic and anticonvulsant activities, and some anti-apomorphine activity [95]. The nonpolar extract also decreased the spontaneous activity in mice, but with a concomitant loss of muscle control, marked hypnosis, analgesia and some local anaesthetic effect. Furthermore, it also reversed the tetrabenazine-induced ptosis. Thus, most of the pharmacological activities appear to reside in the lactones contained in the nonpolar extract.

The effects of kava extract and its pure isolates, methysticin and dihydromethysticin (**14**), were studied on ischemic brain damage in mice and rats, in which focal cerebral ischemia was induced by micro-bipolar coagulation of the left middle cerebral artery [96]. The kava extract and both its isolates protected against the cerebral damage to an extent comparable to the effect of a reference compound, memantine. Kavain (**20**), dihydrokavain (**21**) and yangonin (**1**) failed to show this protection. This study suggests that the neuroprotective activity of kava may be due to methysticin and its dihydro congener.

A synthetically produced kava-pyrone, (±)-kavain, was shown to specifically inhibit the voltage-dependent Na^+ channels in synaptosomes of the rat cerebral cortex. A pre-incubation of the cells with the pyrone prevented the accumulation of intracellular Na^+ in the veratridine-activated channels [97]. Gleitz et al. [98] indirectly determined the anticonvulsant activity of (±)-kavain by studying its effects on 4-aminopyridine-stimulated cerebrocortical synaptosomes (a model of repetitively firing neurons resulting in glutamate release) and its binding to the epitopes of voltage-dependent Na^+ and Ca^{2+} channels in the synaptosomal membrane. Their data suggested a clear interaction of kavain with the ion channels leading to a suppression of the glutamate release. Since convulsions are believed to be due to overactive and rapidly discharging neurons, the study supports the anticonvulsive activity of kavain.

The effect of (±)-kavain on voltage-activated inward currents of Na^+ and Ca^{2+} in the dorsal root ganglion cells of newly born rats was studied, using a patch clamp technique [99]. The kavain, applied extracellularly, reduced the voltage-activated ion currents within 3–5 min, which was enhanced when DMSO was added to increase the water solubility of kavain. Dose-dependently, it also reduced the guinea-pig ileum contractility induced by carbachol, BAY K-8644 or substance P [100]. In another smooth muscle preparation (murine tracheal chain), kavain pretreatment reduced both carbachol- and KCl-induced contractions. This spasmolytic effect, however, did not involve NO-mediation or the prostaglandin pathway. The authors concluded that the synthetic lactone most likely binds to the muscarinic receptors [101].

Schmitz et al. [102] studied the effects of methysticin (13) on *in vitro* seizure models, using extracellular recordings in the slices of rat temporal cortex containing hippocampus and entorhinal cortex. Elevating extracellular K^+ and lowering extracellular Ca^{2+} and Mg^{2+} levels in separate experiments induced Epileptiform activities. Methysticin in a concentration range of 10 to 100 μM reversibly blocked all the induced seizures.

Kavain and dihydromethysticin, possessing anticonvulsant, analgesic and anxiolytic activities, were tested on the field potential (fp) changes induced by omitting the extracellular Mg^{2+} in the guinea pig hippocampal slices [103]. The recordings were made from the CA1 and CA3 areas of the slices.

Both the constituents of kava reduced the frequency of fp in a dose-dependent manner. When tested in combination, the two showed additive effects.

The naturally occurring (+)-kavain was tested for its presumed antithrombotic activity deduced from its ability to inhibit arachidonic acid (AA)-induced platelet aggregation, ATP release, and production of prostaglandin E2 (cyclo-oxygenase, COX, activity) and thromboxane A2 (thromboxane synthase, TXS, activity). Extracellular application of kavain 5 min prior to AA treatment dose-dependently reduced the platelet aggregation, ATP-release and the prostaglandin as well as thromboxane syntheses [104]. The primary target for kavain responsible for its antithrombotic activity appears to be the TXS, because thromboxane A2 is known to induce platelet aggregation.

2.4 Mechanisms of action

Several studies have focused on the possible mechanism(s) of actions of kava and its constituents on the central nervous system. Davies et al. [105] were among the early investigators who studied the interactions of kava extract and its pure isolates with the GABA and benzodiazepine binding sites in the murine cerebral synaptosomal membrane receptors. A relatively weak binding was found to occur with the binding sites studied. The conclusion of these investigators was that the centrally mediated pharmacological activities of kava and/or its constituents do not involve GABA or benzodiazepine binding sites. However, subsequent elaborate studies on GABA receptors in the membranes of synaptosomes from various regions of the brain revealed that kavapyrones might actually produce their sedative effects through mediation of the GABA-A receptors [106]. A lactone-rich kava extract was found to enhance the binding of ^{3}H-muscimol to GABA-A receptors, the maximum effect occurring in the hippocampus, followed in order by the amygdala and medulla oblongata. A minimal effect on the muscimol binding was observed in the cerebellum and the frontal cortex.

Others have suggested the involvement of ion channels in the mediation of kavain effects on the central nervous system. Fast and specific inhibition of voltage-dependent sodium channels by the synthetic kavain was proposed by Gleitz et al. [97, 98]. Anoxia generally stimulates anaerobic oxidation of glucose, leading to lactic acid production and a decrease in ATP levels. In studies with the rat brain vesicles rendered anoxic, a concomitant increase in the intracellular sodium and calcium, that increased further by veratridine treatment, was observed. However, a pretreatment of the vesicles with the sodium channel blockers, tetrodotoxin and (±)-kavain, reduced the anoxic influx of the ions, prevented the veratridine-induced enhancement of the ionic influx, and reduced the lactate production [107]. These data further support the theory that the ion channel blockade by kavain may mediate its central effects.

Involvement of the serotonin 1-A receptor in the mediation of the central activity of kavalactones has been proposed by Walden et al. [108], based on their studies on the guinea-pig hippocampal slices. Ipsapirone, a serotonin-1A receptor agonist, increases the field potential in the CA1 and CA3 regions of the hippocampus, which is blocked by N-allyl-normetazocine (NANM), a ligand for sigma and *N*-methyl-D-aspartate (NMDA) receptors [109]. The extracellular applications of dihydromethysticin and kavain also reduced the ipsapirone-induced increase in the field potentials. Since the serotonin receptors are implicated in anxiety, the anxiolytic activity of kava may involve the blockade of these receptors. Walden's group has also suggested that kavalactones may block NMDA receptors as well as calcium ion channels [103].

The naturally occurring (+)-methysticin and (+)-kavain, as well as the synthetic (±)-kavain, were found to block the reuptake of ^{3}H-noradrenaline in the synaptosomes obtained from the cerebral cortex and hippocampus of rats, with the following order of potency: (±)-kavain > (+)-kavain > (+)-methysticin [110]. This too may contribute toward the mechanism of psychotropic actions of kava.

Since antidepressants exhibit monoamine oxidase-B (MAO-B) inhibitory activity, a lactone-rich kava extract and several of its isolates were also tested for this activity and compared to amitriptyline, imipramine and brofaromine [111]. The enzyme was obtained from human platelets. The extract was found to be a reversible inhibitor of MAO-B. The order of potency was desmethoxy-yangonin > (±)-methysticin > yangonin > (±)-dihydromethysticin > (±)-dihydrokavain > (±)-kavain. Thus, the MAO-B inhibition extrapolated from the thrombocytes to the central nervous system has also been proposed as a possible mechanism of central actions of kava.

Langosch et al. [112] found that (±)-kavain in a concentration-dependent manner reduced the amplitudes of extracellular fp enhancement evoked by electrical stimulation of the CA1 region of guinea-pig hippocampal slices. They suggested that kavain is an effective drug capable of modulating excitatory signals in the hippocampus, the major portion of the limbic system responsible for the emotional component of behavioral expression. Based on ^{3}H-bicuculline binding to GABA-A receptors, which is enhanced by various kavalactones, Boonen and Haberlein [113] concluded that the kava products show their effect on this receptor independent of their interaction with the benzodiazepine receptor.

The effect of kava extract and its isolated pyrones on the neurotransmitter levels in the nucleus accumbens has been studied, using *in vivo* microdialysis of the mesolimbic reward system of the rat [114]. A 20 mg/kg i.p. dose of the extract changed both the animal behavior and the dopamine (DA) levels. Larger doses increased the DA levels in the nucleus accumbens. Among the individual compounds, (±)-kavain in low doses induced a decrease in the DA levels and, in high doses, either an increase or no change. Yangonin decreased DA below detection limits, whereas desmethoxyyangonin increased the DA levels. Dihydrokavain, dihydromethysticin and methysticin did not show any effect on this neurotransmitter. However, (±)-kavain and other kavapyrones decreased the serotonin levels in the nucleus accumbens. These investigators suggested that activation of the dopaminergic neurons in the mesolimbic system may be responsible for the relaxing and euphoric actions of kava.

By using fluorescence correlation spectroscopy, Boonen et al. [92] have shown for the first time that kavain possesses a specific affinity for the human cortical neurons. Kavain was labeled with a fluorescent dye. Human cortical neurons cultivated in Nunc® chambers were incubated with the dye-labeled kavain. The binding data plotted on Scatchard and sigmoid Hill plots indicated several binding sites for kavain in the cortical neurons, but with different binding affinities.

From all these mechanism-of-action studies on kava and its products, it is difficult to specifically pinpoint how kava acts. Until and unless all of the individual bioactive constituents have been pharmacologically characterized, a large volume of controversial and widely spread data is likely to continue to accumulate. Over 50 years of experience with well-known allopathic psychotropic drugs reveals that, in the absence of complete knowledge of biochemical parameters at the molecular level underlying the affective disorders, it is extremely difficult to define the exact mechanism of action of any psychotropic drug, let alone kava, which itself is far from being fully characterized both chemically and pharmacologically.

2.5 Clinical studies

In a double-blind crossover study, 12 volunteers were given oxazepam and kava extract by turn, and a comparison of the two treatments was made in their respective effects on the volunteers' recognition and memory [115]. The subjects were asked to identify, within a list of words, those that were shown for the first time and those shown repeatedly. Oxazepam decreased the subjects' ability to recognize both new and repeated words, whereas kava-treated subjects showed an increase in the recognition. In another randomized, placebo-controlled, double-blind trial, two groups of 29 patients each, suffering from anxiety unrelated to affective or psychic disorders, were treated with 3 daily doses of 100 mg of kava extract WS 1490 (Laitan®) or a placebo for 4 weeks [116]. The Hamilton Anxiety Scale (HAMA) for assessing main outcome variables, the Clinical Global Impression (CGI) for assessing secondary target variables and the Adjective Check List (ACL) were used to assess therapeutic efficacy at 1, 2 and 4 weeks of the treatment. Both HAMA and CGI data showed a significant reduction of anxiety syndrome at week 1 in the kava group compared to the placebo group. This difference increased with longer periods of treatment. No adverse reactions were noticed during the treatment period. This study, if confirmed in a larger trial, would clearly support the anxiolytic effectiveness of kava.

Volz and Kieser [117] carried out a multicenter, randomized, placebo-controlled, double-blind trial on 101 outpatients suffering from anxiety not related to psychic disorder. The kava extract WS 1490 was given orally to the patients for 25 weeks. The HAMA scale showed a significant improvement in the kava-treated patients over the placebo group from week 8 onward. The CGI and other scores also showed a distinct anxiolytic effectiveness of kava. No significant adverse reaction was observed in the patients. Any side-effects seen were evenly distributed among the treatment and the placebo groups. In another observational study involving 52 outpatients with anxiety of nonpsychotic etiology, kava treatment showed a "very good" or "good" improvement in 80% of the patients, with only rare and mild adverse effects [118]. Both these studies also support the theory that kava may be a good alternative to benzodiazepines and antidepressants currently used for treating anxiety disorders.

Pittler and Ernst [119] reviewed seven reported clinical trials on kava and rendered a meta-analysis. All the trials showed that kava was superior to placebo in alleviating anxiety. Three of the seven well-conducted trials clearly showed the anxiolytic effectiveness of kava by all instruments of assessment available.

An interesting study has been reported on the detection in human urine of metabolites of kavalactones following ingestion of aqueous kava extract [120]. Seven major and several minor lactones of kava were isolated by HPLC and identified with the help of methane chemical ionization GC-MS. The biotransformations observed included the reduction of the 3,4-double bond, demethylation of the 4-methoxy alpha-pyrone ring system, demethylation of 12-methoxyyangonin, and C-12 hydroxylation of desmethoxy yangonin. It is not clear as to why one would study the metabolism of a crude extract of a plant or its part containing a large number of known as well as unknown compounds. However, this study could have forensic application in detecting kava consumption by subjects. Although the lactones are claimed to be present in the nonpolar extracts of kava, there must be enough quantities in the aqueous extracts as evident from this study and the fact that islanders drink the root powder suspended in water for psychotropic effects.

Thus, based on the clinical investigations on kava with the currently available methodology, as well as centuries of its usage in folk medicine practiced in the Pacific islands and the Northern Territory of Australia, kava and/or its lactones should be acceptable at least as an anxiolytic alternative to the benzodiazepines that exhibit both tolerance and adverse side-effects. However, there is a need for large-scale, well-controlled and standardized clinical trials on the individual bioactive constituents of kava in order to arrive at the best drug choice in terms of clinical efficacy and safety.

2.6 Adverse reactions

Ruze [121] interviewed and examined 200 heavy drinkers of kava in the Tonga Islands who exhibited a pellagroid dermopathy suggestive of niacin deficiency. A scaly rash, possibly due to acquired ichthyosis, and eye irritation were present in some of the subjects. Of these subjects, 29 were treated with either 100 mg of oral nicotinamide or a placebo daily for 3 weeks. Five subjects in each of the two groups showed some improvement, ruling out the niacin deficiency theory. A history of kava dermopathy has been summarized with the suggestion that the peculiar scaly rash may be due to interference with cholesterol metabolism in the chronic heavy kava consumers [122]. Jappe et al. [123] have also noted a sebotropic drug reaction resulting from kava therapy. A dermatomyositis-like illness following kava ingestion by a 47-year old white woman was examined [124]. She had a rash and proximal muscle weakness two weeks after ingestion. Her creatine level was elevated to 8654 U/L. Her electromyograph showed a myopathic pattern. Skin and muscle biopsies revealed changes similar to dermatomyositis. Predinisone treatment and discontinuation of kava ingestion improved her condition. Whether or not this myositis-like pathology results from the effect of kava on the cerebellar cortex or is a direct effect on the muscle cells remains to be determined.

3 Garlic

Allium sativum L (family Liliaceae, common name garlic) is a perennial plant that has been cultivated since ancient times. While its origin is unknown, some believe that it originated in the Kirgiz desert region of Siberia, then spread to the Mediterranean area, becoming naturalized in the process. The use of garlic has been mentioned ~4000 BC in the "Ayurvedic Medicine" and ~1500 BC in the "Papyrus Ebers". It has been used in the diets of early Romans, Greeks and Egyptians. Today, it is a common ingredient of soups, stews and pickles around the world. Garlic is one of the best-selling herbal dietary supplements in the US. In 1995, the US exported nearly 3.6 milllion kg of dehydrated garlic worth ~$8.5 million.

In folk medicine, garlic has been used as an antibacterial and hypocholesteremic agent, and to treat intestinal parasites such as pinworms. Garlic is used in Ayurvedic medicine as an antiseptic for cleaning wounds and ulcers. The sulfur-containing compounds of garlic give the herb its pungent, spicy aroma, and are also responsible for many of its claimed pharmacological properties. Specifically, they lower cholesterol by stimulating the release of bile by the gall bladder and by decreasing the production of cholesterol in the liver. In addition, garlic compounds have been shown to lower blood pressure. Garlic also stimulates the immune system and enhances the activity of macrophages that phagocytose viruses, bacteria and fungi. Furthermore, garlic increases the activity of the helper-T lymphocytes. The sulfur and selenium compounds are potent antioxidants that protect cell membranes and DNA from damage [125–128].

3.1 Chemistry

Garlic bulbs are a veritable store-house of a variety of organic compounds. Semmler and Wertheim [129, 130] were the first to carry out scientific investigations of *A. sativum* and to identify sulfides in distilled garlic oil. Cavallito et al. [131, 132] reported that allicin is the active principle for its antibacterial activity. Garlic contains organic sulfur compounds predominantly, but several amino acids, L-glutamyl peptides, enzymes, carbohydrates, phospholipids, glycosides, and trace elements have also been identified. The dried bulbs contain ~13% protein [133].

The sulfur compounds isolated from garlic can be divided into four groups:

(a) The characteristic odor of garlic is due to allicin (**44**), a strong oxidant that produces free radicals. However, allicin is only one of the compounds formed by very rapid combination of unstable intermediates when garlic is cut. As many as nine analogues of allicin with typical garlic aroma and taste are formed. Although all these aroma-bearing compounds can be prepared in pure form, they are unstable at room temperature and may be stored only at sub-zero temperatures.

b) Allyl sulfides, e.g., diallyldisulfide (**45**), are obtained by steam distillation of garlic whereas extraction with aqueous EtOH at room temperature gives allicin, the oxide of **45**.

c) A sulfur-containing amino acid, alliin (**46**), can be obtained by extraction of garlic with pure EtOH at temperatures below 0 °C. It is the main odorless component in raw garlic. As soon as a clove of garlic is cut or crushed, the hydrolytic enzyme allinase is released to convert alliin into allicin. Very little is known about the intermediates that are formed when garlic cloves are chopped as they disappear in a fraction of a second after being formed and cannot be stored even at low temperatures. The stable odorless derivatives of L-cysteine (**47**), the natually occurring sulfur-containing amino acids, are found in unbroken garlic cloves and bulbs.

d) More stable products are formed when allicin and the allied compounds are subjected to heat. During cooking, allicin produces the oil-soluble ajoenes (**48**, **49**), diallyl-disulfide (**45**), methyl ajoene (**50**), and dithiins, the products that are stable at room temperature.

On prolonged storage, alliin (**46**) and allicin (**44**) are converted to water-sol-

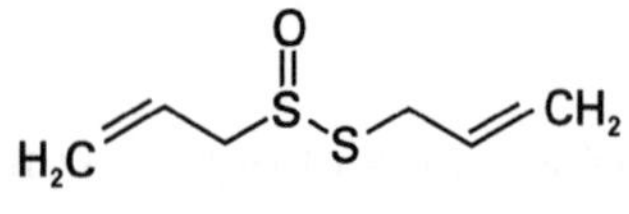

Allicin (**44**)

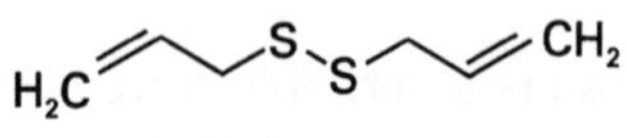

Diallyldisulfide (**45**)

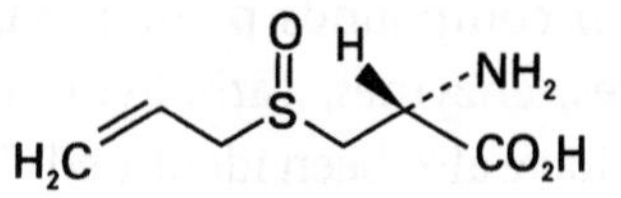

Alliin (**46**)

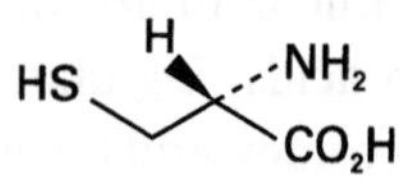

L-Cysteine (**47**)

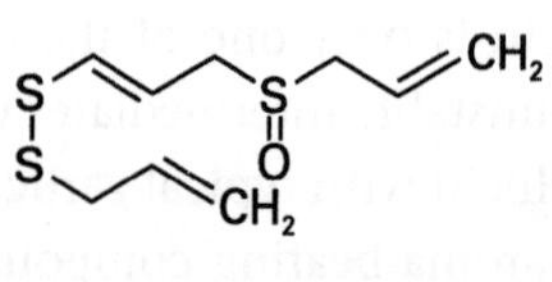

E-Ajoene (**48**)

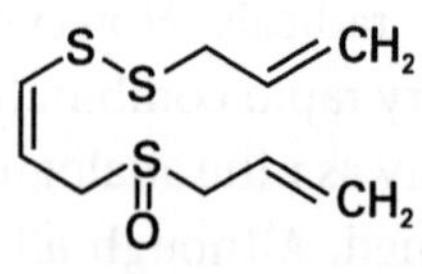

Z-Ajoene (**49**)

uble compounds such as S-allyl-L-cysteine (**51**) and S-allylthio-L-cysteine (**52**), which have little odor, are stable and survive cooking.

3.1.1 Alliin and alk(en)ylcysteine sulfoxides

Stoll and Seebeck isolated alliin (2-propenyl-L-cysteine sulfoxide) (**46**), mp 164–5 °C, $[\alpha]_D + 63.5°$, by gentle extraction with EtOH at < 0 °C, and determined its structure by degradation and synthesis [134]. The characteristic flavor and odor of *Allium* species is attributed to the presence of alliin and other cysteine sulfoxides. Allicin, the predominant thiosulfinate formed by the action of allinase on S(+)-allyl-L-cysteine sulfoxide (**55**), is formed from two molecules of 2-propenesulfenic acid. Two different routes have been used for the synthesis of alliin [135, 136]. S-Allyl-L-cysteine (**51**), the biogenetic precursor of **46**, has been isolated from garlic [137]. The chemistry of garlic with special reference to the biological activity of alliin and allicin has been reviewed [138].

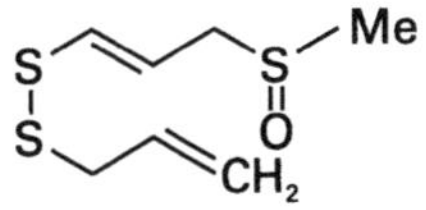

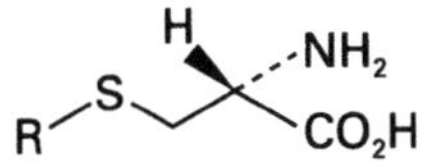

E-Methylajoene (**50**)

(+)-S-Allyl-L-cysteine (**51**) R = H_2C

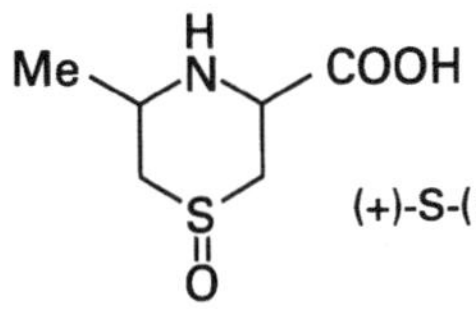

(+)-S-Allylthio-L-cysteine (**52**) R = H_2C

(+)-S-(*trans*-l-Propenyl)-L-cysteine (**54**) R = Me

Cycloalliin (**53**)

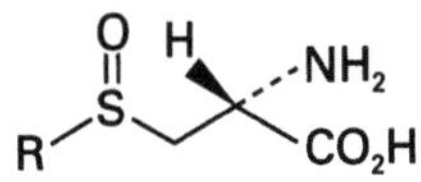

S-Allyl-L-cysteine sulfoxide	(**55**) R = H_2C CH_2
(+)-S-Methyl-L-cysteine sulfoxide	(**56**) R = Me
(+)-S-Butyl-L-cysteine sulfoxide	(**57**) R = n-Bu
(+)-S-(*trans*-1-Propenyl)-L-cysteine sulfoxide	(**58**) R = Me

Table 2 lists the various alk(en)yl cysteines and alk(en)yl cysteine sulfoxides isolated from *A. sativum*. A biosynthetic pathway has been proposed for alk(en)yl cysteine-sulfoxides by feeding labeled sulfate to the leaves of *A. sativum* [139]. Cycloalliin has been isolated from *A. sativum* and *A. cepa* and its structure established as 3-methyl-1,4-thiazine-5-carboxylic acid S-oxide (53) [140–142].

Some investigations have shown that the propyl analogues of alliin, propylsulfides and propyl sulfinates are not present in garlic [146].

3.1.2 γ-Glutamyl peptides

γ-Glutamyl peptides are formed by a carboxamide bond between γ-glutamic acid and another amino acid [18, 23]. These peptides (Tab. 3) were isolated by extraction of garlic with aqueous MeOH and subsequent purification by various chromatographic procedures.

Table 2.
Alk(en)yl cysteines and alk(en)yl cysteine sulfoxides isolated from *A. sativum* [143–145].

(+)-S-Allyl-L-cysteine (**51**)
(+)-S-Allylthio-L-cysteine (**52**)
(+)-S-(*trans*-1-Propenyl)-L-cysteine (**54**)
(+)-S-Allyl-L-cysteine sulfoxide (**55**)
(+)-S-Methyl-L-cysteine sulfoxide (**56**)
(+)-S-Butyl-L-cysteine sulfoxide (**57**)
(+)-S-(*trans*-1-Propenyl)-L-cysteine sulfoxide (**58**)

Table 3.
γ-Glutamyl peptides isolated from *A. sativum* [148–151]

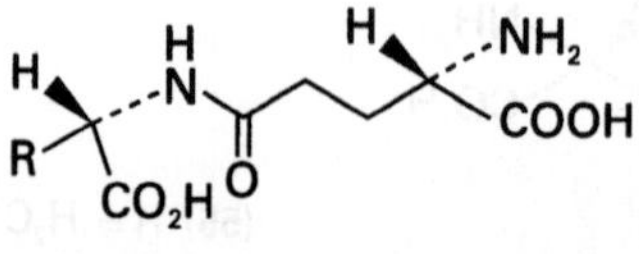

γ-L-Glutamyl-L-leucine (**59**) R = $(Me)_2$–CH–CH–CH_2–
γ-L-Glutamyl-L-isoleucine (**60**) R = Me–CH_2–CH (Me)–
γ-L-Glutamyl-L-valine (**61**) R = $(Me)_2$–CH
γ-L-Glutamyl-L-methionine (**62**) R = $(Me)_2$–CH_2–S–CH_2–CH_2–
γ-L-Glutamyl-L-phenylalanine (**63**) R = Ph–CH_2–

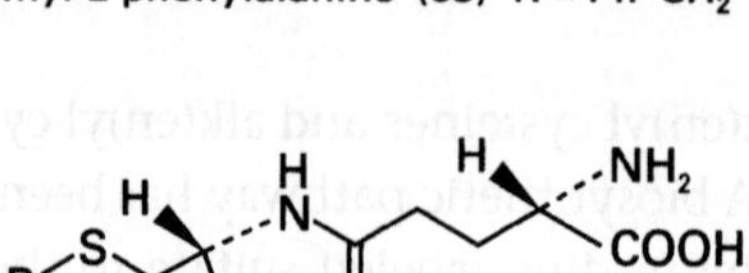

γ-L-Glutamyl-S-methyl-L-cysteine (**64**) R = Me

γ-L-Glutamyl-S-(*trans*-1-propenyl-L-cysteine (**65**) R = Me 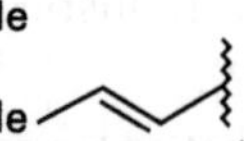

γ-L-Glutamyl-S-allyl-L-cysteine (**66**) R = H_2C 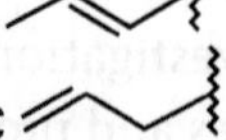

γ-L-Glutamyl-S-allylthio-L-cysteine (**67**) R = H_2C 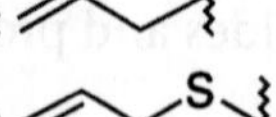

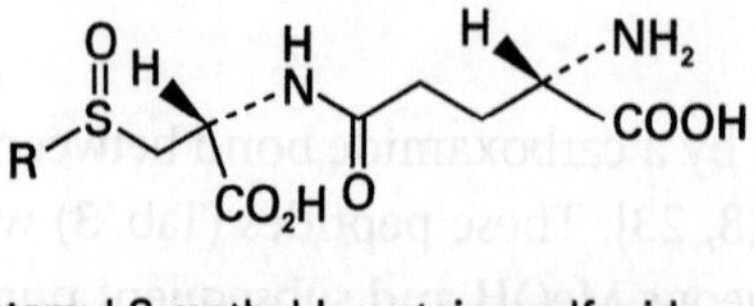

γ-L-Glutamyl-S-methyl-L-cysteine sulfoxide (**68**) R = Me
γ-L-Glutamyl-S-(*trans*-1-propenyl)-L-cysteine sulfoxide (**69**) R = Me

3.1.3 Dipeptides

An aqueous extract of garlic was fractionated by ion exchange and gel filtration to yield fractions having angiotensin-I converting enzyme (ACE) inhibitory activity. Fractions with high ACE inhibitory activity when combined and further chromatographed on a reverse-phase column afforded seven dipeptides with ACE inhibitory activity [152]. The structures of these peptides, derived by sequence analysis and fast bombardment (FAB) MS were Ser-Tyr, Gly-Tyr, Phe-Tyr, Asn-Phe, Ser-Phe, Gly-Phe, and Asn-Phe.

3.1.4 Allicin and other thiosulfinates

Allicin (**44**) is the predominant thiosulfinate formed by the action of allinase on S(+)-allyl-L-cysteine sulfoxide (**55**) when dimerization of two molecules of 2-propenesulfenic acid occurs. Isolated by maceration of garlic with EtOH at room temperature, allicin is a yellowish oil with a garlic odor and it decomposes at 20 °C within 20 h to give diallyl disulfide (**45**) as the major product, and diallyl trisulfide (**70**), diallylsulfide (**71**) and traces of cyclic 3-vinyl-4H-1,2-dithiin (**72**) and 2-vinyl-4H-1,3-dithiin (**73**) as minor products.

Allicin and other thiosulfinates can be synthesized by oxidation of the corresponding disulfides with H_2O_2. Allicin is the most important biologically active compound of garlic. Using paper and TL chromatography, Fujisawa et al. [153] separated the following thiosulfinates from the garlic extract: allyl methyl-CH_2=$CHCH_2SS(O)Me$, methyl allyl-Me-SS(O)CH_2CH=CH_2 and *trans*-1-propenyl-MeCH=CHSS(O)CH_2CH=CH_2. Also, dimethyl-, methyl allyl-, dipropyl-, propyl allyl-, propyl methyl-,1-propenyl allyl-, methyl 1-propenyl-, 1-propenyl methyl-, and allyl 1-propenylthiosulfinates have been isolated by others [148]. All the sulfur-containing compounds of garlic are derived from allicin (**46**). The mechanisms for their formation have been proposed by Block et al. [154].

3.1.5 Ajoenes and vinyldithiins

The *E* and *Z* isomers of ajoene (4,5,9-trithiododeca-1,6,11-triene-9-oxide) (**48**, **49**) are formed as secondary degradation products of allicin (**44**), *via* allyl

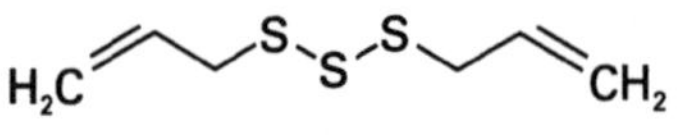

Diallyltrisulfide (**70**)

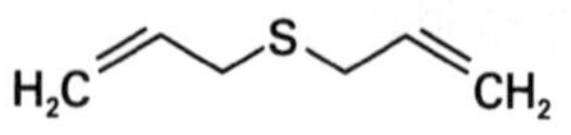

Diallylsulfide (**71**)

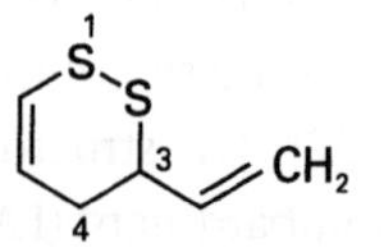

3-Vinyl-4H-1,2-dithiin (**72**)

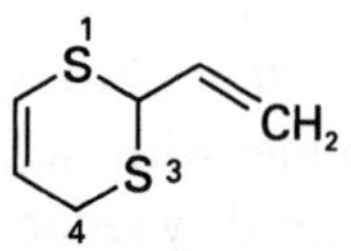

2-Vinyl-4H-1,3-dithiin (**73**)

sulfenic acid that attacks another molecule of **44**, followed by a Cope-type elimination and re-addition of 2-propenesulfenic acid. The structures of the ajoenes have been established [154]. *E*-Methylajoene (**50**) and *E*-dimethylajoene (**75**) have also been isolated from garlic [143]. Allicin decomposes during GC to afford the cyclic compounds 3-vinyl-4H-1,2-dithiin (**72**) and 2-vinyl-4H-1,3-dithiin (**73**) [155, 156]. The dithiins have been synthesized by the dimerization of thioacrolein (**74**) [157].

3.1.6 Organosulfides

Distilled garlic oil and water extracts stored for long periods contain methanethiol, allylthiol, alkyl sulfides such as dimethylsulfide, dimethyldisulfide and dimethyltrisulfide, allyl and methylallyl sulfides like diallylsulfide, diallyldisulfide (**45**), dipropyldisulfide, diallyltrisulfide (**70**), diallyltetrasulfide, methylallylsulfide, methylallyldisulfide, propenylallyldisulfide, and methylallyltrisulfide. These can be isolated from garlic oil by high vacuum fractional distillation [130, 144, 146, 158–161].

3.1.7 Organoselenium compounds

Wang et al. [162] isolated seleno-proteins and Yang et al. [163] isolated seleno-polysaccharides from garlic. Using GC with atomic-emission detection, dimethyselenide, methanesulfenoselenoicacid methylester, dimethyl diselenide, bis(methylthio)selenide, allyl methyl selenide, 2-propenesul-

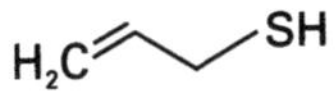

Thioacrolein (**74**)

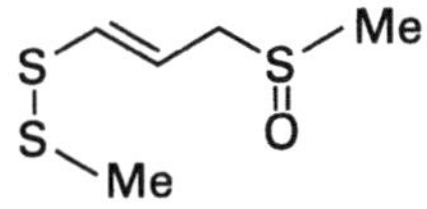

Dimethylajoene (**75**)

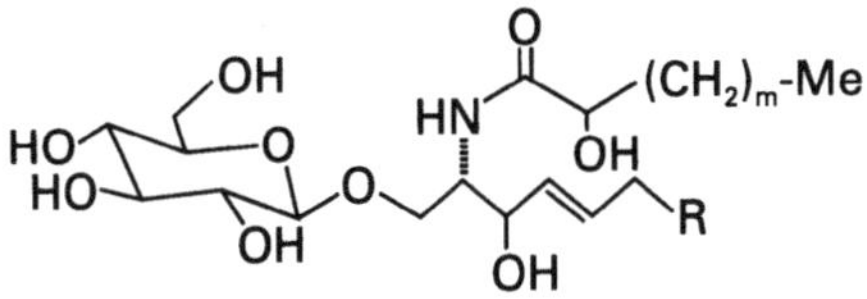

AS-1-1 (**76**) m =11R =
AS-1-2 (**77**) m =12R =
AS-1-3 (**78**) m =12R =
AS-1-4 (**79**) m =13R =
AS-1-5 (**80**) m =13R =

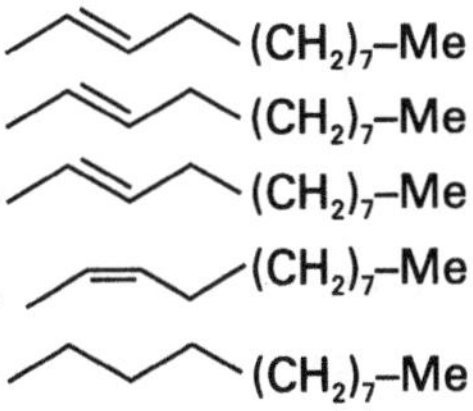

fenoselenoic acid methylester, 1-propenesulfeno-selenoicacid methylester, (allylthio) (methylthio) selenide, and bis(allylthio)selenide have also been identified in the garlic extracts [164]. By similar techniques, seleno-cysteine ($HSeCH_2CH(NH_2)$-COOH), and seleno-methylselenocysteine (SeCys-Se-Me), have been identified as the major seleno-amino acids of garlic [165].

3.1.8 Miscellaneous compounds

Five cerebrosides, AS-1-1 (**76**), AS-1-2 (**77**), AS-1-3 (**78**), As-1-4 (**79**) and AS-1-5 (**80**), have been obtained from the $CHCl_3$-MeOH extract of garlic. The structures of these compounds have been elucidated based on mass and ^1H and ^{13}C NMR spectroscopic data [166].

Allixin (**81**), a stress compound, was isolated from garlic bulbs and its structure was determined as 3-hydroxy-5-methoxy-6-methyl-2-pentyl-4H-pyran-4-one [167]. Synthesis of allixin, the anti-tumor component of garlic, has been accomplished *via* a 2-methyle-netetrahydropyran derivative (**82**) [168].

A novel amino acid glycoside, (–)-N-(1′-deoxy-1′-β-D-fructopyranosyl)-S-allyl-L-cysteine sulfoxide (**83**), (+)-S-allyl-L-cysteine sulfoxide (**55**), (+)-S-

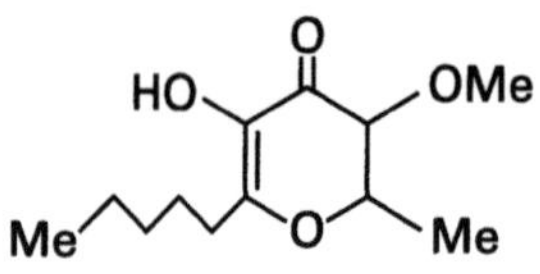

Allixin (**81**)

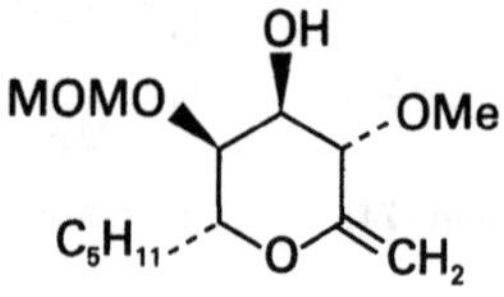

(**82**)

methyl-L-cysteine sulfoxide (**56**) and (+)-S-(*trans*-1-propenyl)-L-cysteine sulfoxide (**58**) were isolated from the hydrophilic extract of garlic leaves, and their structures established by IR, FABMS, ^{1}H- and ^{13}C-NMR spectral studies [169].

A high molecular weight fructan was isolated and its structure determined by enzymatic, chemical and extensive high-resolution NMR spectral studies. The fructan has a (2 → 1)-linked-β-D-Fru*f* backbone with (2 → 6)-linked-β-D-Fru*f* side chains. The structure model with a degree of polymerization of ~ 58 was substantiated using endoinulase-purified *Aspergillus ficuum* and by ^{1}H- and ^{13}C-NMR spectroscopy [170].

Several amino acids other than S-aminoacids and cysteine sulfoxides have been identified by paper and TL chromatography, including arginine, aspartic acid, glutamic acid, methionine and threonine [171–173]. S-(2-Carboxy-n-propyl)-glutathione (**84**), apparently an intermediate in the metabolic pathway of the odor-producing compounds, was also isolated from garlic [137, 174].

Stoll and Seebeck [134] isolated allinase (S-alkylcysteine sulfoxidylase), a pyridoxylphosphate enzyme, from garlic. It has been further purified and characterised [175, 176]. Other enzymes isolated include adenosinetriphosphatase (ATPase), glutamyltrans-peptidases [177], deoxyribonucleases, catalases, hexakinases, invertases, lipases, lysozymes, arginases, polyphenoloxidases, transfructosidases and superoxide-dismutases [178].

Mannose-binding lectins in a dimeric form with molecular weight of ~ 25,000 D [179], arachidonic-, linoleic- and -linoleic-acids [180], prostaglandins A2, F2, E2 and D2 [181, 182], neutral lipids, glycolipids, and phospholipids [183] have also been identified in garlic. From MeOH-extracts of garlic, Matsuura et al. [184, 185] isolated furostanol glycosides, and aglycones, protoeruboside B, eruboside B, sativosides B1, R1, R2, desgalactotigo-

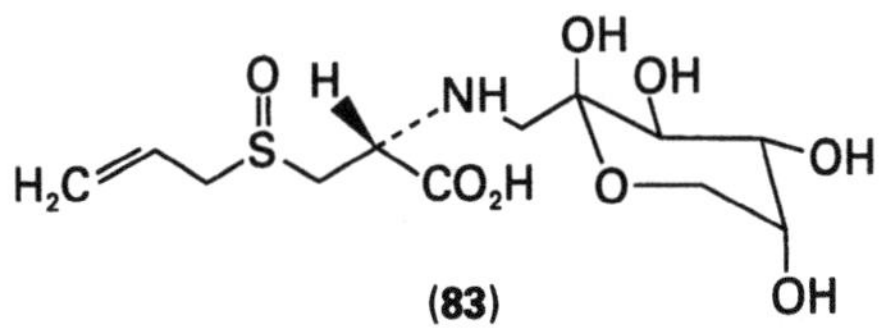

(83)

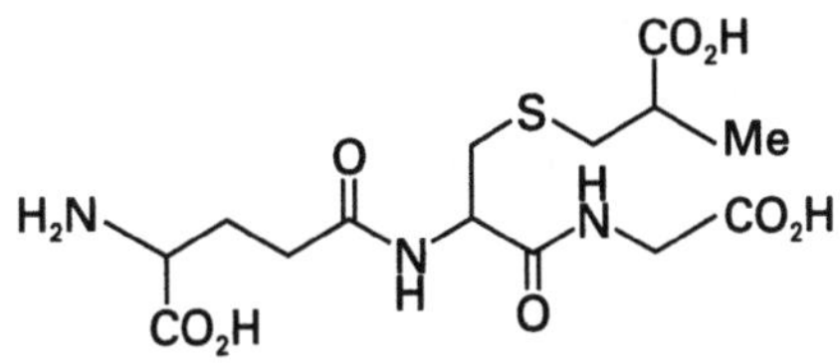

S-(2-Carboxy-n-propyl)glutathione (**84**)

nin, proto-desgalactotigonin and spirostanoglycosides. Six compounds were isolated from fresh garlic bulbs and their structures were elucidated as proto-iso-eruboside B, eruboside B, isoeruboside B, sativioside C, adenosine and tryptophane [186]. Three steroidal saponins ampeloside BS1, Bf1 and Bf2, have been identified in garlic extracts [187]. Finally, the elements Al, Ca, Co, Cu, Cr, F, Fe, Ge, I, K, Mg, Mn, Mo, P, Na, Se and Zn have been identified in garlic [133].

3.2 Analysis and quality control

A steadily increasing number of garlic preparations in the market during the past few years has resulted in a high interest in practical analytical methods to determine the active constituents. A TLC method has been developed to distinguish alliin from amino acids and cysteine sulfoxides [188]. To determine the biologically active constituents of garlic, a number of analytical methods such as GLC and HPLC have been developed. The contents of allymethyl sulfide and dipropyldisulfides in the ether extracts of garlic were studied by GLC and MS [189].

A GC-MS analytical method has been developed to assign the various constituents of garlic, and the results indicate that the computerized GC analysis can be effectively used to identify the allium constituents [190]. A GC method having excellent resolution capability, accuracy and reliability has been developed for the determination of S-alk-(en)ylcysteine sulfoxides. This is based on isolation of the amino acid fraction by ion-exchange chromatography followed by derivatization with ethylchloroformate and reduction of the S-alk-(en)ylcysteine sulfoxides by NaI [191]. An HPLC-^{1}H-NMR method has been developed for the reliable qualitative and semi-quantitative separation and identification of garlic constituents [192]. A simple vacuum distillation procedure facilitates the qualitative analysis of volatile constituents. The method allows both qualitative and quantitative determinations of the polar compounds. It has been shown that the GC involving high temperatures gives erroneous results.

The major thiosulfinate of garlic is allicin (**44**) present up to 0.3% of the fresh weight. The major unsymmetrical thiosulfinates are MeS(O)S-CH_2-CH=CH_2 and MeSS(O)-CH_2-CH=CH_2 found in the ratio of 2:1. A reversed-phase HPLC has been developed for S-alk(en)yl-L-cysteine(+)-S-allyl-L-cysteine sulfoxide, L-glutamyl-S-allyl-L-cysteine and L-glutamyl-S-(*trans*-1-propenyl)-L-cysteine [193]. A high-throughput method for the determination of alliin in garlic powders and dry extracts has also been developed. It is based on immobilized allinase which is combined with a two-channel flow injection analyzer coupled to an ammonia-detecting device [194]. Supercritical fluid (CO_2) extracts of *A. sativum* when examined by HPLC and chemical ionization MS enabled the identification of thiosulfinates MeS (O) SMe, MeS (O) SAll, MeSS (O) All, MeS (O) S1-propenyl-(*E, Z*), MeSS (O) 1-propenyl-(*E*), n-PrS (O) SAll, n-PrSS (O) All, AllS (O) S1-propenyl-(*E, Z*), and AllSS (O) 1-propenyl-(*E*) [195].

3.3 Pharmacology

Garlic has been investigated extensively with over a thousand references, but has had a controversial history in the scientific and clinical literature relative to its usefulness as a hypolipidemic agent. Although several other biological activities have been attributed to it, this review is purposely limited to its claimed cardiovascular effects and some of the more recently discovered interesting activities.

3.3.1 Cardiovascular effects

The cardioprotective action of garlic against ischemia- and reperfusion-induced arrhythmia was studied on the isolated perfusing rat hearts [196]. Garlic powder was added (1%) to standard chow and fed to the animals for 10 weeks prior to isolation of the heart. The incidence of ventricular tachycardia (VT) and fibrillation (VF), produced by partial ligation of the left descending coronary branch, in the garlic-fed rat hearts vs. controls were reduced significantly (0% vs. 35% and 50% vs. 88%, respectively). The lag time for onset of extrasystoles and VT or VF was also prolonged in the garlic group.

Martin et al. [197] determined that a garlic dialysate suppresses premature ventricular contractions (PVCs) and VT in ouabain-intoxicated anaesthetized dogs. The dialysate also reduced the arrhythmia of an electrically driven rat isolated left atrium rendered arrhythmic by isoproterenol and aconitine. It blocked both the chronotropic and inotropic activities of isoproterenol in a dose-dependent manner. The authors suggested that garlic dialysate possesses significant anti-arrhythmic activity in ventricular as well as supraventricular arrhythmias. In another study using varying concentrations of calcium and its blockers in the bath solution of isolated rat atrial preparations, the same group concluded that the negative inotropic effect of the dialysate might be due to its ability to restrict intracellular calcium [198]. The calcium manipulations did not modify the negative chronotropic effect of the garlic dialysate.

The antihypertensive effect of garlic has been demonstrated in the two-kidney-one-clip Goldblatt model hypertensive rat [199]. In this model, there is a rennin-induced activation of ACE that converts angiotensin-I to the potent vasoconstrictor angiotensin II causing hypertension. A single oral dose (0.5 ml) of an aqueous extract of garlic produced a maximum antihypertensive response in 4–6 h after dosing, the residual effect lingering on for up to 24 h. Multiple doses further confirmed the hypotensive activity of garlic.

Garlic in a dose-dependent fashion relaxed the isolated rat aorta analogous to the effects of acetylcholine and L-arginine [200]. Endothelial denudation attenuated but did not totally abolish the vasodilatory activity. Based on this observation, the authors suggested that vasodilation caused by garlic might explain its claimed antihypertensive property. A chromatographically purified fraction of garlic elicited a dose-dependent diuretic-natriuretic response in anaesthetized rabbits, which peaked 60 min after i.v. administration of the fraction [201]. If further substantiated, this activity could also contribute to the hypotensive effect of garlic.

Based on lack of confirmed evidence for a hypolipidemic effect of garlic, Berthold and Sudhop [202] stated that prophylactic use of garlic in atherosclerosis is questionable. They also warned that other claimed effects of garlic, e.g., vasodilatory, antithrombotic, etc., should await confirmation through well-designed clinical studies. This created a barrage of comments and controversial dialogue among investigators globally.

Orekhov and Grunwald [203] reviewed publications on garlic supporting its hypolipidemic activity that appeared prior to 1997. They concluded that garlic reduces hyperlipidemia, hypertension and deposition of atheromatous plaque on the intima of the arteries, and that its value in preventing or reducing atherosclerosis may be established only after the then ongoing clinical trials are completed.

3.3.2 Anticancer potential

Bignall [204] cited earlier studies carried out in Italy and China, which claimed that garlic consumption might protect against gastric cancer, since organosulfides contained in garlic had inhibited experimental mutagenesis. Milner [205] also discussed the anticancer potential of garlic and its sulfides. However, the actual experimental evidence more recently comes from the data suggesting that garlic can inhibit cancer cell implants in mice, and also chemically induced carcinogenesis in rats. An aged garlic extract was found to significantly inhibit the growth of Sarcoma-180 (allogenic) and LL/2 lung carcinoma (syngenic) cells transplanted into mice [206]. Diethylnitrosoamine was used to induce hepatocarcinogenesis in the control and the garlic-treated (20 mg powder/kg/day) groups of Wistar rats [207]. A 48–50% reduction in the number as well as area of glutathione S-transferase (placental form) positive foci was observed in the garlic group compared to the controls that received distilled water. These probably are the first sets of experimental evidence supporting the carcinostatic potential of garlic.

3.3.3 Immunomodulation

Kyo et al. [206] studying the carcinostatic effect of aged garlic extract in mice observed that it stimulated the proliferation of spleen cells as well as the release of cytokines, including interleukin (IL-2) and the tumor necrosis factors (TNFα and γ). It also increased the phagocytic activity of macrophages and reactivity of cytotoxic-T lymphocytes to cytokines. In another study, they observed that the extract prevented the immunosuppression caused by psychological stress [208]. Mice subjected to 4 days of stress in a communication box showed a decrease in the hemolytic plaque-forming cells (PFC) and the weight and number of cells of the spleen. All these effects of stress were prevented by the aged garlic extract.

Three compounds occurring in garlic, diallylsulfide (DAS) (**71**), diallyldisulfide (DADS) (**45**) and allylmethylsulfide (AMS), were tested for their immunomodulatory effect in BALB/c mice [209]. After giving 20 mg/kg daily dose of each compound for 5 days, white blood cell count and antibody titers were monitored. Spleen and bone marrow were examined at the end. Out of the sulfides studied, DADS showed the highest white count (17,900/mm^3) on day 6, the highest antibody titer on day 12, and the highest number of PFC (1409/106 spleen cells). The number of α-esterase positive cells was also significantly increased compared to the controls. All these data indicate an immunostimulant effect of the garlic sulfides.

Based on the immunostimulatory and possible anticancer evidence, Lamm and Riggs [210] have proposed that garlic should be given a serious consideration for the clinical trials as an alternative therapy for prevention and/or treatment of bladder cancer.

3.3.4 Enzyme inhibition

Extracts of different parts of *A. ursinum* (wild species) and garlic with standardized sulfide contents were tested *in vitro* for their comparative inhibitory activities on 5-lipoxygenase (LOX), cyclo-oxygenase (COX), ACE and thrombocyte aggregation (TA) [211]. The IC_{50} values for the extracts from both the species showed a good correlation with the concentration of the major sulfur compounds, thiosulfinates and ajoenes. Garlic extracts were slightly more potent than the extracts of the wild species on both LOX and COX, but there was no difference in their activities on the TA. On the ACE, however, the leaf extract of the wild species containing glutamylpeptides was the most potent inhibitor, followed by the garlic leaf and the bulbs of both plants. These results show the enzyme-inhibiting activities of garlic and the possible clinical utility of the wild species as a substitute for garlic.

In vitro inhibition of cytochrome-P_{450} (c-P_{450}) reductases from pig-liver microsomes by an aqueous extract of garlic was found to correlate well with the inhibition exhibited by an HPLC-purified preparation of alliin (**46**), suggesting that the enzyme inhibition shown by garlic may be due to the active principle alliin [212]. Garlic and onion extracts were shown to inhibit adenosine deaminase (ADA) in a dose-dependent manner [213]. The authors claimed the procedure as a tool for monitoring quality control of garlic products for clinical assessment and for bioequivalence control of pharmaceutical products derived from garlic. Several fructose polymers (fructans) isolated from fresh garlic cloves were tested for ADA inhibition [214]. Those composed of 9 to 14 fructose monomers appeared to have the highest potency. Larger polymers had little or no enzyme-inhibiting property. The inhibition was found to be of a competitive nature, suggesting a close conformational relationship between adenosine and the lower polymeric fructans.

3.3.5 Other activities

Antithrombotic activities of flavonoids, which inhibit phosphodiesterase that hydrolyses cyclic nucleotides, and of garlic have been reviewed [215]. (Z)-ajoene (**49**), isolated from garlic, was found to inhibit histamine release from peritoneal mast cells and block the passive-cutaneous anaphylaxis in the rat [216]. This antiallergic activity has been claimed to be due to the ability of the ajoene to block the release of histamine and an H-like substance.

Doxorubicin, an anthracycline derivative and a potent anticancer drug that acts through intercalation with DNA to disrupt transcription and translation, possesses cardiotoxicity due probably to the production of free radicals. Based on the claimed antioxidant and free-radical scavenging activity of sulfur compounds of garlic, Mostafa et al. [217] tested S-allyl-L-cysteine (SAC) (**51**) for its effect on doxorubicin-induced toxicity in mice. A dose of 30 mg/kg, i. p., was injected into mice daily for 5 days. On day 3, a single i.p.

injection of 15 mg/kg of doxorubicin was given. Deaths were recorded daily, body weight was measured on alternate days, and serum creatine phosphokinase (CPK) levels and histopathology of the heart and the liver were determined 6 days after the doxorubicin injection. The mortality in the SAC-treated group was only 30%, compared to 58% in the control group receiving only doxorubicin. The loss of body weight caused by doxorubicin was also prevented by SAC. The serum CPK levels in the SAC group was 1923 + 635 i.u./L, compared to 5472 + 570 i.u./L in the control group. Histological examination also revealed a protective action of SAC against cardio- and hepatotoxicity. If these activities are confirmed in clinical trials, garlic and/or its constituents may be a very useful adjuvant to anthracycline drugs in cancer treatment.

Allyl mercaptan (AM) and several other constituents of garlic were tested for cytotoxicity and their effect on cholesterol biosynthesis and release in Hep-G2 cells in culture [218]. At concentrations up to 50 ng/ml, no cytotoxicity was seen with any of the compounds, but those above 250 ng/ml drastically reduced cell viability. At 25 ng/ml concentrations of the compounds, the ^{3}H-acetate incorporation into cholesterol was significantly blocked, as was also the secretion of cholesterol by the cells. No effects by the garlic compounds were seen on the incorporation of the labeled acetate into fatty acids or of the tritiated glycerol into triglycerides. This activity would place these garlic sulfides in the category of inhibitors of endogenous cholesterol synthesis, but with none of the toxic effects observed with the currently used cholesterol-lowering allopathic drugs.

3.4 Clinical studies

The earliest double-blind, controlled and randomized clinical trials on garlic in hyperlipidemic patients were reported in Germany [219]. Two studies were carried out with a 6-week period on placebo and a similar period for treatment. In one study, 34 patients were given 3 × 198 mg/day of dried garlic, whereas the second group of 51 patients received a 3 × 450 mg dose/day. Total cholesterol, high-density lipoprotein (HDL), low-density lipoprotein (LDL), triglycerides, apolipoproteins A and B, and several clotting parameters were measured every 3 weeks. Both doses of dried garlic failed to show any significant effect on the lipid profile.

A review of all clinical trials reported prior to 1989 found problems with those trials in either the design or methodology or execution [220]. Several open trials, however, appear to have shown the hypolipidemic activity in the fresh garlic. A placebo-controlled, double-blind study using 800 mg/day dose of dry garlic powder demonstrated a significant inhibition of TA with a concomitant decrease in diastolic blood pressure [221]. The first placebo-controlled, double-blind trial in patients with intermittent claudication showed that garlic therapy could increase the patients' pain-free walking by 50% [222].

Twenty-four healthy volunteers with HDL of less than 10 mg/dl (men) and 15 mg/dl (women) in a randomized, placebo-controlled, double-blind trial were fed a fatty test meal containing 100 g butter [223]. Three brand-named garlic tablets per day, equivalent to 900 mg of dried garlic powder, were given to the treatment group for 6 weeks. Lipid parameters were measured at 0, 3 and 5 h postprandial on day 1, 22 and 43 of the treatment. The data revealed a 35% reduction of the postprandial triglyceride levels and an increase in the HDL levels in the garlic-treated group compared to the placebo group. The number of subjects was obviously too small to draw meaningful conclusions from this study.

The first meta-analysis of all the clinical trials prior to 1993 was carried out by Warshafsky et al. [224], who could find only 5 out of a total of 28 that qualified as standardized and well-conducted trials. They concluded from all the data analyzed that garlic reduced the blood cholesterol levels by 9% compared to placebo. However, Isaacsohn et al. [225] in the US found no significant hypolipidemic effect in randomized 50 hypercholesteremic patients given either placebo (n = 22, mean age 57) or 3 × 300 mg of garlic powder (n = 28, mean age 58), all patients receiving a relatively low-fat diet for 12 weeks. No significant differences were seen in the two groups in any lipid parameters monitored. This trial was relatively larger and perhaps better controlled in terms of dietary intake and actual monitoring. Another double-blind, randomized and cross-over study, published 9 days after the US study but carried out in Germany, also failed to detect any hypolipidemic effect of garlic in 25 mild hyperlipidemic patients (mean age 58) [202]. A trial on pediatric hypercholesteremic patients also failed to detect any significant lipid-lowering property in garlic [226]. Likewise, a relatively large (n = 115), well-designed and executed randomized trial in UK [227] and a smaller but well-designed crossover Australian study [228] both failed to show any significant hypolipidemic activity in garlic.

Interestingly, a 12-week Canadian study on 46 hypercholesteremic patients, using garlic alone (900 mg/day) as well as in combination with fish oil (12 g/day), showed a clear hypolipidemic effect of garlic [229]. Garlic alone and in combination with fish oil lowered total cholesterol (TC) by about 12% while fish oil alone had no effect on TC. Garlic alone also lowered LDL by 14% while fish oil alone raised it. The triglycerides, however, decreased 34% with the combination and 37% with fish oil alone. The HDL levels showed a trend toward increase in all the fish oil-receiving groups. The risk ratios TC/HDL and LDL/HDL both were reduced significantly in the garlic and garlic-fish oil groups, but not in those receiving fish oil alone. This study raises a serious question about the fish oil results, for a large body of evidence over the past half a century suggests that fish oil rich in ω-3 fatty acids significantly lowers cholesterol and LDL.

Of great interest is the recent German study in which the atheroslerotic plaques in the carotid and femoral arteries were measured non-invasively by B-mode ultrasound [230]. Claimed as a randomized, double-blind and placebo-controlled trial over 4 years on 152 probationers using continuous garlic intake, the study showed a 6–13% reduction in the plaque buildup by garlic. Should this observation be confirmed on further trials on atherosclerotic patients, garlic may be the first drug demonstrating a prevention, and perhaps a regression or reversal, of the atherosclerotic process.

The most recent meta-analysis on 13 randomized clinical trials in hypercholesteremic patients confirms the cholesterol-lowering ability of garlic, but questions its overall value as a remedy for treating hypercholesteremia or hyperlipidemia [231]. Morelli and Zoorob [232], while reviewing alternative therapies for congestive heart failure and hypercholesteremia, state: "Despite the many early promising studies and meta-analyses evaluating garlic's effect as a lipid-lowering agent, more recent, rigorous studies have failed to substantiate these benefits. There is no current role for garlic as an antihyperlipidemic agent". However, they based their opinion on only two meta-analyses: one pediatric study and one study that uses garlic oil and not the dried powder or fresh garlic that would have many water-soluble components as well. The meta-analyses cannot be used as scientific evidence and can be skewed in conclusion, depending on publications appearing in the period reviewed that are in favor of a claim vs. those against.

Tyler [233] in March 2001 reported on the highlights of the annual Congress of the Society for Medicinal Plants Research held in Zurich, Switzerland during September 2000. Ajoene, a decomposition product of the major constituent of garlic, allicin, was reported to show potential as an anticancer drug through its ability to produce apoptosis (cell death), analogous to the well-known anticancer drugs doxorubicin and paclitaxel. Both these drugs, however, are extremely cardiotoxic compared to the time-tested safe garlic. Furthermore, garlic has been shown to have protective activity against doxorubicin-induced cardiotoxicity [217].

Another original claim for garlic's benefit is its hypotensive activity. A meta-analysis of three acceptable trials on hypertensive patients showed only slight reduction in the diastolic but greater effect on the systolic pressure in the garlic-treated patients compared to placebo [234]. The overall data were insufficient to draw any serious conclusions and warranted further large-scale, well-controlled trials.

An interesting clinical investigation was carried out to assess the effect of garlic on oxidative stress in 25 healthy volunteers [235]. A daily dose of 900 mg of garlic tablets, with a standardized alliin content of 1.3% and an allicin content of 0.6%, was given to the subjects for 2 months. The levels of malondialdehyde (MDA), reduced glutathione (GSH) and its oxidation product GSSG were measured as stress biomarkers initially and at the end of garlic treatment. The treatment showed a 60% reduction of the initial value of MDA. The GSH levels in the erythrocytes were increased while the GSSG levels showed no significant change from the initial values. Thus the GSSH/GSH ratio showed a significant decrease after the garlic treatment, an indicator of the protective nature of garlic against stress.

3.4.1 Drug-drug interactions

In view of the antithrombotic activity of garlic and its components [215, 221], patients taking warfarin sodium or aspirin-like products on a chronic basis should avoid consumption of garlic. The ability of garlic and its constituents to inhibit COX, LOX and ACE enzymes [211], c-P_{450} [212], and ADA [213] suggests that garlic may be a general enzyme inhibitor. Such agents are known to alter the pharmacokinetics of other drugs, especially their elimination half-life. Physicians and pharmacists should be aware of this potential drug-drug interaction between garlic and those drugs that are metabolized by a mixed-function oxidase involving c-P_{450}. With ACE-inhibitors being widely used for treating hypertension, garlic would have an additive, if not synergistic effect. The same would also hold for the latest anti-arthritic drugs such as COX and LOX inhibitors. In all these cases, garlic could be beneficial in that the dosage of the respective drugs, some of which have serious side-effects, may be reduced.

In conclusion, the equivocal issue of garlic's cardiovascular effects can be settled only by large-scale, well-controlled, double-blind trials, not by meta-analyses which actually add to confusion and controversy. However, its anti-stress and potential anticancer properties currently beg more attention from investigators. These potentials must be further explored to harness garlic's value in health and medicine.

4 Ginger

Zingiber officinale Roscoe (family Zingiberaceae; common name ginger, known in Sanskrit as *Ardraka* or *Sunthi* when dried, Sheng jiang or Gan jiang in Chinese when dried, and Kankyo in Japanese if steamed and Shoukyo when dried) is a perennial herb with aromatic rhizomes. The genus *Zingiber* includes about 85 species, of which *Z. officinale* R. (hereafter referred to as ginger) has been cultivated for millennia in both India and China. Ginger reached the West at least two thousand years ago.

Ginger is a household remedy for indigestion, dyspepsia, flatulence and colic. It is also soothing for cough, colds, flu and other respiratory problems. It has been used in anorexia, arthritis, chest congestion, chicken pox, cholera, chronic bronchitis, cold extremities, diarrhoea, dropsy, fever, disorders of gallbladder, hyperacidity, hypercholesterolemia, hyperglycemia, morning sickness, nausea, rheumatism, sore throat, and vomiting [236, 237]. In Ayurvedic practice, the fresh and dried roots are considered distinctly separate products having differing medicinal properties. Ginger has been extensively studied for a broad range of biological activities [238, 239]. In Germany, ginger products are marketed for treatment of dyspepsia and prophylaxis of motion sickness, the average daily dose being 2 g of the dried rhizome [240]. In recent years, both fresh and dried ginger have become increasingly popular. The US imported more than 4,000 metric tons of ginger in the nineties. World annual production of ginger on a dry-weight basis is estimated at 100,000 tons. The major producers are India, China, Australia, Jamaica, Nigeria and Vietnam [241, 242]. Several reviews have been published on various aspects of ginger [243–245]. However, this review deals specifically with its bioactive principles and their well-tested pharmacological, clinical and mechanistic studies.

4.1 Chemistry

Guenther [246] has summarized the chemical investigations carried out on the essential oils of ginger before 1953. Steam distillation of semi-dried ginger gives pale yellow oil consisting mainly of mono- and sesquiterpene hydrocarbons and their oxygenated products. The oleoresins and non-volatile components of ginger are usually obtained by solvent extraction with CH_2Cl_2 or MeOH and purification by chromatography. Ginger oleoresin contains the pungent gingerols, gingidiols, gingerdiones, and shogaols that are twice as pungent as gingerols. Dried ginger consists of ~ 40–60% starch, 10% protein, 10% fat, 5% fiber, 6% inorganic material, 10% moisture and 1–4% essential oil.

4.1.1 Essential oils

Ginger is valued for its volatile aromatic compounds . The composition of its oil depends on the variety, method of cultivation, the age at harvest, and the geographical location of ginger, as well as the distillation method used. However, the major factor that determines the commercial value of ginger in the international market appears to be its origin [247]. Govindarajan claimed that the hydroxylated terpenes contribute to the aroma of ginger [243]. Recently developed sophisticated techniques of isolation and structure determination have immensely increased the number of identifiable compounds in ginger. Lawrence in 1983 had identified more than 200 volatile compounds in ginger oil [248]. The composition of ginger oil from Vietnam (2.7%) was determined by GC, GC-MS and ^{13}C-NMR spectra. The oil is a complex mixture of ~ 300 peaks, of which 77 most prominent components were identified by MS recorded earlier. The essential oil consisted of 28% monoterpene hydrocarbons, 37% oxygenated monoterpenes, 25% sesquiterpene hydrocarbons, 8% oxygenated sesquiterpenes, and 2% non-terpenoid compounds. The major component was geranial (16%, **85**). The other compounds identified included allo-aromadendrene (0.14%, **86**), β-bisabolene (**87**), camphene (12.6%, **88**), α-D-curcumene (**89**), *p*-cymene-8-ol, 2,6-dimethylhept-5-enal (0.06%), D-limonene (2.1%, **90**), methylisoeugenol, γ-muurolene, neral (8.1%, **91**), β-phellandrene (5.7%, **92**), α-pinene (3.5%, **93**), xanthorrhizol (0.1%) and α-zingiberene (9.2%, **94**) [249]. The chemical composition of the essential oil (2.4%) of Nigerian ginger, also determined by GC and GC-MS, consisted of 64% sesquiterpenehydrocarbons, 6.6% carbonyl compounds, 5.6% alcohols, 2.4% monoterpenehydrocarbons, and 1% esters. The main components were zingiberene (29.5%, **94**) and β-sesquiphellandrene (18.4%, **95**). A number of previously unreported compounds identified included acetic acid, cadinol, α- and γ-calcorene, α-cubebene, 2,6-dimethylhepten-1-ol, eremophilene (**96**), (*E,E*)-α-farnesene (**97**), geranic acid, geranoic acid, geranyl propionate, α-gurjunene (**98**), α-himachalene (**99**), isovaleraldehyde, linalool oxide, n-methylpyrrole, γ-muurolene (**100**), 2-pentenone, pinanol, and α-santalene (**101**). The GC analysis showed a total of 266 peaks, of which 89 constituents were identified by comparing the retention times and MS with reference samples [250]. The hydrocarbons and the oxygenated compounds of the essential oil have been classified as shown in Table 4. Davon, Scott and others [251] have provided a valuable resource for many of the structures and physical constants of mono- and sesquiterpenoids.

Bisabolene-type sesquiterpene zingiberene (**94**) is the major constituent of the essential oil. Eschenmoser and Schinz [252] established the structures of zingiberene while Arigoni and Jeger [253] proved the 7*S* configuration of the side chain stereocentre. The 4*S*,7*S* stereochemistry was confirmed by X-ray crystallography of isozingiberene dihydrochloride, a bicyclic derivative of zingiberene [254]. The total synthesis of (±) zingiberene [255] and 4*S*,7*S* zingiberene have been reported [256, 257], though as a mixture of double bond isomers and/or diastereomers. The diastereomer of zingiberene, 7-*epi*zingiberene, has also been isolated from wild tomato leaves [258]. Treatment of a sesquiterpene-enriched fraction of ginger oil with 4-phenyl-1,2,4-triazolo-3,5-dione to afford a Diels-Alder adduct followed by hydrolysis has been described for a rapid isolation of zingiberene [259]. By isotopic labeling experiments, the biosynthesis of the sesquithujane skeleton has been shown to occur by 1,2-hydrogen shift [260]. Several sesquiterpenes of ginger were shown to possess antirhinoviral activity and the most active compound was shown to be β-sesquiphellandrene (**95**) [261]. Free and glycosidically bound

Table 4.
Classification of the constituents of Nigerian ginger essential oil

Aliphatic	(alcohols)	2,6-dimethylheptane-1-ol, 2-ethyl hexanol, n-heptane-2-ol
	(aldehydes)	n-butylaldehyde, hexanal, isovaleraldehyde, 2-methylbutanal, *trans*-2-octanal
	(ketones)	acetone, 2-methyl-2-hepten-6-one, methyl-n-heptylkerone, methylnonyl ketone, methylundecyl ketone, pentanone
	(acids)	acetic, lauric
Aromatic	(hydrocarbons)	*p*-cymene, toluene
	(phenols)	α-eugenol, *trans*-isoeugenol
Monoterpenes	(hydrocarbons)	camphene, limonene, myrene, α-phellandrene, β-phellandrene (**92**), α-pinene (**93**), β-pinene, sabinene, δ-terpinene, terpinolene
	(alcohols)	borneol (**102**), citronellol (**103**), geraniol, linalool, limonen-10-ol, α-terpineol
	(ketones)	geranylacetone
	(acids)	geranic acid, geranoic acid
	(esters)	citronellyl acetate, geranyl acetate, geranyl propionate, isobornyl acetate, neryl acetate
	(oxides)	1,8-cineole, linalool oxide (**104**)
Sesquiterpenes	(hydrocarbons)	alloaromadendrene (**86**), bergametene, α-calacorene, calamenene, camphor, β-caryophyllene, α-copaene, α-cubebene, β-elemene, γ-elemene, δ-elemene, eremophilene (**96**), farnesene, (*E*)-farnesene, (*E,E*) α-farnesene (**97**), (Z)-β-carnesene, germacrene D, α-gurjumene (**98**), α-himachalene (**99**), α-humulene, γ-muurolene (**100**), perillene, santalene (**101**), β-selinene, β-sesquiphellandrene (**95**), vetivinene, α-ylangene, zingiberene (**94**)
	(alcohols)	α-bisabolol, cadinol, elemol, eudesmol, α-eudesmol, γ-muurolol , nerolidol, pinanol, β-sesquiphellandrol
	(ketones)	ionone
	(oxides)	caryophylline oxide
Others		acetyl furan, *N*-methyl pyrrole

aliphatic alcohols, monoterpenealcohols, aldehydes and acids of ginger juice were isolated and separated on an Amberlite column [262]. The glucosides of citronellol (2*E*,6*E*) and (2*E*,6*Z*)-3,7-dimethyl–8-hydroxyoctadiene-1-ol, 1,8-epoxy-p-menthane-3-ol, geraniol, 2-heptanol, 5-hydroxyborneol, *R*-linalool, and nerol, have also been isolated from ginger. An 80% MeOH extract was

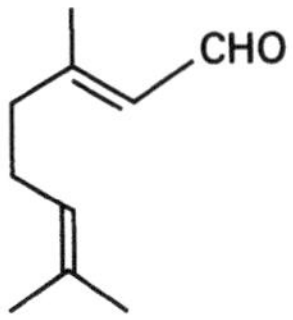
Geranial (**85**)

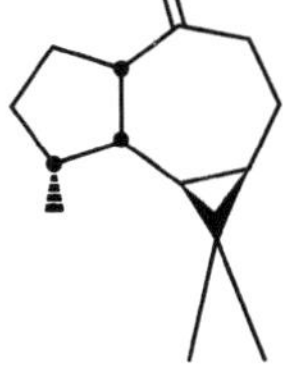
Alloaromadendrene (**86**)

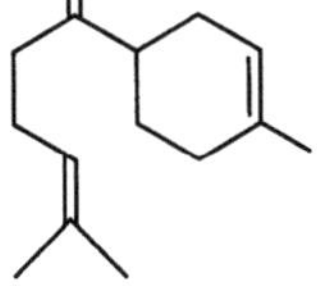
β-D-Bisabolene (**87**)

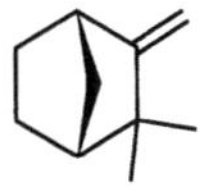
D-Camphene (**88**)

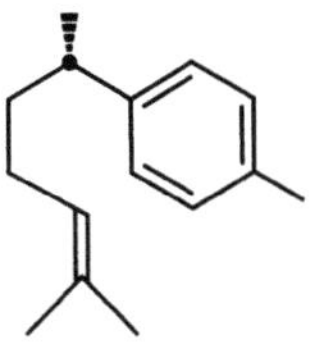
α-D-Curcumene (**89**)

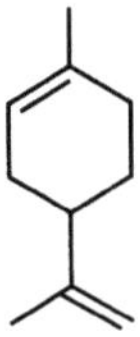
D-Limonene (**90**)

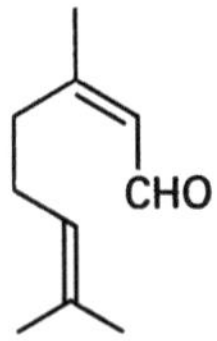
Neral (**91**)

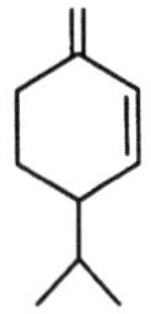
β-D-Phellandrene (**92**)

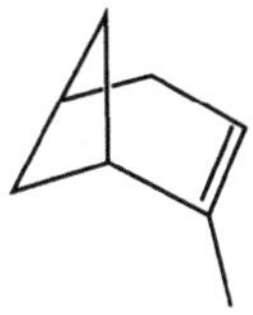
α-Pinene (**93**)

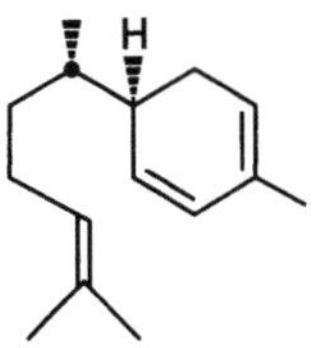
α-Zingiberene (**94**)

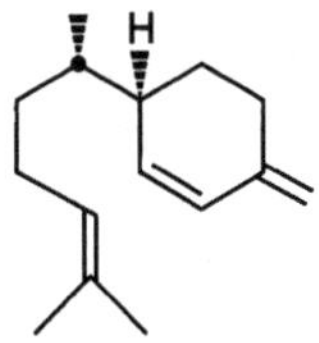
β-Sesquiphellandrene (**95**)

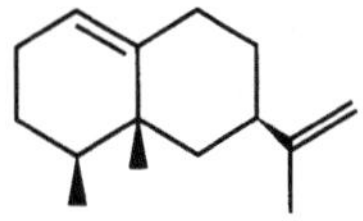
Eremophelene (**96**)

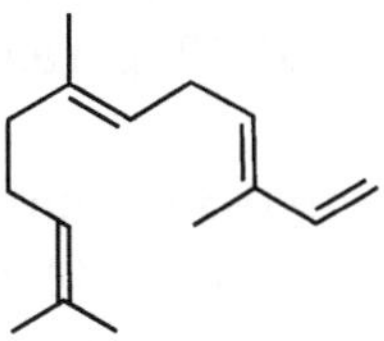
α-Farnesene (**97**)

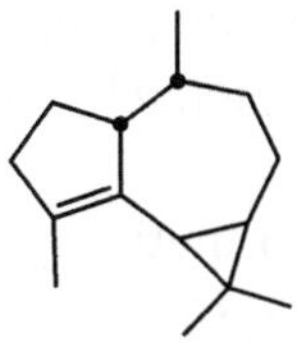
α-L-Gurjunene (**98**)

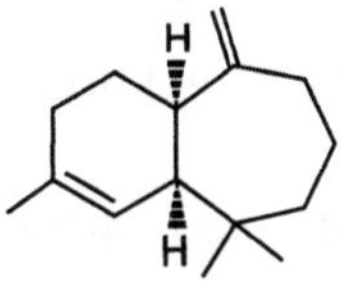
α-Himachalene (**99**)

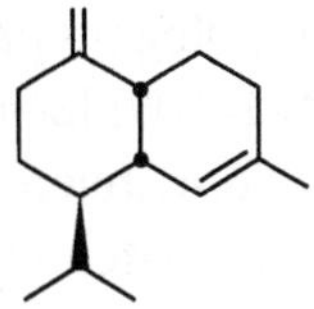
γ-Muurolene (**100**)

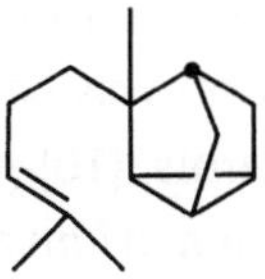
α-Santalene (**101**)

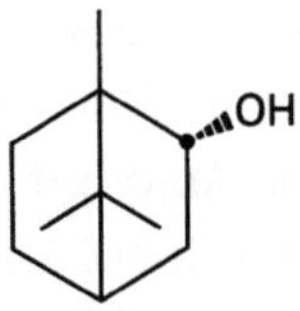
D-Borneol (**102**)

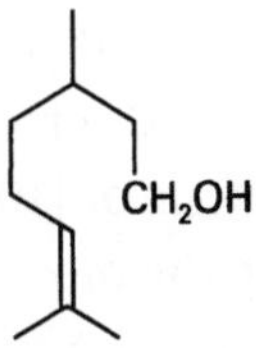
D-Citronellol (**103**)

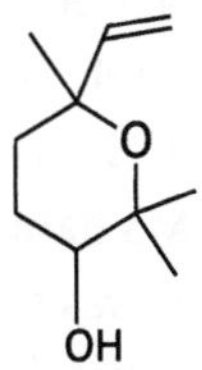
Linalooloxide (**104**)

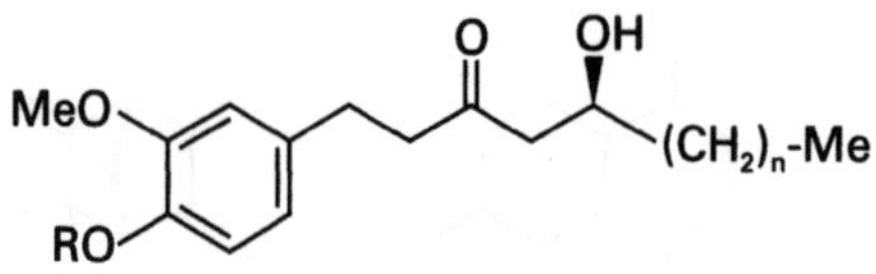

		n	R
[4]-Gingerol	**(105)**	2	H
[6]-Gingerol	**(106)**	4	H
[8]-Gingerol	**(107)**	6	H
[10]-Gingerol	**(108)**	8	H
[12]-Gingerol	**(109)**	10	H
[3]-Gingerol	**(110)**	1	H
Me[6]-Gingerol	**(111)**	4	Me

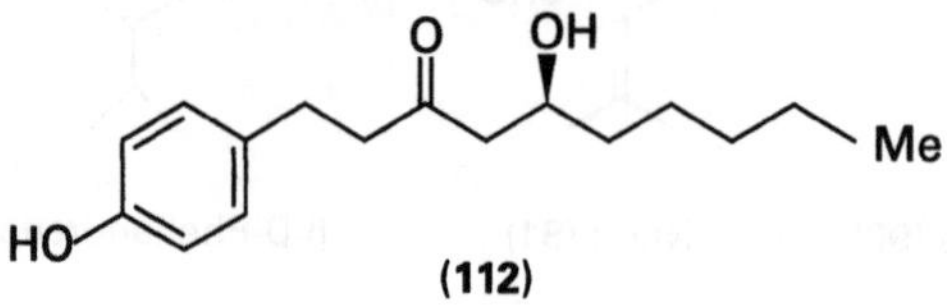

(112)

purified by HPLC and hydrolyzed with glucosidase to yield aglycones, indicating that these glucosides are the aromatic precursors of fresh ginger [263].

4.1.2 Gingerols

The major oily constituents responsible for the pungent taste of ginger are homologous phenolic ketones known as {4}-, {6}, {8}-, {10}- and {12}-gingerols (**105–109**) [264].

{6}-Gingerol {5-hydroxy-1-(4-hydroxy-3-methoxyphenyl)-3-decanone} was isolated in the (*R*) and (*S*) forms. {3}- (**110**), {4}-, {5}-, {8}- and {10}-gingerols have been isolated. Me{6}-gingerol (**111**) is a crystalline compound, mp 65 °C [265]. The gingerols have been synthesized [266, 267]. From a MeOH extract of ginger {6}-, {8}-, and {10}-gingerols were isolated as the anti-emetic principle [268]. {6}-, {8}-, and {10}-gingerols were isolated by fractionation of the CH_2Cl_2 extract of fresh ginger and HPLC. The identification was based on MS data and synthesis of {10}-gingerol. Amongst the gingerols, {10}-gingerol was shown to be the most active inhibitor of *Mycobacterium avium* and *M. tuberculosis in vitro* [269]. Six gingerols (**105–108**, **111**, **112**) were isolated and their structures were elucidated by chemical and spectroscopic evidence.

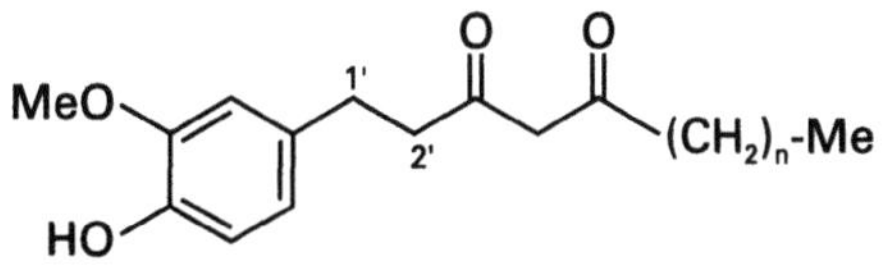

		n
[6]-Gingerdione	(**113**)	4
[8]-Gingerdione	(**114**)	6
[10]-Gingerdione	(**115**)	8
[12]-Gingerdione	(**116**)	10

Most of the compounds showed greater antioxidant effect than α-tocopherol [270, 271]. By a radient elution reversed-phase HPLC separation and HPLC-UV-electrospray-MS for identification, {4}-, {6}-, {8}-, {10}- and Me{6}-gingerols have been identified in ginger extracts [272].

4.1.3 Gingerdiones

A series of enolized homologous β-diketones, {6}-, {8}-, {10}- and {12}-gingerdiones (**113–116**) that are strong prostaglandin inhibitors have been isolated as constituents of ginger. The corresponding 1'2'-dehydro analogues of {6}-, {8}-, {10}-gingerdiones were also obtained [273-275]. {6}-gingerdione was shown to possess a strong antioxidative effect [271, 276]. {10}-gingerdione was detected by HPLC-electrospray-MS [272, 277].

4.1.4 Gingediols

The homologous {4}-, {6}-, {8}-, {10}-gingerdiols (**117–120**) were found to be minor constituents of ginger. The 3,5-diacetate of {4}-gingediol was also isolated [278–280]. {6}-Gingediol and the corresponding diacetate were obtained and their antioxidant properties examined [270]. {6}-Gingediol and four analogues, (3*R*,5*S*)-5-acetoxy-1-(4-hydroxy-3-methoxyphenyl)decane (**121**), (3*R*,5*S*)-3-acetoxy-5-hydroxy1-(4-hydroxy-3-methoxyphenyl)decane (**122**), (3*R*,5*S*)-3,5-diacetoxy-1-(4-hydroxy-3-methoxy-phenyl)-decane (**123**) and (3*R*,5*S*)-3,5-diacetoxy-1-(3,4-dimethoxyphenyl)decane (**124**) were also iso-

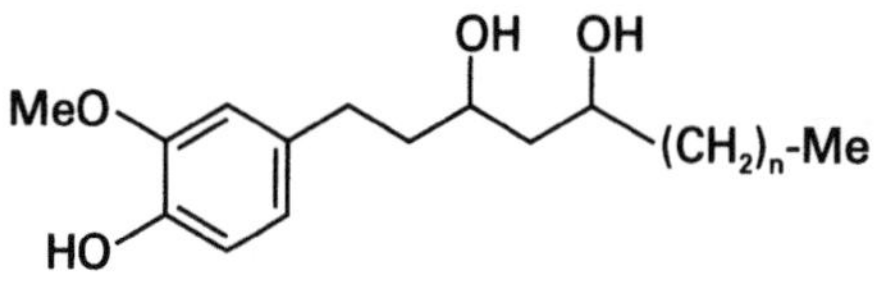

		n
[4]-Gingediol	(**117**)	2
[6]-Gingediol	(**118**)	4
[8]-Gingediol	(**119**)	6
[10]-Gingediol	(**120**)	8

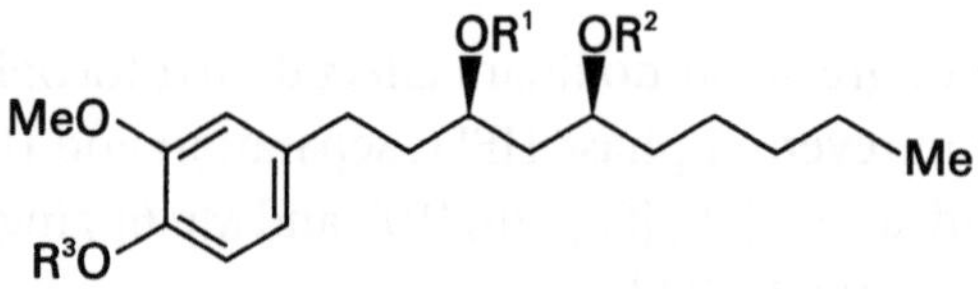

	R^1	R^2	R^3
(**121**)	H	Ac	H
(**122**)	Ac	H	H
(**123**)	Ac	Ac	H
(**124**)	Ac	Ac	Me

lated and their structures were elucidated by chemical and spectral studies. To determine the stereochemistry at C-3 and C-5 of gingediol (**118**), {6}-gingerol (**107**) was reduced with $NaBH_4$, the two epimeric alcohols separated and, by suitable derivatization and ^{1}HNMR spectral studies, the stereochemistry at C-3 and C-5 of the natural gingediol (**118**) was established as 3*R*,5*S* [271, 281]. The absolute stereochemistry of optically active compounds structurally related to the (n)-gingerols-(6) and diols-(7) was established by the highfield ^{1}H-NMR application of Mosher's method [282]. Using reversed-phase HPLC separation and HPLC-UV-electrospray-MS for identification {6}-, {8}-, {12}- and Me{12}-gingediols have been identified in ginger extract [272]. Two novel glucosides of {6}-gingediol were isolated from fresh ginger. Their structures were determined as 1-(4-*O*-β-D-glucopyranosyl-3-methoxyphenyl)decane (**125**) and 5-*O*-β-D-glucopyranosyl-3-hydroxy-1-(4-hydroxy-3-methoxyphenyl)decane (**126**) by HRFAB-MS, and ^{1}H and ^{13}C-NMR analysis. The absolute configuration of both aglycones was identified as 3*S*,5*S* by comparison with synthetic compounds [283].

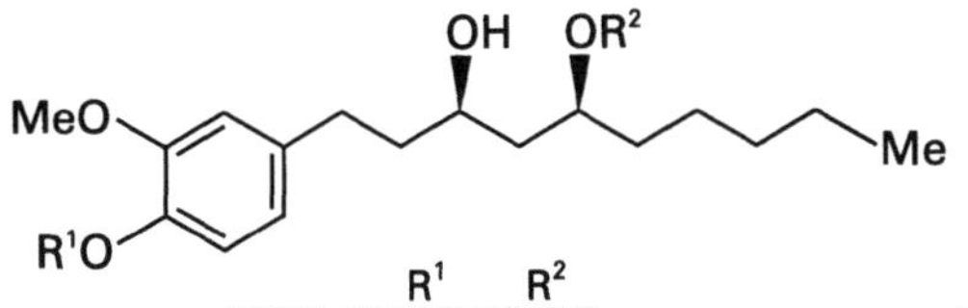

	R¹	R²
(**125**)	Glu	H
(**126**)	H	Glu

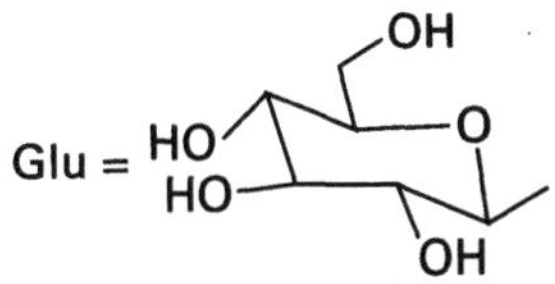

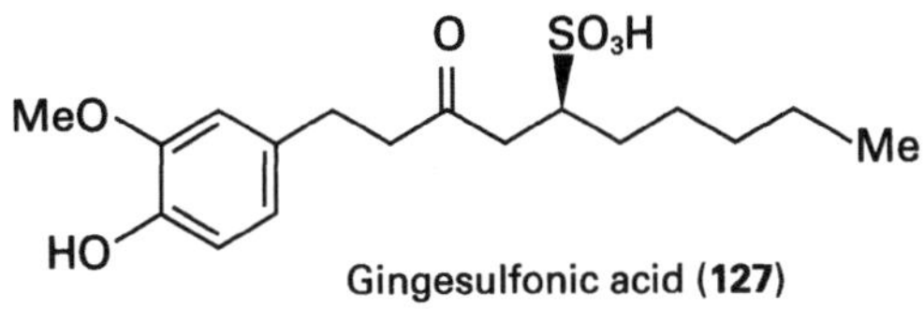

Gingesulfonic acid (**127**)

4.1.5 Gingesulfonic acid

A new anti-ulcer principle designated as gingesulfonic acid was isolated from the MeOH-extract of ginger and further fractionated between EtOAC-H_2O. Reversed-phase column chromatography of the H_2O soluble portion gave 6-gingesulfonic acid (**127**) in 0.0013% yield. The structure was determined by FAB-MS, ^1H, ^{13}C-NMR spectral and chemical correlational studies [284, 285].

4.1.6 Shogaols

The shogaol series of compounds, the dehydration products of the corresponding gingerols formed by heating or on long storage, are even more pungent than the gingerols [286, 287]. From the CH_2Cl_2 extract of ginger and chromatographic purification on silica gel, Sephadex LH-20 and preparative HPLC, six shogaol-type compounds were isolated and characterized from chemical and ^1H, ^{13}C-NMR spectral evidence [270]. {6}-, {8}-, and {10}-shogaols were isolated from the MeOH extract [267]. {6}-, {8}-, and {10}- and Me{6}-shogaols (**128–131**) were isolated by reversed-phase HPLC and MS determination [272]. The structure of 6-gingesulfonic acid was determined by chemical correlation with 6-shogaol [284, 285].

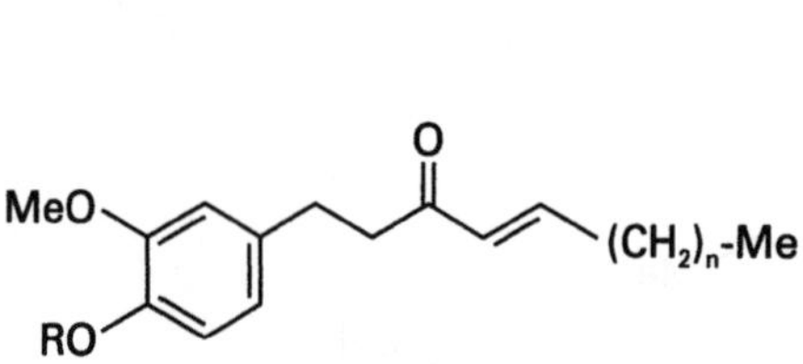

		n	R
[6]-Shogaol	(**128**)	4	H
[8]-Shogaol	(**129**)	6	H
[10]-Shogaol	(**130**)	8	H
Me[6]-Shogaol	(**131**)	4	Me

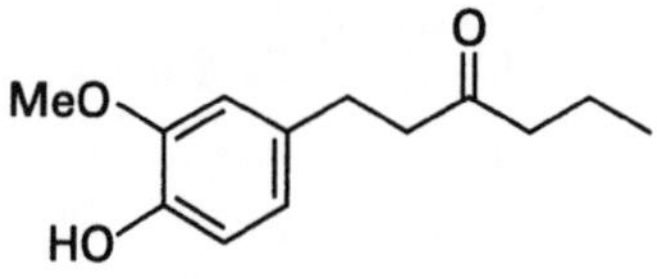

[4]-Gingerone (**132**)

{6}-Shogaol showed greater antioxidant effect than 6-gingerol (**106**) [276]. A high-yield multigram synthesis of {4}-gingerone (**132**) and {6}-shogaol (**128**) has been reported. Both these compounds are prepared by the addition of organolithium reagents to 3-(4-hydroxy-3-methoxyphenyl)-N-methoxy-N-methylpropionamide, which in turn was prepared from ferulic acid. Subsequent addition of MeLi gave **132** while addition of heptynyllithium followed by Cr(II) reduction of the resulting alkyne gave **128** [288]. By monitoring with anti-ulcer effects in rats, the sesquiterpenes β-sesquiphellandrene, β-bisabolene, α-D-curcumene, α-zingiberene, {6}-gingerol and {6}-shogaol were found to be the active components of ginger [289]. The structures of these compounds as {6}-, {8}-, and {10}-dehydroshogaol were established by spectroscopic analysis. The n-dehydroshogaols were synthesized from vanillin by aldol condensation with an alkanol in presence of $LiN(TMS)_2$ [290].

4.1.7 Diarylheptanoids

Four gingerenones, designated as gingerenone-A, -B and -C and isogingerenone-B, were isolated as oils, and their structures were determined as (**133–136**), respectively, by ^{1}H, ^{13}C-NMR spectra [291]. Two diarylheptanoids, meso-3,5-diacetoxy-1,7-bis(4-hydroxy-3-methoxyphenyl)heptane (**137**) and

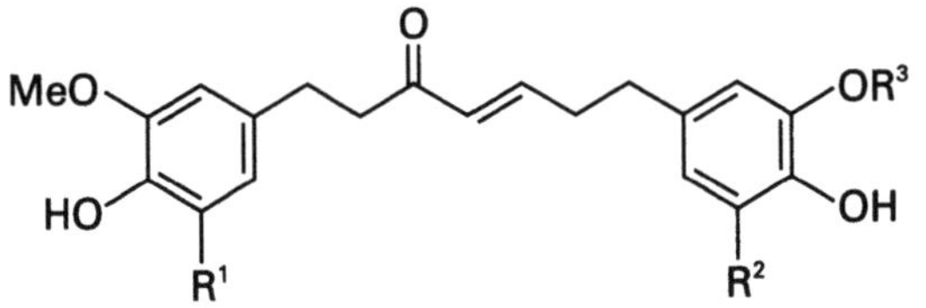

		R^1	R^2	R^3
Gingerenone A	(**133**)	H	H	Me
Gingerenone B	(**134**)	H	OMe	Me
Gingerenone C	(**135**)	H	H	H
Isogingerenone B	(**136**)	OMe	H	Me

3,5-diacetoxy-1-(4-hydroxy-3,5-dimethoxypheyl)-7-(4-hydroxy-3-methoxyphenyl)-heptane (**138**), together with gingerenone-A and hexahydrocurcumin, were also obtained from ginger. The structures of these compounds were elucidated based on chemical and spectroscopic evidence. Spectral and optical rotation data indicated a symmetrical skeleton for **137**. The stereochemistry of hexahydrocurcumin at C-5 was shown to be 5*S* [292]. Eight diarylheptanoids, 5-hydroxy-7-(4-hydroxyphenyl)-1-(4-hydroxy-3-methoxy phenyl)-3-heptanone (**139**), 3,5-diacetoxy-7-(3,4-dihydroxyphenyl)-1-(4-hydroxy-3-methoxyphenyl)heptane (**140**), 5-hydroxy-1-(4-hydroxy-3, 5-dimethoxyphenyl)-1-(4-hydroxy-3-methoxyphenyl)-3-hepta-none (**141**), 5-hydroxy-7-(4-hydroxy-3,5-dimethoxyphenyl)-1-(4-hydroxy-3-methoxyphenyl)-3-heptanone (**142**), (3*R*, 5*S*)-3,5-dihydroxy-1,7-bis(4-hydroxy-3-methoxyphenyl)heptane (**143**), (3*S*,5*S*)-3,5-diacetoxy-1,7-bis(4-hydroxyphenyl)heptane (**144**), 7-(3,4-dihydroxyphenyl)-1-(4-hydroxy-3-methoxyphenyl)-hept-4-en-3-one (gingerenone C) (**135**), and (3*S*,5*S*)-3,5-dihydroxy-1,7-bis(4-hydroxy-3-methoxyphenyl)heptane (**145**) were isolated from ginger. Their structures were established based on chemical and extensive NMR spectroscopic evidence [293]. The absolute stereochemistry of **143** as 3*S*,5*S* was established making use of the dibenzoate chirality method [311]. Eight diarylheptanoids were isolated from the more polar fractions of ginger and their antioxidant properties were evaluated [271]. Five cyclic diarylheptanoids (**146–150**) were isolated from a CH_2Cl_2 extract of ginger. Detailed MS, NMR spectroscopic and chemical studies elucidated their structures. These compounds were oxygenated at C-1, C-3 and C-5 on the heptane chain and

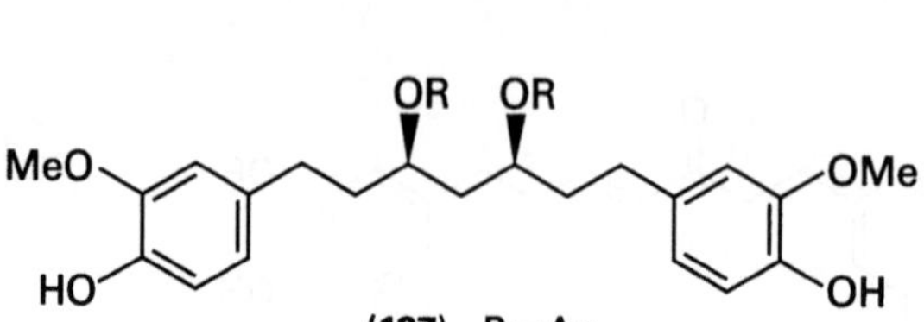

(137) R = Ac
(143) R = H

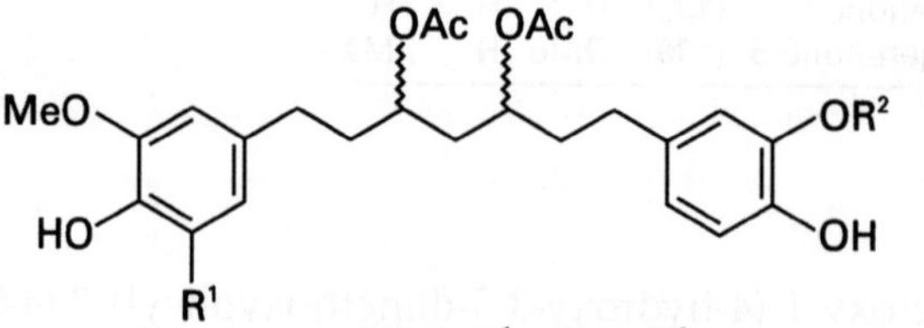

(138) R^1 = OMe, R^2 = Me
(140) R^1 = R^2 = H

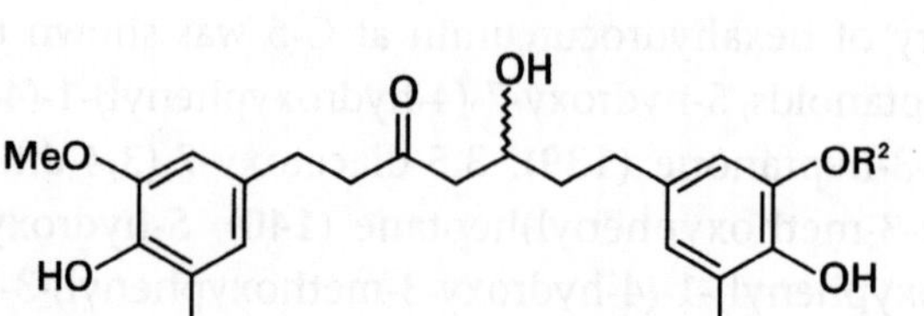

	R^1	R^2	R^3
(139)	H	H	H
(141)	OMe	OMe	H
(142)	H	OMe	OMe

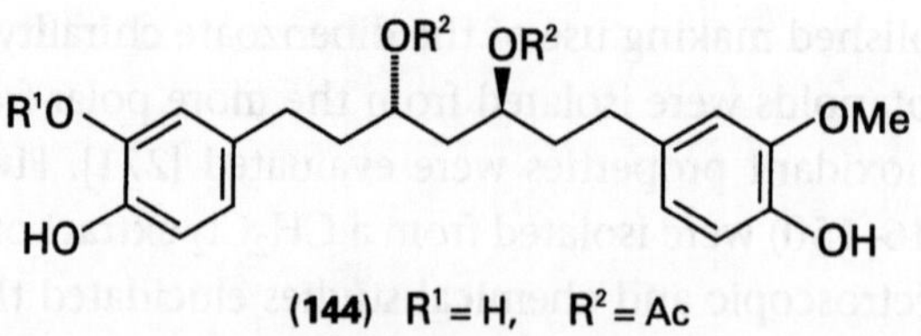

(144) R^1 = H, R^2 = Ac
(145) R^1 = Me, R^2 = H

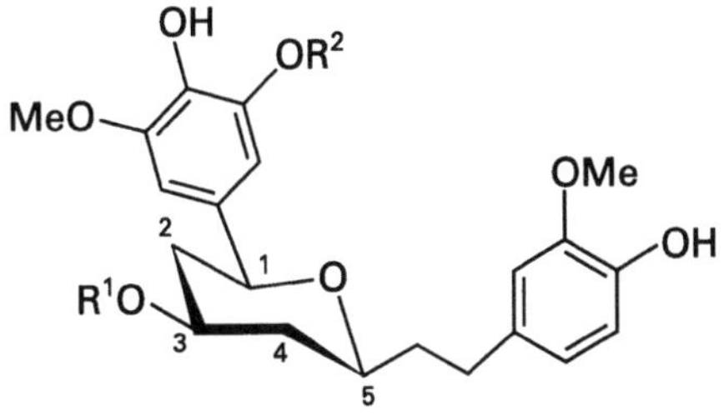

(146) $R^1 = Ac, R^2 = H$
(147) $R^1 = R^2 = H$
(148) $R^1 = H, R^2 = Me$

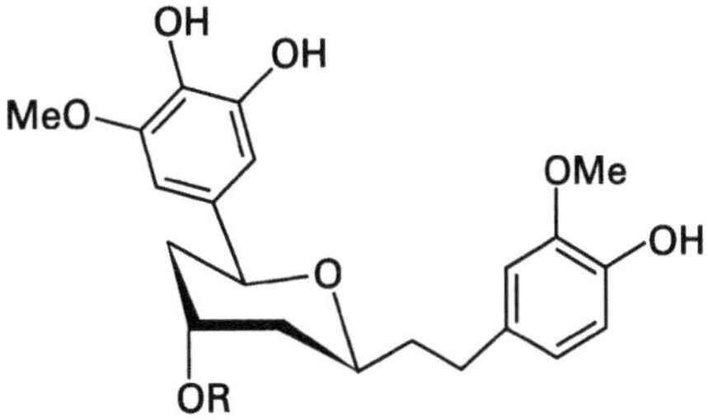

(149) R = Ac
(150) R = H

cyclized between C-1 and C-5 through oxygen. The compounds **146** and **147** are epimers of **149** and **150**, respectively, at C-3 [294].

4.1.8 Miscellaneous compounds

Diterpenes

An acetone extract of ginger and its fractions has been reported to possess anti-serotonergic effects. Analysis of one of the fractions showed that galanolactone (**151**) [295], a diterpenoid, is one of the active constituents. The results show that the anti-5-HT effect of galanolactone is related to antagonism of the 5-HT3 receptor [296].

Gingerglycolipids

From the MeOH extract of dried ginger cultivated in Taiwan an anti-ulcer constituent, 6-gingesulfonic acid, and three monoacyldigalactosylglycerols, gingerglycolipids A, B and C (**152–154**), together with (+)-angelicoidenol-2-*O*-β-D-glucopyranoside (**155**), were isolated, all in ~ 0.0013% yield. Based on chemical reactions and ^{1}H, ^{13}C-NMR spectral evidence, the structures of gingerglycolipids A, B and C were determined. In addition, the absolute stereostructure of (+)-angelicoidenol-2-*O*-β-D-glucopyranoside was clarified based on its synthesis from *d*-borneol. {6}-Gingesulfonic acid showed weaker pungency and more potent anti-ulcer activity than 6-gingerol and 6-shogaol [285, 297].

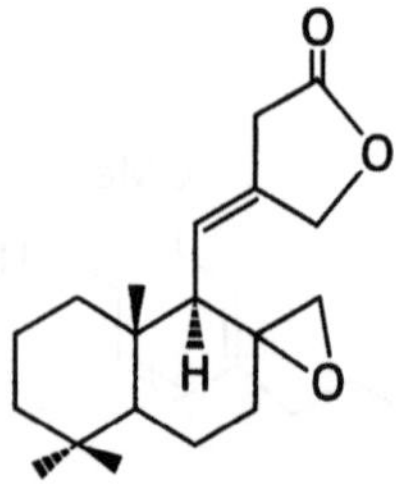

Galanolactone (**151**)

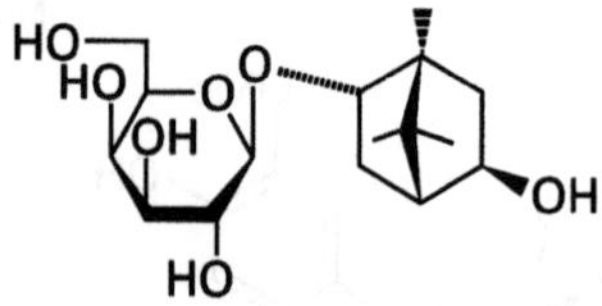

(**155**)

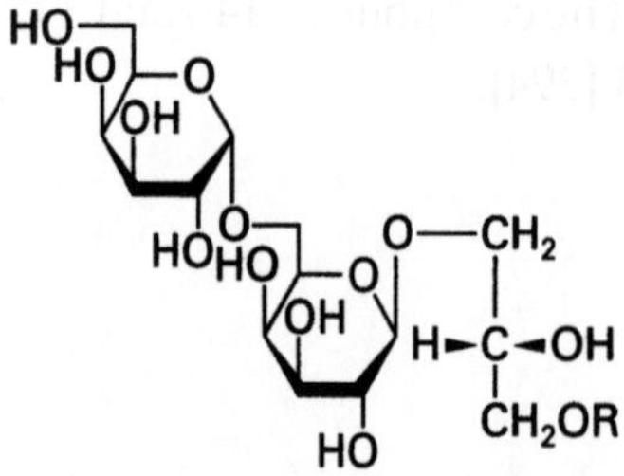

Gingerglycolipid A (**152**) R =

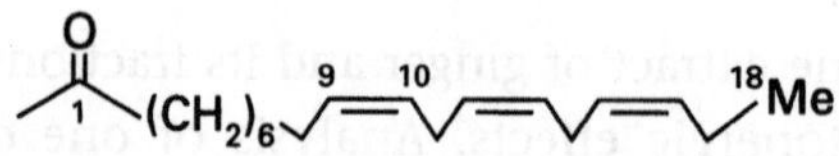

Gingerglycolipid B (**153**) R =

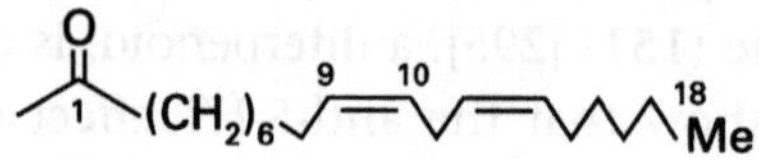

Gingerglycolipid C (**154**) R =

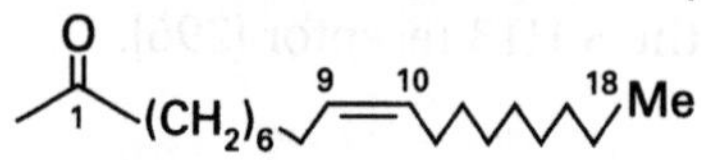

Gingerproteases

Proteases from ginger were reported by Ichikawa et al. [298] and shown to have a high proteolytic activity against casein, bovine serum albumin and collagen [299, 300]. These proteases have been separated by DEAE cellulose chromatography to afford protease I (GP-I) and protease II (GP-II). Complete amino acid sequences of both GP-I and GP-II have been determined. The enzyme GP-II is a 221 amino acid glycoprotein. The three-dimensional X-ray crystallographic structure of GP-II has been determined [301].

4.2 Analysis and quality control

A rapid method for the isolation of {6}-, {8}-, and {10}-gingerols in quantities between 40–500 mg from powdered ginger using counter-current chromatography has been developed [302]. Two rapid techniques of column chromatography, flash chromatography and vacuum liquid chromatography, together with solvent systems differing in polarity, have been used to separate the pungent principles, gingerols and shogaols, of ginger extract [303]. Qualitative and quantitative analysis of bioactive principles of ginger by means of HPLC and GC have been performed for the isolation and characterization of {6}-, {8}-, and {10}-gingerols, {6}-, {8}-shogaols, {6}-dehydrogingerdione and galanolactone [277]. Supercritical fluid (CO_2) can be used to extract components with the least amount of degradation. The volatile components responsible for the flavor of Australian ginger have been determined using supercritical CO_2. Analysis of the extract by GC-MS indicated that the major components are neral, geranial, zingiberene, α-bisabolene and β-sesquiphellandrene. Forty mono- and sesquiterpenes were quantitatively identified from the extract [304]. An oxygenated hydrocarbon fraction of fresh ginger extract was analyzed by capillary GC and eluate-sniffing to identify the characteristic odorants. Twenty-two compounds were detected with a high flavor dilution (FD) factor and analyzed by GC-MS. Compounds with a high FD were linaleol, geraniol, neral, isoborneol, borneol, 1,8-cineol, 2-pinen-5-ol, geranyl acetate, (*E*)-2-octenal, and (*E*)-2-dodecenal. In addition, (*E*)-2-alkenals, 2-octyl acetate, 2-(2′, 3′-epoxy-3′-methylbutyl)-3-methylfuran, and (*E*)- and (*Z*)-3,7-dimethyl-3, 6-octadienal were identified [305]. Isolation of the pungent compounds of Australian ginger by supercritical extraction and identification by electrospray-MS showed that it contains ~ 70 g/kg {6}-gingerol and less than 2 g/kg {6}-shogaol [306, 307]. The major pungent compounds and essential oils of West Indian ginger were identified and quantified by liquid chromatography on silica gel [308].

4.3 Pharmacology

Ginger has been used liberally as a food spice by over half the world's population, which should at least vouch for safety in its consumption. Traditionally, as well as from experimental evidence, it has been considered as anti-inflammatory and a stimulant of gastrointestinal (GI) motility, the carminative effect having been attributed to its pungent gingerols [309] that stimulate the GI tract and bile secretion [310]. This review includes only selective recent literature relating to these effects and largely to the newly discovered antihyperlipidemic and anticancer activities of ginger and some of its constituents.

4.3.1 Gastrointestinal activities

Several constituents of ginger, including β-bisabolene (**87**), α-D-curcumene (**89**) and [6]-shogaol (**128**), were found to be anti-ulcer in the ethanol/hydrochloric acid (HCl)-induced stomach ulcers in rats [311]. Subsequently, [6]-gingesulfonic acid (**127**) was shown to be a less pungent but more potent anti-ulcer compound than [6]-gingerol (**106**) and [6]-shogaol [312].

Based on the effects of test substances on copper sulfate-induced vomiting in leopard- and ranid frogs, several gingerols and shogaols isolated from ginger were found to be anti-emetic [313]. The anticancer drug cisplatin produces nausea as one of its adverse side-effects. Relatively non-polar extracts, but not aqueous extracts, of dry ginger showed a dose-dependent protective action against the cisplatin-emesis in dogs [314]. The active extracts, however, were far less effective than granisetron, a serotonergic receptor (5-HT3) antagonist. The ginger extracts did not show any anti-emetic activity against the apomorphine-induced emesis in dogs. The authors of these studies have suggested that ginger could be a cheap and effective adjuvant in cancer chemotherapy.

Cisplatin also causes an inhibition of peristalsis and gastric emptying time. Ginger juice and acetone and/or alcohol extracts of dry ginger were found to counter the cisplatin-induced gastric emptying in rats [315]. The juice, however, appeared to possess more potent activity than the 5-HT3 receptor antagonist ondansetron.

4.3.2 Anti-inflammatory activity

Since ginger has been used as a condiment for millennia and found to be quite safe for human consumption, far more clinical than animal studies have been carried out and published. Jain et al. [316] reported on the anti-inflammatory, antipyretic and analgesic activities of ginger in rats. Eugenol and ginger oil were shown to possess potent anti-inflammatory activity in severe chronic arthritis in the paw and knee of the rat induced by injecting 0.05 ml of a fine suspension of dead *Mycobacterium tuberculosis* in liquid paraffin (5 mg/ml) [317]. A significant suppression of the experimental arthritic inflammation was seen when the rats were pretreated for 26 days with oral doses of 33 mg/kg of eugenol and ginger oil. In other similar experiments, the same investigators observed a significant decrease ($p < 0.01$) of the plasma kallikrein levels in the synovial fluid compared to that in the non-treated rats [318].

4.3.3 Anticancer activity

Gingerol and several other substances isolated from plants of Zingiberaceae family showed a strong inhibition of tumor promoter-induced activation of Epstein-Barr virus *in vitro* [319]. In dimethylbenzene-initiated SENCAR mice, the skin tumor-promoters, e. g., 12-*O*-tetradecanoylphorbol-13-acetate (TPA), induce epidermal ornithine decarboxylase (ODC), COX and LOX enzymes. Pre-application of an ethanolic extract of ginger to the skin of mice, prior to TPA administration, significantly reduced this enzyme induction caused by TPA [320]. Furthermore, the extract also reduced the TPA-induced epidermal edema and hyperplasia, as well as the number of tumors, compared to the non-ginger-treated control mice. Epidermal growth factor (EGF) too is a tumor promoter. It induces skin cell transformation and the activation protein-1 (AP-1) that has a critical role in tumor promotion. 6-Gingerol and 6-paradol both were found to be effective blockers of the EGF-induced AP-1 activation [321].

The pungent vanilloid constituents of ginger, 6-gingerol and 6-paradol, inhibited the viability of and DNA synthesis in the human leukemia HL-60 cells in culture [322].TPA-induced activation of Epstein-Barr virus in Raji cells was inhibited by extracts of ginger and several other Zingiberacaea plant rhizomes [323]. This blockade/inhibition of tumor promotion was observed in the Raji cells, with no cytotoxicity caused by the extract. Finally, ginger was recently reported to exhibit a clastogenic effect in mice treated with colchicine to induce chromosomal damage [324]. The bone-marrow cell preparation was used to examine the damage. The aqueous extract of ginger showed some protection against chromosomal damage but ginger oil showed more chromosomal aberrations, indicating that the aqueous extract contains substance(s) that suppress clastogenesis. All these various laboratory studies are suggestive of the potential anticancer activity in ginger and its constituents, and have led to a number of clinical investigations.

4.3.4. Other activities

Thermogenic activity of crude extracts of fresh and dried ginger, and of their constituents, gingerols and shogaols, was determined in the perfusing rat hindlimb by analyzing the oxygen consumption by the limb tissue corresponding to the perfusion pressure and lactate production [325]. The extracts increased the oxygen consumption while also increasing both the perfusion pressure and lactate formation. On a molar basis, the gingerols were more potent than the corresponding shogaols, but 6-gingerol was the most potent constituent, causing a 21% increase in oxygen consumption, 30% increase in the perfusion pressure and 87% increase in lactate production. With higher doses of gingerols, the oxygen consumption reached an optimum and began to decline, whereas the perfusion pressure kept on increasing. The pressure increase appeared to be mediated *via* vasoconstriction of the limb that is not related to α- or β-adrenergic blockade. However, zingeronolol, an alcohol prepared by reduction of zingerone, produced a dose-dependent bradycardia in anaesthetized normotensive rats [326]. It also blocked the isoproterenol-induced tachycardia (β-adrenergic) but not the phenylephrine-induced hypertension (α-adrenergic). The binding of ^{3}H-dihydroalprenolol to guinea pig ventricular cell membranes was inhibited by zingeronolol, its IC_{50} being 5.2 +1.1, compared to the IC_{50} values for the well-known β-blockers propranolol and atenelol as 0.009 + 0.002 and 6.5 + 1.0, respectively. However, zingeronolol showed a mild cardio-depression at high doses, but did not show any sympathomimetic activity as is present to some extent in other β-adrenergic blockers.

In a totally different vein, (*E*)-8-β,17-epoxylabd-12-ene-15,16-dial (ZT), isolated from ginger, was found to lower plasma-cholesterol levels in the Triton WR-1339-induced hypercholesteremic mice [327]. Adding ZT to homogenized rat liver decreased cholesterol biosynthesis. Interestingly, no other pharmacological activity was observed with this compound in the usual pharmacological laboratory screen. Ethanolic extract of ginger proved hypocholesteremic in atherofed hypercholesteremic rabbits, the atherogenic index decreasing from 4.7 to 1.2. Both the total and the LDL cholesterol levels were lowered [328]. The fecal excretion of cholesterol appeared to increase, indicating perhaps that components in the ginger extract interfered with the enteric absorption of cholesterol while increasing its biliary excretion. In another similar study, the ethanolic ginger extract was shown to be antihyperlipidemic in the cholesterol-fed rabbits, the effect being comparable to that of gemfibrozil currently prescribed for treating hyperlipidemic patients [329]. Ginger powder at 35 and 70 mg/kg daily doses as a suspension in water was administered orally daily for 10 weeks to rats on a high-fat feed. The control group received water in place of ginger suspension. The cholesterol, triglyceride and phospholipid levels in the organs and serum were significantly decreased in the ginger-treated rats compared to the controls [330]. The LDL and very low-density lipoproteins (VLDL) were also decreased while the HDL showed an increase in the ginger group.

In relatively well-designed and well-conducted experiments in apolipoprotein E-deficient mice fed atherodiet, ginger extract in 1.1% ethanol in water at two different oral doses for 10 weeks showed a clear hypolipidemic profile [331]. The aortic atheroslerotic lesions were reduced 44% ($p < 0.01$) in the group receiving 250 mg dose of ginger, compared to the placebo group. The treated group showed a reduction of 27% ($p < 0.01$) in plasma cholesterol, 29% ($p < 0.01$) in triglycerides, and of 33 to 58% in LDL and VLDL. This lipid-lowering profile was associated with a 76% reduction in the cholesterol biosynthesis in the peritoneal macrophages obtained from the ginger-treated mice. Interestingly, these cells had a 45 to 60% reduction in their capacity to oxidize LDL. This oxidation has been found essential for progression of atherosclerosis, and antioxidants interfering with this process have proven to be beneficial in attenuating atherosclerotic development. Thus, ginger appears to possess an anti-atherogenic effect as well as lipid lowering activities.

4.3.5 Mechanisms of action

Ascorbate/iron-induced lipid peroxidation in rat liver microsomes was inhibited by zingerone from ginger, though at relatively higher concentrations than eugenol from clove and curcumin from turmeric [332]. If other ginger constituents are also found to protect peroxidation, especially at low concentrations, ginger would emerge as a protector of polyunsaturated fatty acids known to be beneficial in preventing atherogenesis but highly susceptible to peroxidation.

A high-fat diet fed to rats for 10 weeks resulted in significantly higher levels of hydroperoxides and thiobarbiturate-reactive substances (TBARS), decreased catalase and superoxide dismutase (SOD) activities, and lower levels of GHS as well as vitamins C and E [333]. However, when ginger was simultaneously fed to the animals, the levels of TBARS and hydroperoxide decreased while those of GSH, vitamins C and E increased. There was also an increase in the activities of SOD and catalase. Based on these data, the authors concluded that ginger could reduce the free radical-mediated oxidative stress to cells. Another recent study on malathion-induced lipid peroxidation causing oxidative stress in rats also revealed the protective action of ginger against this stress [334].

Gingerols and diarylheptanoids from ginger were found to inhibit biosyntheses of PG-E2 and LT-B4 involving COX and LOX enzymes, respectively. This effect on biosynthesis was found to be due to the enzyme inhibition by the ginger products [335]. Prostaglandin-E2 and LT-B4 produced by COX and LOX enzymes, respectively, are believed to be the mediators of the inflammation process. Ginger extracts have shown anti-platelet aggregation activity, but six different gingerols isolated from ginger did not account for this activity [336]. Consequently, two labdane-type diterpene dialdehydes from ginger were found to be strong inhibitors of platelet aggregation comparable to indomethicin, but did not inhibit prostaglandin endoperoxide synthase in the arachidonic acid cascade. However, these dialdehydes are also potent inhibitors of LOX. Synthetic gingerol-induced potentiation of the maximal contractile response of mouse mesenteric vein to PG-F2α, but not when the vein was de-endothialized, was totally abolished by COX inhibitors, aspirin and indomethicin [337]. The LOX inhibitors did not block this effect. This would suggest that the potentiation is COX-dependent and may be due to some vasoconstrictor substance other than PG-E2, since gingerol has been shown to inhibit PG-E2 synthesis.

4.4 Toxicity

Since ginger has been consumed globally as a condiment in half the world and for centuries, the question of its toxicity has remained moot. It is only last year that a few reports appeared in the literature. Weidner and Sigwart [338], in three different studies in rats, tested the effect of a standardized ginger extract on blood pressure, blood glucose, heart rate and coagulation. No significant effect was observed on any of the parameters examined. This would reconfirm the generally held belief that ginger is pharmacologically safe.

Ginger tea in folk medicine is a common morning-sickness remedy. Therefore, a study was undertaken to determine the effect of ginger tea on fetal development in pregnant Sprague-Dawley rats [339]. Two different doses of ginger tea mixed with drinking water were given to the rats from day 6 to 15 of gestation, and the rats were sacrificed on day 20 to examine the fetuses. Although no maternal toxicity was seen, the embryonic loss in the ginger-treated group was twice that in the controls. However, no gross morphological malformations were seen in the surviving fetuses, which were actually more robust with advanced skeletal development than those of the controls.

The most recent teratogenic study on a patented ginger extract (EV.EXT 33) was carried out in 3 groups each of 22 Wistar rats, given 0.1, 0.33 and 1 g/kg of the extract in sesame oil orally from day 6 to 15 of gestation [340]. The fourth control group received the vehicle only. Body weight and food intake were monitored throughout the treatment period and the animals were sacrificed on day 21 of gestation. The extract was well tolerated and no deaths or adverse reactions were observed in the treatment groups. The fetuses revealed no malformations. Thus, ginger extract caused no maternal or developmental toxicity in the rats even at 1 g/kg dose.

4.5 Clinical studies

In a placebo-controlled, double-blind crossover trial in 8 healthy volunteers, the effect of ginger powder was studied on vertigo and nystagmus following caloric stimulation of the vestibular system [341]. Based on the results of 48 vertigo scores and the same number of electronystagmograms, ginger was found to significantly reduce the induced vertigo compared to the placebo. However, there was no effect on the nystagmus. In another double-blind, randomized, placebo-controlled trial conducted in the open sea on 80 naval cadets unaccustomed to sailing in rough seas, ingestion of 1 g ginger powder resulted in significantly reduced ($p < 0.05$) nausea, vertigo and cold sweating, compared to the symptoms observed in the placebo-treated subjects [342]. The overall number of vomits was also considerably reduced in the ginger-treated subjects.

The effectiveness of British Pharmacopoeia (BP)-ginger in protecting against postoperative nausea was studied in a double-blind, randomized and placebo-controlled trial on 108 patients undergoing gynecological laparoscopic surgery under general anaesthesia [343]. The BP-ginger at 0.5 and 1.0 g oral doses failed to prevent post-operative nausea. A literature analysis in 1998 concluded that ginger may be beneficial as an alternative therapy for nausea and vomiting in early pregnancy [344]. An update on pathophysiology, prophylaxis and therapy of motion- and seasickness included ginger as an available treatment option, along with the well-known antimuscarinics and antihistamines [345]. In other trials relative to the effects of ginger on the gastro-intestinal tract, ginger was found not to affect the gastric emptying rate in a randomized, placebo-controlled, crossover study [346]. Orally given ginger was found to increase gastro-duodenal motility in both fasting and postprandial states in 12 healthy volunteers [347]. A systematic review of randomized clinical trials on ginger for nausea and vomiting revealed that, collectively, ginger was superior to placebo [348]. This conclusion was based on 6 studies that met the criteria for inclusion set forth by the reviewers.

A few trials have been carried out to study the effect of ginger on arthritic and musculo-skeletal disorders. In one open study, 28 patients with rheumatoid arthritis, 18 with osteoarthritis and 10 with muscular discomfort used oral ginger powder for their ailments for a period of 3 to 30 months [349]. Among the arthritis patients, over 75% experienced varying degrees of pain relief and a decrease in inflammation, whereas all of the muscular discomfort group experienced pain relief. No adverse side-effects were reported during the ginger consumption. In another trial that was a randomized, placebo-controlled, double-blind, crossover study, ginger extract was compared with ibuprofen and placebo in osteo-arthritic patients [350]. The crossover data showed no significant differences between the ginger- and the placebo-treated groups, although the data of the three treatments in sequence showed the efficacy order as ibuprofen > ginger > placebo.

In an open study on 20 healthy males, dietary supplementation of 100 g butter per day for 7 days significantly increased the platelet aggregation from the baseline value, but 5 g ginger powder in two divided doses added to the fatty meal significantly inhibited ($p < 0.001$) the fat-induced aggregation [351]. In 10 volunteers, the adenosine diphosphate (ADP)-induced platelet aggregation was also inhibited. In another placebo-controlled trial on ginger and fenugreek, the subjects included healthy individuals, patients with coronary artery disease (CAD), and non-insulin-dependent diabetics (NIDD) with or without CAD [352]. In the CAD patients, 4 g of oral ginger powder daily for 3 months did not affect the ADP- and epinephrine-induced platelet aggregation, or the fibrinogen levels and the fibrinolytic activity. However, a single dose of 10 g significantly reduced the drug-induced aggregation. There was no effect on the blood glucose and lipid levels.

In conclusion, both experimental and clinical evidence is emerging to suggest several potential therapeutic uses of ginger and/or its constituents. However, far more rigidly controlled and well-designed clinical studies on a large scale are warranted before the fate of ginger in medical practice can be decided. Fortunately, there is little evidence for its toxicity. Therefore, it should be safe and easily permissible by the US FDA to conduct such trials in the US.

References

1a P.N. Kaul: Progr. Drug. Res. *47*, 151 (1996).

1b B.S. Joshi and P.N. Kaul: Progr. Drug. Res. *56*, 1 (2001).

1 J.M. Watt, in: T. Swain (ed.): *Plants in the Development of Modern Medicine*, Harvard University Press, Cambridge, 1972; W. Emboden: *Narcotic plants*, Studio Vista, London, 1979.

2 Y.N.Singh: J. Ethnopharmacol. *37*, 13 (1992).

3 J. Cook: A Voyage to the Pacific, London, *2*, 145, 155 (1785).

4 L. Lewin: *Phantastica; Narcotic and Stimulating Drugs*. Rutledge and Kegan Paul, 1964, 215; J.A. Duke: *CRC Handbook of Medicinal Herbs*, CRC Press, Inc. Boca Raton, Florida, 1985, 381.

5 V.E. Tyler, in J. Janick (ed.): *Perspectives on New Crops and New Uses*. ASHS Press, Alexandria, VA, 1999, 442; M.T. Murray, in: *The Healing Power of Herbs*, Prima publishing, 2nd ed., Rocklin, CA, 1995, 210.

6 M. Blumenthal, W.R. Busse and A. Goldberg (eds.): *The Complete Commission E Monographs: Therapeutic Guide to Herbal Medicines*. Boston, MA: Integrative Medicine Communications, 1998, 156.

7 A.T. Shulgin: Bull. Narc. *25*, 59 (1973); M. Grieve: *A Modern Herbal*, Reprint, 1974, Hafner Press, New York, 1931, 916; V. Lebot, M. Merlin and L. Lindstrom: *Kava: The Pacific Drug*, New Haven, Yale University Press 1992; S.J. Dentali: *Herb Safety Review: Kava, Piper methysticum Forster f. (Piperaceae)*, Boulder, Co, Herb Research Foundation 1997.

8 G. Cuznet: Revue Coloniale (Paris) 2nd Series, *15*, 582 (1856) ; Compt. Rend. *52*, 205 (1861).

9 M. Gobley: J. Pharmazie, 3rd Series, *32*, 19 (1860).
10 W. Borsche and C..K. Bodenstein: Chem. Ber. *62*, 2515 (1929).
11 W. Borsche: Chem. Ber. *60*, 982 (1927).
12 W. Borsch and B.K. Blount: Chem. Ber. *63*, 2418 (1930); ibid. 65, 822 (1930).
13 W. Borsche and B.K. Blount: Chem. Ber. *66*, 803 (1933); ibid. 66, 1792 (1933),
14 W. Borsch and M. Gerhardt: Chem. Ber. *47*, 2902 (1914)
15 W. Borsch, C.H. Meyer and W. Pietzsch: Chem. Ber. *60*, 2113 (1927).
16 W. Borsche and W. Pietzsch: Chem. Ber. *62*, 360 (1929).
17 W. Borsche and W. Pietzsch: Chem. Ber. *62*, 368 (1929).
18 W. Borsche and W. Pietzsch: Chem. Ber. *63*, 2414 (1930).
19 W. Borsche, W. Rosenthal and C.H. Meyer: Chem. Ber. *60*, 1135 (1927).
20 W. Borsche and A. Roth: Chem. Ber. *54*, 2229 (1921).
21 W. Borsche and C. Walter: Chem. Ber. *60*, 2112 (1927).
22 *Review of Chem. Pharm and Hist. Sketch*, U.S.Public Health Service Publ. No. 1645, D.H. Efron (ed): 1967, 103; L. Lewin: *Über Piper methysticum (Kawa)*, A. Hirschwad, Berlin, 1886.
23 I. Chmielewska, J. Cieselak: Roczniki Chem. *28*, 38 (1954); I. Chmielewska, J. Cieselak, K. Gorzcynska, B. Kontnik and K. Pitakowska: Tetrahedron *4*, 36 (1958).
24 J.D. Bu'Lock and H.G. Smith: J. Chem. Soc. *502* (1960).
25 R. Hänsel and L. Klapworth: Arch Pharm (Weinheim Ger.) *299*, 503 (1966); R. Hänsel, H. Sauer and H. Rimpler: Arch Pharm (Weinheim Ger.) *299*, 507 (1966); Z. Macierewicz: Roczniki Chem. *24*, 144 (1939).
26 B. Talapatra, D.K. Pradhan and S. Talapatra: Indian J. Chem. *14B*, 300 (1976).
27 P. Beak and H. Abelson: J. Org. Chem. *27*, 3715(1962).
28 C.P. Dutta, L.P.K. Ray and A. Chatterjee: Phytochemistry *11*, 2891 (1972).
29 T.M. Harris and C.S. Combs Jr: J. Org. Chem. *33*, 2399 (1968).
30 F. Paulino, F. Hipolito,J. Muradian, and W.B. Mors: Rev. Latinoam. Quim. *8*, 79 (1977); Chem. Abs. 87, 53025 q (1977).
31 P. Engel and W. Nowacki : Z. Crystallogr. Krystallogeom. Krystallphys. Krystallchem. *134*, 180 (1971).
32 A.V. Lopezavila and J. Benedicto: J. High Resolution Chromatogr. *20*, 555 (1997); H. Achenbach, W. Karl and S. Smith: Chem. Ber. *104*, 2688 (1971).
33 N.C. Franca, O.R. Gottlieb and A.M. Puentes Suarez: Phytochemistry *12*, 1182 (1973).
34 Y. Shao, K. He, B.L. Zheng and Q.Y. Zheng: J. Chromatogr. A *825*, 1 (1998).
35 X.G. He, L.Z. Lin and L.Z. Lian: Planta Medica *63*, 70 (1997).
36 C. Pomeranz: Monatsch Chem. *10*, 783 (1889).
37 Y. Murayama and K. Shinozaki: J. Pharm. Soc. Japan, No. *520*, 3 (1925).
38 E. Winzheimer: Arch. Pharm. *246*, 338 (1908).
39 R. Hänsel, H. Sauer and H. Rimpler: Arch. Pharm. *299*, 507 (1966).
40 G. Snatzke and R. Hänsel: Tetrahdron Letters *1797* (1968)
41 R.S. Cahn, C.K. Ingold and V. Prelog: Angew. Chem. *78*, 413 (1966).
42 M.W. Klohs, F. Keller, R.E. Williams, M.R. Toekes and G.E. Cronheim: J. Med. Chem. *1*, 95 (1959).
43 M.W. Klohs, F. Keller and R.E. Williams: J. Org. Chem. *24*, 1829 (1959).
44 H. Achenbach: Chem. Ber. *106*, 2648 (1973).
45 P. Engel and W. Nowacki: Z. Crystallogr. *136*, 437 (1972).

46 W.B. Mors, M.T. Magalhaes and O.R. Gottlieb, in: L. Zechmeister (ed.): *Progress in the Chemistry of Natural Products*, Springer Verlag, New York 1962, 131.
47 F. Keller and M.W. Klohs: Lloydia *26* , 1 (1963).
48 R. Hänsel, D. Weiss and B. Scot: Arch. Pharm. *301*, 369 (1968)
49 Y. Kimura and T. Tamara: Agri. Biol. Chem. *38*, 875 (1974).
50 T. Reffstrup and P.M. Boll: Acta Chem. Scand. B *30*, 613 (1976).
51 H. Achenbach , J. Worth and B. Raffelsberger: Org. Mass Spectrometry *10*, 850 (1975)
52 J. Møller, T. Reffstrup and P.M. Boll: Acta Chem. Scand. B *31*, 671 (1977).
53 T. Izawa and T. Makaiyama: Chem. Letters *161* (1975).
54 Z.H. Israili and E.E. Smissman: J. Org. Chem. *41*, 4070 (1976).
55 S. Castellino: Tetrahedron Letters *25*, 4059 (1984).
56 A.G. Van Veen: Rec. Trav. Chem. Pays-Bas *58*, 521 (1939).
57 M.A. Mpalantinos, R.S. de Moura, J.P. Parente and R.M. Kuster: Phytotherapy Research *12*, 442 (1998).
58 H. Achenbach and N. Theobold: Chem. Ber. *107*, 735 (1976).
59 A. Yoshino: Z. Krstallogr. Kristallgeom. Kristallphys. Krystallchem. *136*, 66 (1972).
60 P. Engel and W. Nowacki: Z. Krstallogr. Kristallgeom. Kristallphys. Krystallchem. *136*, 453 (1972).
61 C.H Hocart, B. Fankhauser and D.W Buckle: Rapid Comm. In Mass Spec. *7*, 219 (1993).
62 H. Achenbach and G. Wittmann: Tetrahedron Letters 3259 (1970).
63 H. Achenbach and H. Huth: Tetrahedron Letters 119 (1974).
64 Y. Arai: J. Org. Chem. *65*, 258 (2000).
65 R.W. Friesen: J. Org. Chem. *61*, 9130 (1996).
66 D. Cheng, R.O. Lidgard, P.H. Duffield, A.M. Duffiels and H. Borphy: Biomed. Environ Mass Spectrometry *17*, 371 (1988).
67 R. Hänsel, P. Bähr and J. Elich: Arch. Pharm. *294*, 739 (1961).
68 R. Hänsel, G. Ranft and P. Bähr: Z. Naturforsch. *18*, 370 (1963).
69 H. Von Sauer and R. Hänsel: Planta Medica *15*, 443 (1967).
70 P. Jossang and D. Molho: J. Chromatogr. 1375 (1967).
71 N.R. Farnsworth, N.A. Pilewski and F.J. Draus: Lloydia *25*, 312 (1962).
72 H. Achenbach and W. Karl: Chem.Ber. *103*, 2535 (1970).
73 R.M. Smith: Tetrahedron *35*, 437 (1979).
74 B.S. Joshi, V.N. Kamat and A.K. Saksena: Tetrahedron Letters 2395 (1968).
75 H. Joggy and H. Achenbach: Planta Medica *58*, 111 (1992).
76 H. Achenbach, H. Frey and R. Waibel: J. Nat. Prod. *54*, 1331 (1991).
77 M. Akasu, H. Itokawa and M. Fujita: Tetrahedron Letters 3609 (1974).
78 R. Hänsel, A. Leuschke, A. Gomez-Pompa: Lloydia *38*, 529 (1975).
79 H. Hänsel and A. Leuschke: Phytochemistry *15*, 1323 (976).
80 S.J. Desai, R.N. Chaturvedi, L.P. Badheka ans N.B. Mulchandani: Indian J. Chem. B *28B*, 775 (1989).
81 R.N. Duve: Anlyst *106*, 160 (1981).
82 R.L. Young, J.W. Hylin, D.L. Plunknett, Y. Kawano and R.T. Nakayama: Phytochemistry *5*, 795 (1966).
83 H. Achenbach, W. Karl and S. Smith: Chem. Ber. *104*, 2688, (1971).
84 A.M. Duffield, R.O. Lidgard and G.K.C. Low: Biomed. Environ Mass Spectrometry *13*, 305 (1986).

85 R.L. Young, J.W. Hylin D.L. Plucknett, Y. Kawano and R.T. Nakayama: Phytochemistry *5*, 795 (966).

86 L. Cauper: Pharmazie 25, 197 (1970); N. DiRenzo: Farmaco, Ed. Pract. *27*, 318 (1972); Chem. Abs. *77*, 66235b (1972).

87 L. Gracza and P. Ruff, J. Chromatogr. *183*, 436 (1980); R.M. Smith, H. Thakrar, T.A. Arowolo and A.A. Shafi: J. Chromatogr. *283*, 303 (1984).

88 R.M. Smith: Phytochemistry *22*, 1055 (1983).

89 K. He, C.B.L. Zheng and Q.Y. Zheng: J. Chromatogr. A *825*, 1 (1998).

90 G. Boonen, M.A. Beck and H. Haberlein: J. Chromatogr. B *702*, 240 (1997); G. Boonen and M.A. Beck: Planta Medica *63*, 63 (1997).

91 M. Ganzera and I.A. Khan: Chromatographia *50*, 649 (1999).

92 G. Boonen, A. Pramanik, R. Rigler and H. Haeberlin: Planta Medica *66*, 7 (2000).

93 A.R. Clough, C.B. Burns and N. Mannungurr: Drug and Alcohol Rev. *19*, 310 (2000).

94 P.H. Duffield, D.D. Jamieson and A.M. Duffield: Arch. Int. Pharmacodyn. Ther. *301*, 81 (1989).

95 D.D. Jamieson, P.H. Duffield, D. Cheng and A.M. Duffield: Arch. Int. Pharmacodyn. Ther. *301*, 66 (1989).

96 C. Backhaus and J. Krieglstein: Eur. J. Pharmacol. *215*, 265 (1992).

97 J. Gleitz, A. Biele and T. Peters: Neuropharmacology *34*, 1132 (1995)

98 J. Gleitz, J. Friese, A. Biele, A. Ameri and T. Peters: Eur. J. Pharmacol. *315*, 89 (1996).

99 K. Schirrmacher, D. Busselberg, J.M. Langosch, J. Walden, U. Winter and D. Bingmann: Eur. J. Neuropsychopharmacol. *9*, 171 (1999).

100 U. Seitz, A. Ameri, H. Pelzer, J. Gleitz and T. Peters: Planta Medica *63*, 303 (1997).

101 H.B. Martin, W.D. Stofer and M. Echinger: Planta Medica *66*, 601 (2000).

102 D. Schmitz, C.L. Zhang, S.S. Chatterjee and U. Heinemann: Naunyn-Schmiedebergs Arch. Pharmacol. *351*, 348 (1995).

103 J. Walden, J. von Vegerer, U. Winter, M. Berger and H. Grunze: Prog. Neuropsychopharmacol. Biol. Psychiatry *21*, 697 (1997).

104 J. Gleitz, A. Biele, P. Wilkens, A. Ameri and T. Peters: Planta Medica *63*, 27 (1997).

105 L.P. Davies, C.A. Drew, P. Duffield, G.A. Johnston and D.D. Jamieson: Pharmacol. Toxicol. *71*, 120 (1992).

106 A. Jussofie, A. Schmiz and C. Heimke: Psychopharmacology *116*, 469 (1994).

107 J. Gleitz, C. Tosch, A. Biele and T. Peters: Neuropsychopharmacology *35*, 1743 (1996).

108 J. Walden, J. von Wagerer, U. Winter and M. Berger: Human Psychopharmacology-Clinical and Experimental *12*, 265 (1997).

109 M. Kumari and M.K. Ticku: Progr. Drug Res. *54*, 151 (2000).

110 U. Jappe, I. Franke, D. Reinhold and H.P. Gollmick: J. Am. Acad. Dermatol. *38*, 104 (1998).

111 R. Ubelback, I. Franke and H.J. Schewe: Pharmacopsychiatry *31*, 187 (1998).

112 Langosch, C. Norman, K. Schirrmacher, M. Berger and J. Walden: Comp. Biochem. Physiol. A Mol. Integr. Physiol. *120*, 545 (1998).

112 G. Boonen and H. Haberlein: Planta Medica *64*, 504 (1998).

113 S.S. Baum, R. Hill and H. Rommelspacher: Prog. Neuropsychopharmacol. Biol. Psychiat. *22*, 1105 (1998).

115 T.F. Munte, H.J. Heinze, M. Matzke and I Steitz: Neuropsychobiol. *27*, 46 (1993).

116 E. Lehmann, E. Kinzler and J. Friedmann: Phytomedicine 3, 113 (1996).

117 H.P. Volz and M. Kieser: Pharmacopsychiatry *30*, 1 (1997).

118 I. Scherer: Advances in Therapy *15*, 261 (1998).
119 M.H. Pittler and E. Ernst: J. Clin. Psychopharmacol. *20*. 84 (2000).
120 A.M. Duffield, D.D. Jamieson, R.O. Lidgrad, P.H. Duffield and D.J. Bourne: J. Chromatogr. *475*, 273 (1989).
121 P. Ruze: Lancet *335*, 1442 (1990).
122 S.A. Norton and P. Ruze: J. Am. Acad. Dermatol. *31*, 9 (1994).
123 U. Jappe, I. Franke, D. Reinhold and H.P. Gollnick: J. Am. Acad. Dermatol. *38*, 104 (1998)
124 S. Guro-Razuman, P. Anand, Q.L. Hu and R. Mir: JCR-J. Clin. Rheumatol. *5*, 342 (1999).
125 S. Foster: *Garlic, Allium sativum*. Botanical Series, No. 311. 2nd. Ed. Austin, Texas: American Botanical Council, 1 (1996).
126 H.P. Koch and L.D. Lawson: *Garlic - The Science and Therapeutic Application of Allium sativum L. and Related Species*, 2nd Ed. Williams & Wilkins, Baltimore 1995.
127 A. Sendl, G. Elbl, B. Steinke, K. Redl, W. Breu and H. Wagner: Planta Medica *58*, 1 (1992).
128 L.D. Lawson, In: A.D. Kinghorn, M.F. Balandrin (eds.): *Bioactive Sulfur Compounds of Garlic and Garlic Products, Human Medicinal Agents from Plants*, ACS Symposium Series 534; American Chemical Society, Washington DC 1993, 306.
129 T. Wertheim: Ann.Chem. Phar. *51*, 289 (1844}.
130 F.W.Semmler, Ann. Pharm. *230*, 434 (1892).
131 C.J. Cavallito and H. Bailey: J. Am. Chem. Soc. *66*, 1950 (1944).
132 C.J. Cavallito, J.S. Buck and D.M. Suter: J. Am. Chem. Soc. *66*, 1952 (1944).
133 H.D. Reuter and A. Sendl, in: H. Wagner and N. Farnsworth (eds.): *Allium sativum and Allium ursinum Chemistry, Pharmacology and Medicinal Applications, Economic and Medicinal Plant Research*, Vol 6,1994, Academic Press, New York..
134 A. Stoll and E. Seebeck: Helv. Chim. Acta *34*, 481 (1951).
135 V. Du Vigneaud, L.F. Audrieth and H.S. Loring: J. Am. Chem. Soc. *52*, 4500 (1930).
136 D. Theodoropoulos: Ann. Chem. Scand. *13*, 383 (1959).
137 T. Suzuki, M. Sugii and T. Kakimoto: Chem. Bull. Japan *9*, 251 (1961).
138 S.S. Singh, S.K. Aggarwal, S. Verma, M.S. Siddiqui and S. Kumar: J. Med. and Aromatic Plant Sci. *20*, 93 (1998).
139 J.E. Lancaster and M.L. Shaw: Phytochemistry *28*, 455 (1989).
140 Suzuki, M. Sugii and T. Kakimoto: Chem. Bull. Japan *9*, 77 (1961).
141 G.C. Freeman, R.J. Whenham, I.A. Mackenzie and M.R. Davey: Plant Sci. Letters *3*, 121 (1974).
142 I. Virtanen and E.J. Matikkala: Acta Chem. Scand. *13*, 623 (1959).
143 A. Sendl and H. Wagner: Planta Medica *57*, 361 (1991).
144 H. Wagner and S. Sendl: Dtsch. Apoth. Ztg. *130*, 1809 (1990).
145 L. Horhammer, H. Wagner, M. Seitz and Z.J. Vejdelek: Pharmazie *23*, 462 (1968).
146 L. Lawson, S. Wood and B.G. Hughes: Planta Medica *57*, 263 (1991); S.J. Ziegler and O. Sticher: Planta Medica *55*, 372 (1989).
147 M. Sugii, T. Suzuki, S. Nagasawa and K. Kawashima: Chem. Pharm. Bull. Japan 12, *1114* (1964).
148 L. Lawason, Z.J. Wang and B.G. Hughes: J. Nat. Prod. *54*, 436 (1991).
149 M. Mütsch-Eckner, B. Meier, A.D. Wright and O. Sticher: Phytochemistry *31*, 2389 (1992).
150 A.I. Virtanen: Phytochemistry *4*, 207 (1965).
151 M. Mazelis: Phytochemistry *2*, 15 (1963).
152 K. Suetsuna, J. Nutritional Biochem. *9*, 415 (1998).

153 M. Fujisawa, M. Yoshimura and S. Tsao: J. Biochem. (Tokyo) *42*, 491 (1933); A. Sendl, M. Schlick, R. Loser, M. Stanislaus and H. Wagner: Atheroscerosis *94*, 79 (1992).
154 E. Block, S. Ahmed, M.K. Jain, R.W. Crecely, R. Apitz-Castro and M.R. Cruz: J. Am. Chem. Soc. *106*, 6295 (1984); E. Block, S. Ahmed, J.L. Castalfamo, M.K. Jain and R. Apitz-Castro: J. Am. Chem. Soc. *108*, 704 (1986).
155 M.H. Brodnitz, J.V. Pascale and L.J. van Derslice: Agri. Food Chem. *19*, 273 (1971).
156 B. Iberl, G. Winkler, B. Müller and K. Knobloch: Planta Medica *56*, 320 (1990).
157 P. Beslin: J. Heterocyclic Chem. *20*, 1753 (1983).
158 D.M. Oaks, H. Hartmann and K.P. Dimick: Anal. Chem. *36*, 1560 (1064).
159 A. Sendl, G. Elbl, B. Steinke, K. Redl, W. Brew and H. Wagner: Planta Medica *58*, 1 (1992).
160 S.J. Brois, J.F. Pilot and H.W. Barum: J. Am. Chem. Soc. *92*, 7629 (1970).
161 G. Barany and A. Mott: J. Org. Chem. *49*, 1043 (1984).
162 W. Wang, J. Tang and A. Pang: Shengwu Huaxue Zazhi *5*, 229 (1989); Chem. Abs. *111*, 95847 (1989).
163 M. Yang, K. Wang, L. Gao, Y. Han, J. Lu and T. Zhan: J. Chin. Pharm. Sci. *1*, 28 (1993); Chem. Abs. *118*, 77092 (1993).
164 X.J. Cai, P.C. Uden, E. Block, X. Zhang, B.D. Quinby and J.J. Sullivan: J. Agri. Food. Chem. *42*, 2081 (1994).
165 X.J. Cai, E. Block, P.C. Uden, X. Zhang, B.D. Quinby and J.J. Sullivan: J. Agri. Food. Chem. *43*, 1754 (1995).
166 M. Inagaki, Y. Harada, K. Yamada, R. Isobe, R. Higuchi, H. Matsuura and Y. Itakura: Chem. Pharm. Bull. Japan *46*, 1153 (1998).
167 Y. Kodera, H. Matsuura, S. Yoshida, T. Sumida, Y. Itakura, T. Fuwa and H. Nishino: Chem. Pharm. Bull. Japan *37*, 1656, (1989).
168 H. Arimoto, S. Asano and D. Uemura: Tetrahedron Letters *38*, 7761 (1997).
169 M. Mütsch-Eckner, C.A. Erdelmeier, O. Sticher and H.D. Reuter: J. Nat. Prod. *56*, 864 (1993).
170 S. Baumgartner, T.G. Dax, W. Praznik and H. Falk: Carbohydrate Research *328*, 177 (2000).
171 K. Parthasarathy and C. Sastry: Indian J. Pharm. *21*, 282 (1959).
172 T. Perseca and M. Parvu: Contrib. Bot. 255 (1986).
173 T. Kasai, T. Nishitoba, Y. Shiroshita and S. Sakamura: Agri. Biol. Chem. *48*, 2271 (1984).
174 A.I. Virtanen and E.J. Mattikala: Hoppe Seyler's Z. Physiol. Chem. *322*, 8 (1974).
175 L.P. Nock and M. Mazelis: Arch. Biochem. Biophys. *249*, 47 (1986); Plant Physiol. *85*, 1079 (1987).
176 R.A. Kazaryan and E.V. Goryachenkova: Biochemistry *43*, 1502 (1978).
177 S. Schwimmer and S. J. Austin: J. Food Sci. *36*, 807 (1971).
178 H.P. Koch and G. Hahn (eds.): *Knoblauch I.* Urban & Schwarzenberg, Munich-Vienna-Baltimore (1980).
179 E. van Damme, I. Goldstein and N. Peumans: Phytochemistry *30*, 514 (1991).
180 G.R. Fenwick and A.B. Hanley: CRC Critical Reviews in Food Sciences and Nutrition, Vol. 22, *199*, 273 (1985).
181 S.A. Al-Nagdi, M.O. Abdel-Rahman and H.I. Heiba: Phytother. Res. *2*, 196 (1988).
182 M. Ali, M. Afzal, R. Hassan. A. Farid and J. Burka: J. Gen. Pharm. *21*, 273 (1990).
183 V.S. Kamanna and M. Chandrasekhara: J. Am. Oil. Chem. Soc. *57*, 236 (1980).
184 H. Matsuura, T. Ushiroguchi, Y. Itakura, Y. Hayashi and T. Fuwa: Chem. Pharm. Bull. Japan *36*, 3659 (1988).

185 H. Matsuura, T. Ushiroguchi, Y. Itakura and T. Fuwa: Chem. Pharm. Bull. Japan *37*, 2741 (1989).
186 J.P. Peng, H. Chen, Y.Q. Quiao, L.R. Ma, T. Narui, H. Suzuki, T. Okuyama, H. Kobayashi: Yaoxue Xuebao *31*, 607 (1996).
187 T. Morita, T. Ushiroguchi, H. Hayashi, H. Matsuura, Y. Itakura and T. Fuwa: Chem. Pharm. Bull. Japan *36*, 3480, 3659 (1988).
188 M. Keusgen: Planta Medica *63*, 93 (1997).
189 R.A. Martinlagos, M.F. Serrano and M.D. Lopez: Food Chemistry *53*, 91 (1995).
190 E. Mochizuki, T. Yamamoto, Y. Komiyama and H. Nakazawa: Chem. Pharm. Bull. Japan *46*, 5170 (1998).
191 R. Kubeck, M. Svobodova and J. Velisek: J. Chromatogr. A *862*, 85 (1999).
192 E. Block, S. Naganathan, D. Putman and S.H. Zhao: J. Agri. Food Chem. *40*, 2418 (1992)
193 M. Mütsch-Ecker, O. Sticher and B. Meier: J. Chromatogr. *625*, 183 (1992).
194 M. Keusgen: Planta Medica *64*, 736 (1998).
195 E.M. Calvey, J.E. Matusik, K.D. White, R. DiOrazio, D.Y. Sha and E. Block: J. Agri. Food Chem. *45*, 4406 (1997).
196 B. Rietz and R. Jacobs: Arzneimittel-forschung/Drug Research *43*, 94 (1993).
197 N. Martin, L. Bardisa, C. Pantoja, M. Vargas, P. Quezada and J. Valenzuela: J. Ethnopharmacol. *43*, 1 (1994).
198 N. Martin, L. Bardisa, C. Pantoja, E. Barra, C. Demetrio, J. Valenzuela and M. Barrios: J. Ethnopharmacol. *55*, 113 (1997).
199 K.K. AlQattan, M.A. Alnaqeeb and M. Ali: J. Ethnopharmacol. *66*, 217 (1999).
200 Y. Ozturk, S. Aydin, M. Kosar and K.H. Baser: J. Ethnopharmacol. *44*, 109 (1994).
201 C.V. Pantoja, B.C. Norris and C.M. Contreres: J. Ethnopharmacol. *52*, 101 (1996).
202 H.K. Berthold and T. Sudhop: Curr. Opin. Lipido. *9*, 565 (1998).
203 A.N. Orekhov and J. Grunwald: Nutrition *13*, 656 (1997).
204 J. Bignall: Lancet *341*, 888 (1993).
205 J.A. Milner: Nutrition Review *54*, S83 (1996).
206 E. Kyo, N. Uda, A. Suzuki, M. Kakimoto, M. Ushijima, S. Kasuga and Y. Itakura: Phytomedicine *5*, 259 (1998).
207 M.D.P. Samaranayake. S.M.D.N. Wickramasinghe, P. Angunawela, S. Jayasekera, S. Iwai and S. Fukushima: Phytotherap. Res. *14*, 564 (2000).
208 E. Kyo, N. Uda, M. Ushijima, S. Kasuga and Y. Itakura: Phytomed. *6*, 325 (1999).
209 G. Kuttan: J. Ethinopharmacol. *72*, 93 (2000).
210 D.L. Lamm and D.R. Riggs: Urologic Clinics of North America *27*, 157 (2000).
211 A. Sendl, G. Elbl, B. Steinke, K. Redl, W. Brew and H. Wagner: Planta Medica *58*, 1 (1992).
212 B. Oelkers, H. Diehl and H. Liebig: Arzneimittel-forschung./Drug Research *42*, 136 (1992).
213 H.P. Koch, W. Jager, J. Hysek and B. Korpert: Phytotherap. Res. *6*, 50 (1992).
214 H.P. Koch, W. Jager, U. Groh, J.E. Hovie, G. Plank, U. Sedlak and W. Praznik: Phytotherap. Res. *7*, 387 (1993).
215 A. Beretz and J.P. Cazenave: Planta Medica *57*, S68 (1991).
216 T. Usui, R. Terumo and D. Cent: Natural Medicines *50*, 135 (1996).
217 M.G. Mostafa, T. Mima, S.T. Ohnishi and K. Mori: Planta Medica *66*, 148 (2000).
218 B.S.H. Cho and S.Q. Xu: Comp.Biochem.Physiol.C-Pharmacol. Toxico. Endocrin. *26*, 195 (2000).

219 C. Luley, W. Lehmann-Leo, B. Müller, T. Martin and W. Schwartzkoff: Arzneimittelforschung/Drug Research *36*, 766 (1986).

220 J. Kleijnen, P. Knipschild and G. ter Riet: Br. J. Clin. Pharmacol. *28*, 535 (1989).

221 H. Kiesewetter, F. Jung, G. Pindur, E.M. Jung, C. Mrowietz and E. Wenzel: Int.J. Clin.Pharmacol. Therap. Toxicol. *29*, 151 (1991).

222 H. Kiesewetter, F. Jung, E.M. Jung, J. Blume, C. Mrowietz, A. Birk, J. Koscielny and E. Wenzel: Clinical Investigator *71*, 383 (1993).

223 W. Rotzsch, V. Richter, F. Rassoul and A. Walper: Arzneimittel.-forschung./Drug Research *42*, 1223 (1992).

224 S. Warshafsky, R.S. Kamer and S.L. Sivak: Annals Intern. Med. *119*, 599 (1993).

225 J.L. Isaacsohn, M. Moser , E.A. Stein, K. Dudley, J.A. Davey, E. Liskov, an H.P. Black: Arch. Intern. Med. *158*, 1189 (1998).

226 B.W. McCrindle and E. Helden: Arch. Ped. Adol. Med. *152*, 1089 (1998).

227 H.A.W. Neil, C.A. Silagy, T. Lancaster, J. Hodgeman, K. Vos, J.W. Moore, L. Jones, J. Cohill and G.H. Fowler: J. Royal Coll. Physicians *30*, 329 (1996).

228 L.A. Simons, S. Balasubramaniam, M. von Konigsmark, A. Parfitt, J. Simons and W. Peters: Atherosclerosis *113*, 219 (19195).

229 A.J. Adler and B.J. Holub: Am. J. Clin. Nutr. *65*, 445 (1997).

230 J. Koscieln, D. Kluessendorf, R. Latza, R. Schmitt, H. Radtke, G. Siegel and H. Kiesewetter: Atherosclerosis *144*, 237 (1999).

231 C. Stevinson, M.H. Pittler and E. Ernst: Annals Intern. Med. *133*, 420 (2000).

232 V. Morelli and R.J. Zoorob: Am. Family Physician *62*, 1325 (2000).

233 V.E. Tyler: Prevention *53*, 105 (2001).

234 C.A. Silagy and H.A.W. Neil: J. Hypertens. *12*, 463 (1994).

235 T. Grune, T. Scherat, H. Behrend, E. Conradi, R. Brenke and W. Siems: Phytomed. *2*, (1996).

236 S. Narasimhan, V.S. Govindarajan: J. Food Technol. *13*, 31 (1978).

237 D.W. Connell and R.A. Jordan: J. Sci. Food Agri. *22*, 93 (1971).

238 M.E. Bone, D.J. Wilkinson, J.R. Young, J. McNeil and S. Charlton: Anesthesia *45*, 669 (1990).

239 A.Y. Leung and S. Foster: Encyclopedia of Common Natural Ingredients used in Food, Drug and Cosmetics, 2nd ed. Wiley, New York 1996, 271.

240 M. Blumenthal, W.R. Busse, A. Goldbergs (eds.): *The Complete Commission E Monographs: Therapeutic Guide to Herbal Medicines*. Integrative Medicine Communications, Boston, MA 1998, 135.

241 D.V.C. Awang: Can. Pharm. J. *125*, 309 (1992).

242 N.G. Bisset and M. Wichtl, in: *Herbal Drugs and Phytopharmaceuticals*. Medpharm Scientific Publishers, Stuttgart 1994.

243 V.S. Govindarajan: Crit. Rev. Food Sci. Nutr. *17*, 1, 189 (1982).

244 A.G. Mathew, N. Krishnamurthy, E.S. Nambudri and Y.S. Lewis: Flav. Ind. *4*, 226 (1973).

245 M.M. Lawrence: Perf. Flav. *9*, 2 (1984).

246 E. Guenther: *The Essential Oils*, Vol 5, D. van Nostrand, Toronto 1952.

247 N. Anand: *Selected markets for ginger and derivatives with special reference to dried ginger: Report of the Tropical Products Institute*, G161 vii, London 1982.

248 M.M. Lawrence: *Recent Studies on the oil of Zingiber officinale*, Paper presented at the 9th International Essential Oil congress, Singapore 1983.

249 T.A. van Beek, M.A. Posthumas, G.P. Llelvyeld, H.V. Phiet and B.T. Yen: Phytochemistry *26*, 3005 (1987).

250 P.C. Onyenekwe and S. Hashimoto: European Food and Research Technology *209*, 497 (1999}.

251 T.K. Devon and A.I. Scott: *Handbook of Naturally Occurring Compounds*, Vol 2, Terpenes, Academic Press, New York 1974; J.L. Simonson and D.H.R. Barton: *The Terpenes*, Cambridge University Press, New York 1961, Vol. III, 12; Sukh Dev, A.P.S. Narula and J.S. Yadav, in Sukh Dev (ed.) *CRC Handbook of Terpenoids*, Vols. 1, II, CRC Press Inc. Boca Raton, Florida 1982.

252 E. Eschenmoser and Schinz: Helv. Chim. Acta *33*, 171 (1950).

253 D. Arigoni and O. Jeger: Helv. Chim. Acta *37*, 881 (1954).

254 M.D. Stoffer and L.A. Burke: Tetrahedron Letters *26*, 3543 (1985).

255 S.M. Mehta and N.K. Bhat: J. Amer. Chem. Soc. *75*, 4698 (1957}.

256 G.D. Joshi and S.N. Kulkarni: Indian J. Chem. *6*, 27 (1968). G. Zheng and H. Kakisawa: Chem. Abs. *114*, 43213 (1991).

257 G. Zheng and H. Kakisawa: Chem.Abs. *114*, 43213 (1991}.

258 D.C. Breeden and R.M. Coates: Tetrahedron *50*, 11123 (1994).

259 J.G. Miller: J. Nat. Prod. *61*, 1025 (1998).

260 P.K. Sharma, R.S. Thakur and A. Akhila, Phytochemistry *27*, 3471 (1988).

261 C.V. Denyer, P. Jackson, D.M Loakes, M.R. Ellis and D.A.B. Young: J. Nat. Prod. *57*, 658 (1994).

262 P. Wu, M.C. Kuo and C.T. Ho: J. Agri. Food Chem. *38*, 1555 (1990).

263 Y. Sekiwa, Y. Mizuno, Y. Yamamoto, K. Kubota, A. Kobayashi and H. Koshino: Bioscience, Biotechnology and Biochemistry *63*, 384 (1999).

264 M. Miyazawa and H. Kameoka: Agri. Biol. Chem. *52*, 2961 (1988).

265 D.W. Connell and M.D. Sutherland: Austr. J. Chem. *22*, 1033 (1969}

266 D. Enders, H. Eichenauer and R. Pieter: Chem. Ber. *112*, 3703 (1979); B.P. Giovanni, M. Fabio, P.G. Piero, S. Daniels, B. Achille and B. Simonetta: J. Chem. Soc, Perkin I, 2983 (1982).

267 T. Kawai, K. Kinoshita, K. Koyama and K. Tahkahashi: Planta Medica *60*, 17 (1994).

268 K. Kato, Y. Hamada and T. Shioiri: Chem. Pharm. Bull. Japan *32*, 1679 (1984).

269 R.D. Hiseroudt, S.G. Franzblau and R.T. Rosen: J. Agri. Food. Chem. *46*, 2504 (1998).

270 H. Kikuzaki, Y. Kawasaki and N. Nakatani: Food phytochemicals for cancer prevention II *547*, 237 (1994).

271 H. Kikuzaki and N. Nakatani: J. Food Sci. *58*, 1407 (1993).

272 X.G. He, M.W. Bernart, L.Z. Lian and L.Z. Lin: J. Chromatogr. A *796*, 327 (1998).

273 D.J. Harvey: J. Chromatogr. *212*, 75 (1981).

274 F. Kikuchi, M. Shibuya and U. Sankawa: Chem. Pharm. Bull. Japan *39*, 754 (1982).

275 P. Denniff, I. Macleod and D.A. Whiting: J. Chem. Soc. Perkin I, 82 (1981).

276 H. Kikuzaki, Y. Kawasaki and N. Nakatani: J. Food Sci. *58*, 1407 (1993).

277 A.M. Yashikawa, S. Hatakeyama, N. Chatani, Y. Nishino and J. Yamahara: Yakugaku Zasshi *113*, 307 (1993).

278 T. Murata, M. Miyamato and M. M. Shinohar: Chem. Pharm. Bull. Japan *20*, 2291 (1972).

279 Y. Masada, T. Inoue, K. Hashimoto, K. Fujoka and C. Uchino: Yakugaku Zasshi *94*, 735 (1974).

280 I. Kimura, L.R. Pancho, T. Shioiri and M. Kimura: Japn. J. Pharmacol. *48*, 257 (1988).

281 H. Kikuchi, S.M. Tsai and N. Nakatani: Phytochemistry *31*, 1783 (1992).

282 M. Juch and P. Ruedi: Helv. Chim. Acta *80*, 436 (1997).
283 Y. Sekiwa, K. Kubota and A. Kobayashi: J. Agri. Food Chem. *48*, 373 (2000).
284 M. Yashikawa, S. Hatakeyama, K. Taniguchi, H. Matuda and J. Yamahara: Chem. Pharm. Bull. Japan *40*, 2239 (1992).
285 M. Yoshikawa, S. Yamaguchi, K. Kunimi, H. Matuda, Y. Okuno, J. Yamahara and N. Murakami: Chem. Pharm. Bull. Japan *42*, 1226 (1994).
286 A. Lapworth and F. N. Wykes, J. Chromatogr. *111*, 790 (1971).
287 D.J. Harvey, J. Chromatogr. 212, 75 (1981); G. Hartmann and S. Kostner: Fleischwirtschaft *74*, 313 (1994); R. Wang: J. Food Sci. *59*, 1338 (1994).
288 W.J. Sanders and J.L.Seidel: J. Agri. Food Chem. *40*, 263 (1992).
289 S. Inoshiri, M. Saiki, H. Kohda, H. Otsuka and K. Yamasaki: Phytochemistry *27*, 2869 (1988).
290 T.S. Wu, Y.C. Wu, P.L. Wu, Y.L. Leu and Y.Y. Chan: Phytochemistry *48*, 889 (1998).
291 K. Endo, E. Konno and Y. Oshima: Phytochemistry *29*, 797 (1990).
292 H. Kikuzaki, J. Usuguchi and N. Nakatani: Chem. Pharm. Bull. Japan *49*, 120 (1991).
293 H. Kikuzaki, M. Kobayashi and N. Nakatani: Phytochemistry *30*, 3647 (1991).
294 H. Kikuzaki and N. Nakatani: Phytochemistry *43*, 273 (1996).
295 H. Morita and H. Itikawa: Planta Medica *54*, 117 (1988).
296 Q. Huang, H.T. Iwamoto, S. Aoki, N. Tanaka, K. Tajima, J. Yamahara, Y. Takaishi, M. Yoshida, T. Tomimatsu and Y. Tamai: Chem. Pharm. Bull. Japan *39*, 397 (1991).
297 M. Yoshikawa, S. Hatakeyama, K. Taniguchi, H. Matuda and J. Yamahara: Chem. Pharm. Bull. Japan *40*, 2239 (1992).
298 Y. Ichikawa, H. Sawa and K. Michi: J. Japn. Soc. Food Nutr. *26*, 377 (1973).
299 A. Hashimoto, Y. Takeuti, Y. Kawahara and K. Yasumoto: J. Jpn. Soc. Nutr. Food Sci. *44*, 127 (1972).
300 E.H. Thompson and C.E. Allen: J. Food Sci. *38*, 652 (1973).
301 K.H. Choi, R.A. Laursen and K.N. Allen: Biochemistry. *38*, 11624 (1999).
302 J.E. Farting and M.J. O'Neill: J. Liquid Chromatogr. *13*, 941 (1990).
303 R.S. Zarate and M.M. Yeoman: J. Chromatogr. *609*, 407 (1992).
304 J.P. Bartley and P. Foley: J. Sci. Food and Agri. *66*, 365 (1994).
305 O. Nishimura: J. Agri. Food Chem. *43*, 2941 (1995).
306 J.P. Bartley: J. Sci. Food Agri. *68*, 215 (1995).
307 A.P.Jarvis and D. Morgan: Phytochemical Analysis *8*, 217 (1997).
308 A. Balladin and O. Headley: Renewable Energy *18*, 257 (1999).
309 A. Jansco-Gabor: Acta Physiol Sci. Hung. *66*, 57 (1989)
310 J. Yamahara, K. Miki, T. Chisaka, T. Sawada, H. Fujimura, T. Tomimatsu, K. Nakano and T. Nohora: J. Ethnopharmacol. *13*, 217 (1985).
311 J. Yamahara, S. Hatakeyama, K. Taniguchi, M. Kawamura and M. Yoshikawa: Yakugaku Zasshi *112*, 645 (1992).
312 M. Yoshikawa, S. Yamaguchi, K. Kunimi, H. Matsuda, Y. Okuno, J. Yamahara and N. Murakami: Chem. Pharm. Bull. *42*, 1226 (1994).
313 T. Kawai, K. Kinoshita, K. Koyama and K. Takahashi: Planta Medica *60*, 17 (1994).
314 S.S. Sharma, V. Kochupillai, S.K. Gupta, S.D. Seth and Y.K. Gupta: J. Ethnopharmacol. *57*, 93 (1997).
315 S.S. Sharma and Y.K. Gupta: J. Ethnopharmacol. *62*, 49 (1998).
316 N. Mascolo, R. Jain, S.C. Jain and F. Copasso: J. Ethnopharmacol. *27*, 129 (1989).
317 J.N. Sharma, K.C. Srivastava and E.K. Gan: Pharmacology *49*, 314 (1994).

318 J.N. Sharma, F.I. Ishak, A.P. Yusof and K.C. Srivastava: Asia Pacific J. Pharmacol. *12*, 9 (1997).

319 H. Ohigashi, A. Murakami and K. Koshimizu: Food Phytochemicals for Cancer Prevention II *547*, 251 (1994).

320 S.K. Katiyar, R. Agarwal and H. Mukhtar: Cancer Res. *56*, 1023 (1996).

321 A.M. Bode, W.Y. Ma, Y.J. Surh and Z.G. Dong: Cancer Res. *61*, 850 (2001).

322 E. Lee and Y.J. Surh: Cancer Lett. *134*, 163 (1998).

323 S. Vimala, A.W. Norhanom and M. Yadav: Brit. J. Cancer *80*, 110 (1999).

324 A. Mukherjee: Phytotherap. Res. *14*, 555 (2000).

325 T.P. Eldershaw, E.Q. Colquhoun, K.A. Dora, Z.C. Peng and M.G. Clark: Internl. J. Obes. *16*, 755 (1992).

326 B.N. Wu, W.C. Ho, L.C. Chiang and I.J. Chen: Asia Pacific J. Pharmacol. *11*, 5 (1996).

327 M. Tanabe, Y.D. Chen, K. Saito and Y. Kano: Chem. Pharm. Bull. Japan *41*, 710 (1993).

328 I. Sharma, D. Gusain and V.P. Dixit: Phytotherap. Res. *10*, 517 (1996).

329 U. Bhandari, J.N. Sharma and R. Zafar: J. Ethnopharmacol. *61*, 167 (1998).

330 J.S. Murugaiah, N. Namasivayam and V.P. Menon: J.Clin. Biochem. Nutr. *27*, 79 (1999).

331 B. Fuhrman, M. Rosenblat, T. Hayek, R. Coleman and M. Aviram: J. Nutr. *130*, 1124 (2000).

332 A.C.P. Reddy and B.R. Lokesh: Mol. Cell. Biochem. *111*, 117 (1992).

333 S.M. Jeyakumar, N. Nalini and V.P. Menon: Med. Sci. Res. *27*, 341 (1999).

334 R.S. Ahmed, S. Iwakami, M. Shibuya, F. Hanaoka and U. Sankawa: Chem. Pharm. Bull.Japan *38*, 443 (2000).

335 F. Kiuchi, S. Iwakami, M. Shibuya, F. Hanoaka and U. Sankawa: Chem. Pharm. Bull.Japan *40*, 387 (1992).

336 S. Kawakishi, Y. Morimitsu and T. Osawa: Food Phytochemicals for Cancer Prevention II *547*, 244 (1994).

337 Y. Hata, L.R. Pancho, H. Nojima and I. Kimura: Biol. Chem. Bull. *21*, 792 (1998).

338 M.S. Weidner and K. Sigwart: J. Ethnopharmacol. *73*, 513 (2000).

339 J.M. Wilkinson: Reproductive Toxicol. *14*, 507 (2000).

340 M.S. Weidner and K. Sigwart: Reproductive Toxicol. *15*, 75 (2001).

341 A. Grontved and E. Hentzer: ORL J. Otorhinolaryngol. Relat. Spec. 48, 282 (1986).

342 A. Grontved, T. Brask, J. Kambskard and E. Hentzer: Acta Otolaryngol. *105*, 45 (1988).

343 Z. Arfeen, H. Owen, J.L. Plummer, A.H. Ilsly, R.A. Sorbyadams and C.J. Doecke: Anesthesia and Intensive Care *23*, 449 (1995).

344 M.P. Aikins: Obstet. Gynecol. *91*, 149 (1998).

345 T. Wolffgram: Medizin. Welt *51*, 21 (2000).

346 S. Phillips, S. Hutchinson and R. Ruggier: Anesthesia *48*, 393 (1993).

347 G.H. Micklefield, Y. Redeker, V. Meister, O. Jung, I. Greving and B. May: Int. J. Clin. Pharmacol. Therap. *37*, 341 (1999).

348 E. Ernst and M.H. Pittler: Brit. J. Anesthes. *84*, 367 (2000).

349 K.C. Srivastava and T. Mustafa: Med. Hypothesis *39*, 342 (1992).

350 H. Bliddal, A. Rosetzsky, P. Schlichting, M.S. Weidner, L.A. Andersen, H.H. Ibfelt, K. Christensen, O.N. Jensen and J. Barslev: Osteoarthritis and Cartilage *8*, 9 (2000).

351 S.K. Verma, J. Singh, R. Khamesra and A. Bordia: Ind. J. Med. Res B *98*, 240 (1993).

352 A. Bordia, S.K. Verma and K.C. Srivastava: Prostaglandins Leukotrienes and Essential Fatty Acids *56*, 379 (1997).

Progress in Drug Research, Vol. 57 (E. Jucker, Ed.)

Virus population dynamics, fitness variations and the control of viral disease: an update

By Esteban Domingo[1], Antonio Mas[1], Eloisa Yuste[1], Nonia Pariente[1], Saleta Sierra[2], Mónica Gutiérrez-Rivas[1], and Luis Menéndez-Arias[1]

[1]Centro de Biología Molecular "Severo Ochoa"
Consejo Superior de Investigaciones Científicas
Universidad Autónoma de Madrid
Cantoblanco, 28049 Madrid, Spain
<edomingo@cbm.uam.es>

[2]Institut für Virologie, Universität zu Köln, Fürst-Pückler Str. 56, 50935 Köln, Germany

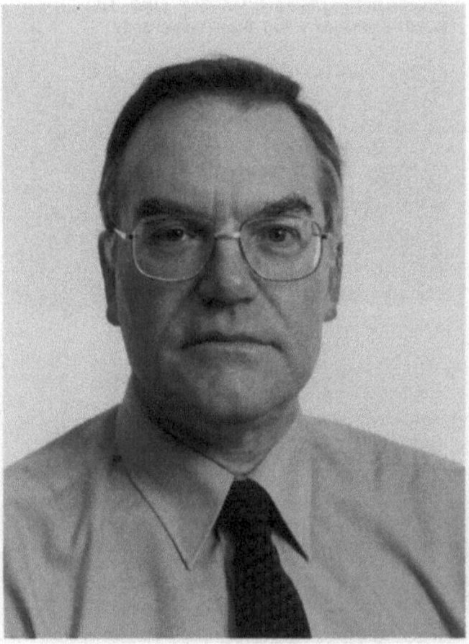

Esteban Domingo

studied Biochemistry at the University of Barcelona (Spain), where he gained a Ph.D. in 1969. His postdoctoral experiences encompass studies of in vitro *transcription at the University of California at Irvine (USA) with Robert C. Warner and research on phage genetics with Charles Weissmann at the University of Zürich (Switzerland). From 1986 to 1992, Domingo was the Spanish representative in the Standing Technical Committee of the FAO. Currently, he is professor at the Spanish Research Council (CSIC) and member of the editorial boards of several renowned virological journals.*

Summary

Viral quasispecies dynamics and variations of viral fitness are reviewed in connection with viral disease control. Emphasis is put on resistance of human immunodeficiency virus and some human DNA viruses to antiviral inhibitors.

Future trends in multiple target antiviral therapy and new approaches based on virus entry into error catastrophe (extinction mutagenesis) are discussed.

Contents

1	Introduction: overview of quasi-species complexity in relation to viral disease prevention and treatment	80
2	HIV variation and strategies for HIV persistence	82
3	Anti-retroviral therapy and development of drug resistance: population dynamics of HIV infection	85
4	Selection of HIV variants resistant to anti-retroviral drugs	88
5	Resistance mutations and their effect on viral fitness	90
5.1	Complex genotypic pathways leading to resistance to multiple nucleoside analogue inhibitors of reverse transcriptase	92
5.2	Resistance to protease inhibitors	94
6	Multidrug-resistant virus: an obstacle to eradication	95
7	Resistance to antiviral drugs specific for other RNA viruses	96
8	Resistance to antiviral drugs specific for DNA viruses	98
8.1	Inhibitors of viral replication of Herpesviridae	99
8.2	Inhibitors of reverse transcription as antiviral drugs for chronic hepatitis B	102
9	Future directions: multiple-target antiviral therapy	105
	Acknowledgements	107
	References	107

Keywords

Virus, quasispecies, HIV, fitness, influenza, herpes, hepatitis B, inhibitor, resistance, extinction mutagenesis

Glossary of abbreviations

CMV, cytomegalovirus; CTL, cytotoxic T lymphocyte; EBV, Epstein-Barr virus; HAART, highly active anti-retroviral therapy; HBV, hepatitis B virus; HCV, hepatitis C virus; HIV-1, human immunodeficiency virus type 1; HSV, herpes simplex virus; PR, protease; RT, reverse transcriptase; TK, thymidine kinase; VSV, vesicular stomatitis virus; VZV, varicella zoster virus.

1 Introduction: overview of quasi-species complexity in relation to viral disease prevention and treatment

Previous versions of this article [1, 2] emphasized the need to design antiviral strategies taking into consideration that RNA viruses are highly heterogeneous and dynamic, rather than constrained genomes that would lend themselves to control by inhibitors and immune responses. It was proposed that a better control of viral replication should be achieved with combination antiviral therapy and multivalent vaccines [1, 2]. As deeper insight into the structure and dynamics of RNA viruses is gained, such proposals find increasing justification. The mutant spectra of many RNA viral quasi-species have been shown to hide mutants with altered biological properties (altered phenotypes). Of immediate relevance to disease control are inhibitor-resistant mutants [3–6], and antibody and cytotoxic T lymphocyte (CTL)-escape mutants [7–12]. The origin of the rich repertoire of genetic and phenotypic variants is a biochemical property of all known RNA-dependent DNA and RNA polymerases: low template-copying fidelity, partly associated with the absence (or very low efficiency) of proofreading-repair activities [13, 14]. By application of genetic and biochemical procedures, mutation rates averaging 10^{-3} to 10^{-5} misincorporations per nucleotide have been determined for several RNA viruses ([15] and references therein). This strong mutational pressure unavoidably yields mutants with different relative replication efficiency (fitness) and thus, different mutants are found at different frequencies in viral quasi-species. Mutation frequencies, measured as the number of mutations in a set of genomes relative to the number of nucleotides screened, range from 10^{-2} to 10^{-5} substitutions per nucleotide. This broad range reflects a complex set of parameters which influence the heterogeneity of a mutant spectrum: duration of an infection (either in cell culture or a natural host), number and extent of environmental perturbations affecting viral multiplication, and many others. Examples of very different mutation frequencies determined in our laboratory under disparate biological circumstances (clonal populations in cell culture *versus* prolongued infections *in vivo*) can be found in ([3, 16, 17]; as a recent general review see also [18]).

These well-documented mutation rates and mutation frequencies render it very likely that a selective pressure directed to a specific locus of a viral genome (or its protein product) will result in the selection of a viral variant capable of overcoming the selective constraint (the isolation of monoclonal antibody-escape mutants is a classical example). Therefore, for statistical reasons, given the population size of replicating viruses – often higher than 10^{11} particles during human hepatitis C virus (HCV) or human immunodeficiency virus (HIV) infections [19–23] – an antiviral treatment must target three or more genetic loci of a virus. The evolution of therapeutic regimens implemented for the control of HIV-1 infections from the middle eighties until the present constitutes a revealing example. Monotherapy resulted in the systematic selection of inhibitor-resistant HIV-1 mutants in infected individuals [5, 24, 25, and many other studies]. In contrast, the so-called "highly active anti-retroviral therapy" (HAART) which involves administration of three or more anti-retroviral drugs targeting two different viral enzymes, has resulted in a generally effective suppression of HIV-1 replication and a reduction of AIDS cases [26–28]. Parallel arguments apply to vaccines [1, 2, 29, 30]. The main demonstration that multi-valent, multi-epitopic vaccines are required for protection against diseases associated with RNA viruses, is that no vaccines consisting of a single synthetic peptide capable of affording protection in a reproducible manner have been produced, despite much investment ([31, 32], among other reports].

Mutant swarms may hide additional types of mutants and their presence may affect viral pathogenesis. Individual components of vesicular stomatitis virus (VSV) quasi-species displayed either a higher or lower capacity to induce interferon than the average population in natural isolates of VSV [33]. For several RNA viruses, mutants with altered host cell tropism have been isolated from the quasi-species swarms [34–36]. In other cases, the presence of critical phenotypic variants may not be readily identified, but the number of different sequences in the mutant distribution may itself have a predictive value. Large quasi-species complexity correlated with a high pathogenic potential of the coronavirus mouse hepatitis virus for mice [37]. Evolution of the HCV quasi-species replicating in patients correlated with the transition from an acute to a chronic infection [38]. Also, despite early contradictory results, when the complexity of HCV quasi-species has been reliably measured by extensive nucleotide sequencing, a high mutant spectrum complexity predicts failure of elimination of the virus by the combined action of interferon α and the nucleoside analogue ribavirin ([39], reviewed in [40]).

Recently, a new feature of quasi-species has been revealed: the presence of memory genomes, as minority components of the mutant spectrum, which reflect those genomes which were dominant at an earlier stage in the evolutionary history of the virus ([17, 41], review in [42]). Memory can be durable provided no genetic bottlenecks intervene during viral replication, showing that memory is a property of the quasi-species as a whole [further discussion in 42]. The presence of memory is a feature of complex adaptive systems, such as the immune system [43]. Its presence in RNA virus quasi-species suggests that adaptation to virology of concepts related to complexity in physics [44] may provide new grounds to study viral population dynamics.

The overview of long-established facts, together with recent observations, on the nature of RNA virus quasi-species suggests that the consensus nucleotide sequence (the one resulting from assigning to each genomic position the most abundant nucleotide found at the corresponding position, for the set of compared sequences) provides only a fragmentary information to guide decisions on antiviral treatment. Insights into complexity and composition of mutant spectra are required. Furthermore, RNA genome complexity has also inspired entirely new antiviral strategies, such as forcing virus replication into error catastrophe, an interesting possibility reviewed in section 9. HIV appears as a viral system where many of these issues have been thoroughly investigated, and here we summarize current knowledge on viral dynamics and molecular mechanisms leading to emergence of mutants escaping the immune response, as well as to the emergence of drug resistance. Finally, drug resistance in other RNA viruses, as well as in DNA viruses, will be discussed in the light of current treatment options.

2 HIV variation and strategies for HIV persistence

Rapid replication rates and high mutation rates are thought to be the engine of HIV-1 genetic diversity. The HIV-1 reverse transcriptase is error-prone, and its error rate has been estimated at between 10^{-4} to 10^{-5} mutations per nucleotide and cycle of replication [45–48]. Mutation rates may also show sequence- or structure-dependent variation; hence, all mutations may not occur with similar rates. If one assumes that 10^{9}–10^{10} virions are produced each day, then they must be the product of at least 10^{7}–10^{8} replication cycles. Given the length of the HIV-1 genome (approximately 10^{4} nucleotides), it is plausible that every single possible point-mutation (and probably many double mutations) will occur at least once each day, in an infected individual. Although specific combinations of multiple mutations may be rare, it is clear that the degree of potential genetic change drives the diversification of HIV-1 in response to the selective pressure of host immune responses or anti-retroviral therapy.

The emergence of mutant forms of HIV results in escape from neutralizing antibody responses and CTLs. Neutralizing antibodies found in sera of infected individuals are directed to the envelope glycoprotein complex. This complex is arranged in a trimeric configuration of heterodimers, each consisting of a gp120 surface subunit non-covalently associated with a gp41 transmembrane subunit. The infection progress is initiated by attachment of the virus to the target cell through the interaction of gp120 with the cellular receptor CD4. The subsequent interactions between gp120 and its coreceptors are complex and require conformational changes induced by binding to CD4 (for a review see [49]). The third variable (V3) loop of gp120 is the principal neutralizing domain, as evidenced by its dominant role in the neutralization of T cell line-adapted HIV-1 strains (i.e., IIIB, SF2, MN) by sera from HIV-1 infected individuals and gp120 vaccine recipients. Binding studies with monomeric gp120-CD4 complexes have demonstrated that monoclonal antibodies to the V3 loop inhibit the interaction of this complex with the coreceptor [50–52]. Neutralizing antibodies emerge only relatively late in the course of infection [53–55] and contribute to the control of viral replication, as shown by passive immunization in animal models, and also by the correlation between titers of neutralizing antibodies and lack of disease progression in long-term survivors of HIV-1 infection [56–58]. The emergence of neutralization escape mutants has been associated with viral persistence *in vivo*, and disease progression [12, 55, 59]. However, escape mutations are not always located in the V3 loop of gp120. It has been shown by many authors that the role of V3-specific antibodies in primary isolate neutralization is insignificant [60–62]. Recently, it has been suggested that neutralization resistance of primary isolates could be considered as an escape mechanism from humoral immune control [63]. This study revealed that the emergence of neutralization-resistant HIV correlated with increased variation in the env gene, and preceded disease development in an individual that was accidentally infected with the T cell line-adapted neutralization-sensitive IIIB isolate.

CTLs constitute an essential component of protective anti-retroviral immunity. HIV-1 can use mutational and nonmutational mechanisms to avoid the CTL response (for recent reviews see [8, 64]). Viral mutation can lead to epitope deletion, failure of antigen processing, loss of major histocompatibility complex class I binding and impaired recognition by the T cell receptor. HIV-1 variants with impaired CTL recognition properties occur during the initial course of infection. Several examples illustrating how HIV can avoid CTL response through variations in T cell epitopes have been described. The first example was found following an attempt to treat an HIV-infected patient by adoptive transfer of a CTL clone, which had been grown to a very large number [65]. The CTL clone recognized an epitope presented by HLA A3. The clinical response was disappointing with no reduction in viral load or rise in $CD4^+$ T cells. The reason for the clinical failure was the emergence of a virus with a deletion in the nef gene, that was devoid of the T cell epitope spanning residues 69 to 78 of Nef. There are two examples of CTL escape occurring during the acute phase of infection. In one of them, the patient developed a strong monospecific response against an epitope (AENLWVTVY) including residues 30 to 38 of the Env protein, and presented by HLA B44 [66]. After a few weeks, variants appeared having Gly, Ala or Lys instead of Glu at the second position of the epitope, and several weeks later, they became predominant in the viral population. These variants escaped the initial CTL response of the patient. A similar case has been described by Price et al. [67], although in this case the T cell epitope includes residues 86 to 93 of Nef (sequence FLKEKGGL), and the CTL escape is associated with mutations at the fifth position of the epitope as well as with its deletion. Escape from CTL has also been observed late in HIV infection. Two patients who maintained a monospecific response to a single epitope in Gag, were found to select a virus with the same mutation as they progressed to AIDS [68]. The mutation changed an Arg to a Lys at position 2 of the epitope (KRWIILGLNK, residues 263–272 of the Gag precursor). The arginine residue was essential for binding of the peptide to HLA B27.

Strong support of the CTL "escape" hypothesis has been recently provided by a series of experiments showing the accumulation of amino acid replacements within CTL epitopes located on the proteins Env and Nef, and arising during the course of simian immunodeficiency virus disease progression in macaques [11]. Further studies revealed that Tat-specific CTLs select for SIV escape variants during the acute phase of infection [69]. The accumulation of mutations in Tat CTL epitopes suggests that responses against viral proteins that are expressed early during the viral life cycle are important to control viral replication.

3 Anti-retroviral therapy and development of drug resistance: population dynamics of HIV infection

Since the discovery of AZT (3'-azido-3'-deoxythymidine, zidovudine) as an effective anti-retroviral agent against HIV [70], a number of potent drugs that inhibit HIV-1 replication *in vivo* have been developed. As of March 2001, there are nine reverse transcriptase (RT) inhibitors and six protease (PR) inhibitors which have been approved for clinical use (Tab. 1). RT inhibitors prevent infection of new cells by blocking the synthesis of proviral DNA using the viral RNA as template, while PR inhibitors act on the late phase, interfering with the production of new infectious virions by infected cells. The obsolete monotherapy with AZT has become unacceptable and has been substituted by more powerful triple and quadruple combinations of drugs including RT and PR inhibitors [26–28]. Their use led to a significant reduction in the level of viral RNA in plasma, thereby indicating that the rate of virus production is impaired as a consequence of the treatment. Recent studies suggest that the half-life of free virus particles is extremely short, on the order of minutes to hours [23]. Analysis of dynamic changes in the level of plasma virus at different stages of disease and in response to anti-retroviral therapy has provided new insights into the mechanism of $CD4^+$ T cell depletion, the reasons for drug failure, the nature of viral reservoirs, and the intriguing possibility that prolonged therapy may lead to virus eradication (for reviews see [71, 72]). Following the initial infection, the immune response to HIV-1 develops, and plasma viral levels fall from a peak of viremia to lower steady-state values that vary in different individuals and are predictive of the rate of disease progression [20]. In untreated asymptomatic patients, the plasma HIV-1 RNA levels are typically in the range of 10^3–10^6 copies/ml in plasma. The viral burden is constant during the asymptomatic phase of infection and tends to be higher in patients showing more rapid declines in $CD4^+$ lymphocyte counts and more rapid progression to AIDS.

The introduction of HAART and sensitive molecular tools to measure HIV-1 RNA in plasma has permitted the kinetic analysis of HIV-1 infection. HIV-1 infection is characterized by rapid viral replication and rapid viral clearance [21–23]. The initiation of potent anti-retroviral therapy produced a very rapid exponential drop in the level of plasma virus. Typically, plasma viral levels decreased 100-fold in two weeks. The corresponding half-life ranges from 1.3 to 3.3 days [21, 22], and results from two different events: the clear-

Table 1.
Reverse transcriptase and protease inhibitors approved by the U.S. Food and Drug Administration for the treatment of HIV infection.[1]

Drugs	Commercial name	Company	Date of approval
Reverse transcriptase inhibitors			
Zidovudine (AZT)	Retrovir	Glaxo Wellcome	March 1987
Didanosine (ddI)	Videx	Bristol Myers-Squibb	October 1991
Zalcitabine (ddC)	Hivid	Hoffman-La Roche	June 1992
Stavudine (d4T)	Zerit	Bristol Myers-Squibb	June 1994
Lamivudine (3TC)	Epivir	Glaxo Wellcome	November 1995
Abacavir	Ziagen	Glaxo Wellcome	December 1998
Nevirapine	Viramune	Boehringer Ingelheim Pharmaceuticals, Inc.	June 1996
Delavirdine	Rescriptor	Pharmacia & Upjohn	April 1997
Efavirenz	Sustiva	DuPont Pharmaceuticals	September 1998
Protease inhibitors			
Saquinavir	Invirase	Hoffman-La Roche	December 1995
Ritonavir	Norvir	Abbott Laboratories	March 1996
Indinavir	Crixivan	Merck & Co. Inc.	March 1996
Nelfinavir	Viracept	Agouron Pharmaceuticals	March 1997
Amprenavir	Agenerase	Glaxo Wellcome	April 1999
Lopinavir	Kaletra[2]	Abbott Laboratories	September 2000

[1]Data shown have been taken from the WWW address: http://www.fda.gov/oashi/aids/virals.html, in March 2001.
[2]Kaletra is an approved oral capsule and solution, including lopinavir plus ritonavir. Other approved combinations of anti-retroviral drugs are Combivir (zidovudine and lamivudine) and Trizivir (zidovudine, lamivudine and abacavir), approved in September 1997 and November 2000, respectively.

ance of infectious virus (whose half-life was around 6 h), and the clearance of productively infected cells (whose half-lives were estimated to be 1.55 days) [23]. The short-lived cells that produce most of the plasma virus are $CD4^+$ T lymphoblasts.

When potent anti-retroviral therapy is maintained, it is possible to observe a slower decay in plasma viral levels that follows the initial rapid clearance of infectious virus and productively infected T lymphocytes. This second phase of decay brings levels of plasma virus down to below the limit of detection of current assays (20–500 copies/ml), and corresponds to the elimination of latently infected cells or long-lived and chronically productive cells, for example, resting $CD4^+$ T cells with unintegrated HIV-1 DNA, infected macrophages or virions trapped on follicular dendritic cells [26, 73, 74]. From the half-lives of these viral reservoirs (8 to 15 days), it was estimated that 2–3 years of HAART would eliminate these viral pools.

However, despite the success of HAART in reducing viremia to undetectable levels in some patients, the recovery of replication-competent HIV-1 was reported for infected individuals who experienced complete suppression of new cycles of replication for the estimated 2–3 years required for the second phase of decay to be complete. Several recent studies suggest that latently infected $CD4^+$ CD45 RO^+ memory T cells with integrated provirus represent a extremely stable reservoir for HIV-1, that may be responsible for the third phase of decay in patients under potent anti-retroviral therapy [75–79]. Memory cells must survive for long periods of time in order to provide protection against a previously encountered pathogen. Sequence analysis of viruses isolated from memory T cells revealed little evidence for the evolution of drug resistance, suggesting that the viruses that persist in this compartment are derived from long-lived cells infected prior to initiation of HAART [78, 79]. Rough estimates of half-lives of these viral reservoirs are difficult to obtain due to the lack of longitudinal samples. The median lifespan of $CD4^+$ memory T cells is estimated to be approximately 200 days [80], but the range may extend for years. If this estimate is correct, then conventional treatment methods would not be effective in eradicating HIV-1.

The contribution of the different pools of infected cells to the re-emergence of the virus after discontinuation of the anti-retroviral treatment is currently under investigation. Thus, using heteroduplex mobility and tracking assays, Chun et al. [81] have shown that the detectable pool of latently infected, resting $CD4^+$ T cells does not account entirely for the early rebounding plasma HIV in infected individuals in whom HAART was discontinued. In the majority of patients examined, the rebounding plasma virus was genetically distinct from both the cell-associated HIV-1 RNA and the replication-competent virus within the detectable pool of latently infected, resting $CD4^+$ T cells. These results point towards the existence of other persistent HIV reservoirs that could prompt rapid emergence of plasma viremia after cessation of HAART. Persistence of replication in lymphoid tissues, albeit at low levels, during seemingly effective treatment has been documented [82]. However, the precise anatomical location of the source of viral rebound remains undefined. Potential reservoirs are specific subsets of susceptible cells (i.e., follicular dendritic cells) [83], or anatomical reservoirs such as the brain, gut-associated lymphoid tissue or the genital tract [84, 85].

4 Selection of HIV variants resistant to anti-retroviral drugs

Current anti-retroviral drug regimens include RT and PR inhibitors (Figs. 1 and 2, respectively). A large number of mutations conferring partial or total resistance to those inhibitors has been observed *in vitro*, and subsequently detected *in vivo* after the examination of sequences obtained from patients failing monotherapy. The role of many of the resulting amino acid substitutions has been further verified by *in vitro* mutagenesis experiments, and large compilations of mutations have been presented in a previous review in this series [2] and elsewhere [86–89].

Development of high-level resistance to specific anti-retroviral drugs can be achieved either through the acquisition of specific mutations or through multiple amino acid substitutions. For example, a single mutation at codon 184 of HIV-1 RT (i.e., M184I or M184V) is sufficient to confer >1,000-fold resistance to lamivudine (3TC). On the other hand, high-level resistance to zidovudine (AZT) requires several amino acid substitutions (typically, M41L, D67N, K70R and T215F or T215Y), and one of them (T215Y) involves two nucleotide substitutions. The low genetic barrier to lamivudine resistance leads to the emergence of a resistant virus in just a few weeks [90], while in the case of zidovudine, its genetic barrier is higher, and the appearance of a resistant virus may take a few months [24]. Other examples of RT inhibitors having a low genetic barrier are nevirapine, delavirdine or efavirenz. In these cases, there are several single-nucleotide substitutions which can confer high-level resistance to the drug. For example, these include K103N, Y181C or G190A in the case of nevirapine, L100I, K103N, Y181C or P236L in the case of delavirdine, and L100I or K103N in the case of efavirenz. Interestingly, some of these mutations can confer cross-resistance to all inhibitors of this class, as occurs with K103N. In the case of PR inhibitors, the acquisition of high-level resistance is usually mediated by at least 3–4 changes. PR inhibitors are substrate analogues which contain a nonhydrolyzable peptidic bond. Resistance to PR inhibitors can be initially achieved through the acquisition of mutations affecting residues involved in substrate/inhibitor binding, such

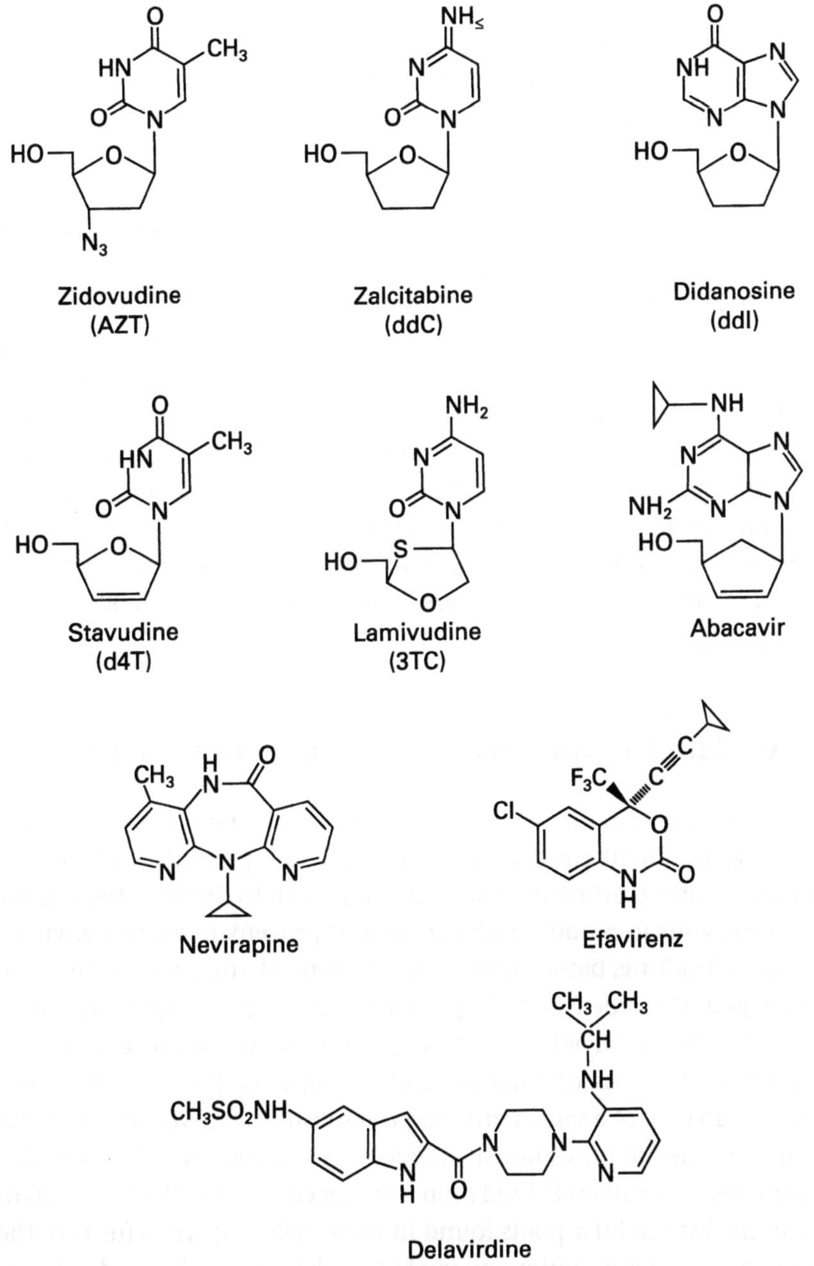

Fig. 1
Structural formulae of approved drugs targeting HIV-1 reverse transcriptase.

as Asp-30, Val-82 or Ile-84. However, these amino acid changes reduce the proteolytic activity of the enzyme, compromising viral fitness, and further mutations appear to recover the viral replicative capacity.

Generally, there are two main processes leading to resistance-related treatment failure: pre-existing resistant strains may be selected by the drugs used, or resistant mutants are generated *de novo* by residual viral replication during treatment. Some genetic variability occurs in the PR and RT coding regions even in the absence of significant selective pressure, which result in sequence polymorphisms. Single mutations related to resistance to RT or PR inhibitors have been shown to pre-exist in the HIV-1 quasi-species of drug-naïve patients [3, 4]. However, the question is still open for a multidrug-resistant virus arising during potent combination therapies, since current methods are not sensitive enough to detect mutants at very low frequencies or are too laborious to be used in clinical practice. Models based on population genetics predict that treatment failure is most likely to be caused by the pre-existence of a multidrug-resistant virus, and they therefore propose that the key to drug resistance lies in the diversity of the viral population at the start of therapy [91].

5 Resistance mutations and their effect on viral fitness

Fitness is a complex parameter aimed at describing the replicative adaptability of an organism to its environment (for reviews see [92, 93]). For HIV (and other viruses), an experimental and useful approach to fitness is the relative ability of the virus to produce stable infectious progeny in a given environment (i.e., cell culture, blood stream, etc.). In general, drug-resistance mutations emerge at the expense of a loss in viral fitness. For example, the substitution of Met-184 by Val or Ile, which confers high-level resistance to lamivudine, leads to the loss of viral replication capacity [94-98]. The lower replication capacity of a virus harboring the substitutions M184V or M184I has been attributed to the diminished processivity of the viral RT [94], which is accentuated in peripheral blood mononuclear cells due to the low levels of dNTPs in the intracellular pools found in these cells [95]. The effects of the lamivudine resistance mutations on viral fitness have been observed not only in the sequence context of a wild-type subtype B HIV-1, but also in the presence of other drug-resistance mutations such as V75I, F77L, F116Y and

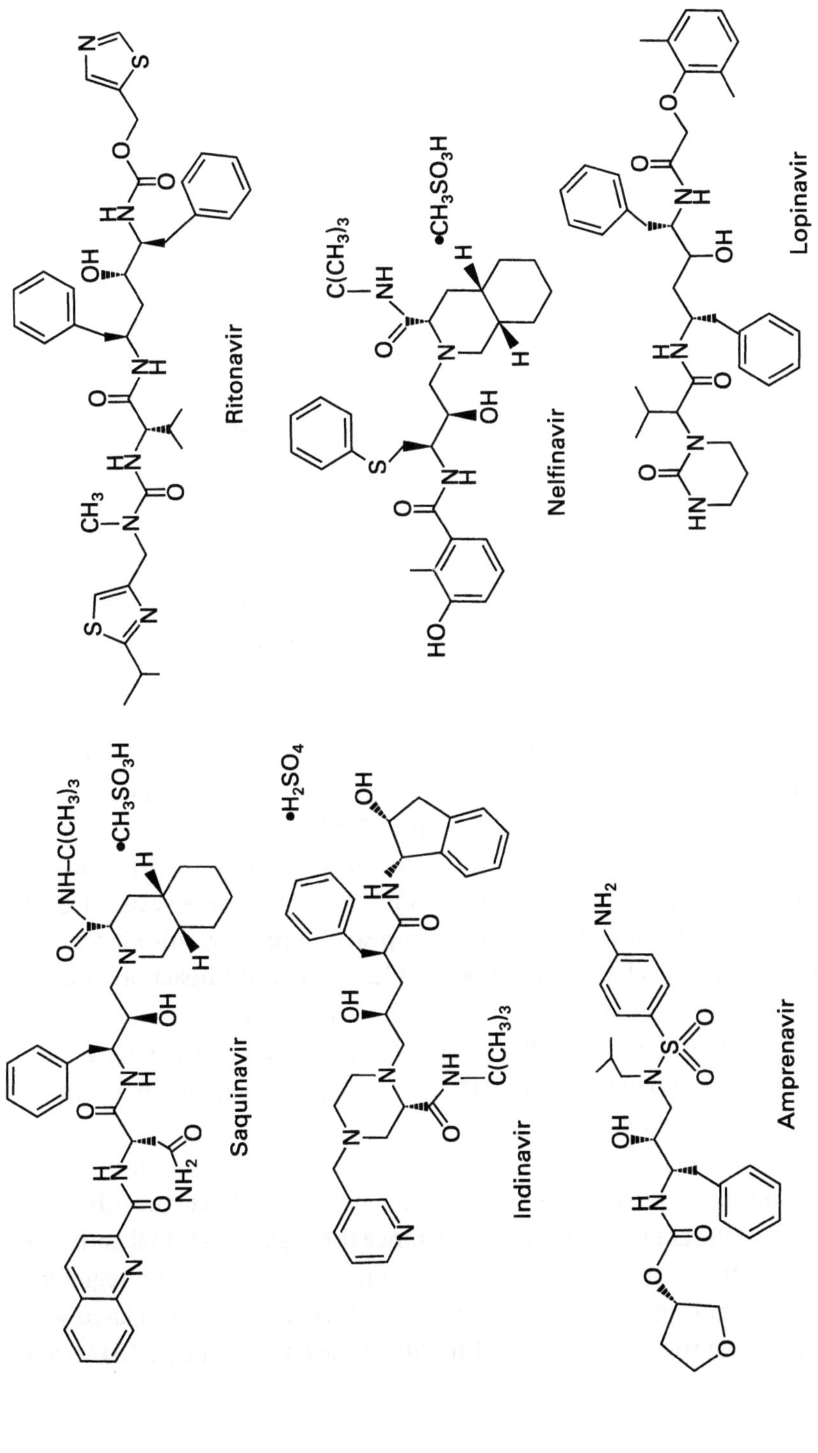

Fig. 2
Structural formulae of approved inhibitors of HIV-1 protease.

Q151M [99]. These results reported for cell cultures are also in good agreement with observations based on clinical experience. It has been shown that once the resistant virus becomes predominant in the viral quasi-species obtained after treatment with lamivudine, drug removal leads to the rapid replacement of the resistant virus by the wild-type. Estimates obtained from population dynamics *in vivo* revealed that in the presence of lamivudine, a virus having the mutation M184V showed only 10% of the fitness value calculated for the wild-type virus in the absence of the drug [100].

5.1 Complex genotypic pathways leading to resistance to multiple nucleoside analogue inhibitors of reverse transcriptase

In those cases in which two or more mutations are required to achieve high-level resistance, the sequential appearance of mutations in the viral population becomes critical. Thus, in the case of zidovudine, high-level resistance is acquired through the acquisition of several mutations including M41L, D67N, K70R, L210W, T215F/Y and K219Q/E. Different levels of resistance are observed depending on the particular combination of resistance-related mutations found in the viral clone. For example, IC_{50} values for zidovudine obtained with HIV-1 clones having the substitutions T215Y, M41L/T215Y, D67N/K70R/T215Y and M41L/D67N/K70R/T215Y are 3 to 16, 31, 33–70, and >100 times higher, respectively, than the values obtained with wild-type virus (reviewed in [87]). Primary mutations for zidovudine resistance are K70R and T215F/Y. The K70R mutation appears frequently, since it requires only one nucleotide change, and does not have a major impact on viral fitness [101]. However, its effect on viral resistance is relatively small [102, 103]. The substitution of Thr-215 by Phe or Tyr implies two nucleotide changes and has a major impact on viral fitness [101, 104, 105], although it has a stronger effect on viral resistance.

The situation becomes more complex in a virus displaying multidrug resistance. Combined therapies with two or more nucleoside analogue inhibitors of RT leads to the emergence of drug resistance through mutational pathways which are different from those obtained with monotherapeutic regimens. Resistance to multiple nucleoside inhibitors of RT has been associated with a substitution at the nucleotide binding site of the enzyme (i.e., Q151M) and with insertions or deletions around positions 67–70 of the RT. The acquisition of resistance through the Q151M pathway was initially observed in the virus isolated from patients receiving zidovudine and didanosine [106]. In this situation, the first amino acid change that appears in the viral population is Q151M, which involves two nucleotide changes. Viral clones harboring this amino acid substitution display moderate resistance to zidovudine and zalcitabine, and low resistance to other nucleoside analogues [106, 107]. However, further acquisition of additional mutations, such as A62V, V75I, F77L, or F116Y led to the appearance of highly resistant virus. Fitness assays involving the determination of replication kinetics or growth competition experiments have shown that the mutations at codons 62, 75, 77 and 116 improve the replication capacity of the resistant virus [108, 109]. The frequency of emergence of Q151M and its related mutations has been estimated as ranging from 3.5% to more than 19% in patients receiving combination chemotherapy with multiple dideoxynucleosides for more than a year [106, 107, 110–112]. Its low frequency is probably related to the requirement of two nucleotide changes to obtain the initial Q151M mutation (from CAG to AUG). In addition, any intermediate step, involving either the substitution of Q151K (CAG to AAG) or Q151L (CAG to CUG), results in a virus whose replication efficiency is very low, as demonstrated by introducing these mutations in proviral HIV clones [109]. The conservative change to Q151L appears to be lethal for viral replication and has been rarely observed *in vivo*. However, a recent study suggests that in the presence of Gly instead of Ser at position 68, this mutant retains some replicative capacity [113], and therefore could facilitate the emergence of multidrug resistance through the Q151M pathway.

An insertion of two amino acids (often Ser-Ser, Ser-Gly or Ser-Ala) between residues 69 and 70 of HIV-1 RT has recently been described in patients subjected to prolonged therapy with AZT, often together with (or followed by) administration of other nucleoside inhibitors [114–120]. The insertion appears to be associated with multiple amino acid substitutions, including AZT-resistance mutations, such as T215Y. The insertion is critical for the acquisition of zidovudine resistance, since it improves the enzyme's ability to unblock and further extend AZT-terminated primers in the presence of ATP [121]. Interestingly, this effect occurs only in the background of a virus having many resistance mutations, where it probably increases its replication capacity. Although the molecular mechanism leading to the emergence of the insertion is not known, it could result from the duplication of a six-nucleotide sequence, after the replacement of Thr-69 by Ser. In any case, this event would be rare, in agreement with frequency estimates of insert-containing strains in patients undergoing potent anti-retroviral therapy, which are usually between 1 and 3% [116, 117, 120, 122].

A deletion at codon 67 (Δ67 mutation) has been recently reported to be associated with multidrug resistance either in the context of mutations of the Q151M pathway [123] or in the presence of known zidovudine resistance mutations (i.e., K70R, T215F or K219Q) and non-nucleoside RT inhibitor resistance mutations (i.e., K103N) [124]. The deletion appears to be associated with a substitution at codon 69 (T69G). An extensive analysis of the fitness of a virus carrying the deletion and/or the T69G mutation in different sequence contexts revealed that the substitution of T69G is critical for the acquisition of high-level resistance to zidovudine, while the Δ67 mutation is important to restore viral fitness in the context of a heavily mutated multidrug-resistant virus [125, 126].

5.2 Resistance to protease inhibitors

Currently approved PR inhibitors share relatively similar chemical structures (Fig. 2), and therefore, cross-reactivity is frequently observed in the clinical setting [25]. Primary resistance mutations involved substitutions at positions of the substrate/inhibitor binding site. Examples are V82A or I84V, among others. A multidrug-resistant virus appearing during prolonged therapy with indinavir bore the substitutions M46I, L63P, V82T and I84V in the PR [25]. Crystallographic studies of the mutant enzyme revealed that the substitutions at codons 82 and 84 were critical for the acquisition of resistance, while the amino acid changes at codons 46 and 63, which are away from the inhibitor binding site, appear as compensatory mutations [127, 128]. In a similar way, saquinavir resistance implies the acquisition of substitutions G48V and L90M [129], where G48V exerts the major influence on resistance, and L90M, which is located away from the substrate/inhibitor binding site, contributes to the stability of the HIV PR.

The analysis of viral fitness of clones bearing PR inhibitor resistance mutations is broadly consistent with the hypothesis suggesting that the acquisition of resistance implies a significant cost in terms of viral replicative capacity. Primary mutations, such as D30N, M46I or M46L, G48V and V82A or V82T, which arise after treatment with nelfinavir, indinavir, saquinavir or ritonavir, respectively, have been shown to have a severe impact on viral fitness [130–134]. In all cases, these substitutions affect residues which are important to stabilize the substrate in its binding pocket.

The acquisition of drug resistance in the case of PR inhibitors usually involves several mutations in the protease gene, as well as in secondary loci of the genome. One example that illustrates this concept comes from a clinical study in which the emergence of indinavir resistance was monitored in patients treated for over a year [135]. Sequential analysis of the genotype of viral isolates obtained at different times after initiation of therapy revealed that the substitution V82A appeared first, but additional mutations in the PR gene emerged shortly afterwards or simultaneously in some patients. These mutations were L10I, M46L and I54V, and are commonly observed as secondary mutations during treatment with other PR inhibitors. It was also observed that several isolates bore an additional change at the cleavage site between the gag-encoded proteins p1 and p6. Further treatment implied additional mutations in the PR coding region (i.e., K20M/R, L24I, G48V, A71V/T, G73S, L89M/P and L90M), and another substitution in one of the amino acids of the cleavage site between the nucleocapsid protein, p7 (NC), and the peptide p1. These results revealed that the virus optimizes its viral fitness through the accumulation of changes in PR, but also through the acquisition of mutations at cleavage sites in precursor polyproteins (in HIV-1, termed as Gag and Gag-Pol), which need to be hydrolyzed by the PR in order to complete viral maturation successfully. Mutations at Gag cleavage sites may increase proteolytic processing and compensate for the functional impairment shown by the PR bearing drug-resistance mutations [135, 136]. An interesting effect of the substitution found at the p1/p6 cleavage site is that it produces a 3- to 11-fold increase in the expression of pol, as a consequence of an increased level of frameshifting [137]. The consequence is that the same mutation improves Gag cleavage and stimulates PR synthesis.

6 Multidrug-resistant virus: an obstacle to eradication

In addition to the enormous variability of HIV derived from the inaccuracy of its RT and the high viral loads involved in the infection, recombination events can also contribute to substantial genetic variation. Recombination between strains resistant to RT inhibitors and to PR inhibitors has been demonstrated *in vitro* as a source of dual resistance [138]. In this scenario, suboptimal therapies, such as the sequential treatment with multiple drugs, may accelerate the appearance of a multidrug-resistant virus through the accumulation of inhibitor-specific drug resistance mutations [139], or through mutational pathways discussed above.

7 Resistance to antiviral drugs specific for other RNA viruses

Influenza is the paradigm of a viral disease in which continued evolution of the virus has an enormous influence in annual epidemics and occasional pandemics of disease in humans. Point mutations (antigenic drift), gene assortment (genetic shift), defective-interfering particles, and RNA recombination are significant contributors to antigenic variation which ultimately leads to viral escape from immune control (reviewed in [140]). Approved drugs for treatment of influenza are amantadine, rimantadine, zanamivir and oseltamivir (Fig. 3) (reviewed in [141]). Amantadine and rimantadine act at an early stage of the viral life cycle, impairing the functionality of the proton channel formed by the viral protein M2. These compounds block the flow of hydrogen ions that goes into the viral particle in the initial steps of viral infection. Inside the virion, the low pH promotes dissociation of the M1 protein from the ribonucleoprotein and triggers initiation of viral replication [142, 143]. Resistant mutants have been isolated *in vitro* and have been recognized in about 25–35% of the treated patients. Escape mutants were usually resistant to both drugs and most of them contained the amino acid substitution S31D at the transmembrane domain of the M2 protein [144].

Neuraminidase is an influenza virus enzyme which allows the virus to penetrate the host cell. The neuraminidase inhibitors, zanamivir and oseltamivir are analogues of N-acetylneuraminic acid (the cell-surface receptor for influenza viruses) [145, 146]. Zanamivir-resistant viruses have been selected *in vitro* [147, 148], although resistance mutations have not been described so far in clinical trials with this drug [149]. In the case of oseltamivir, resistance has been shown to occur in 1.5% of the treated patients [149].

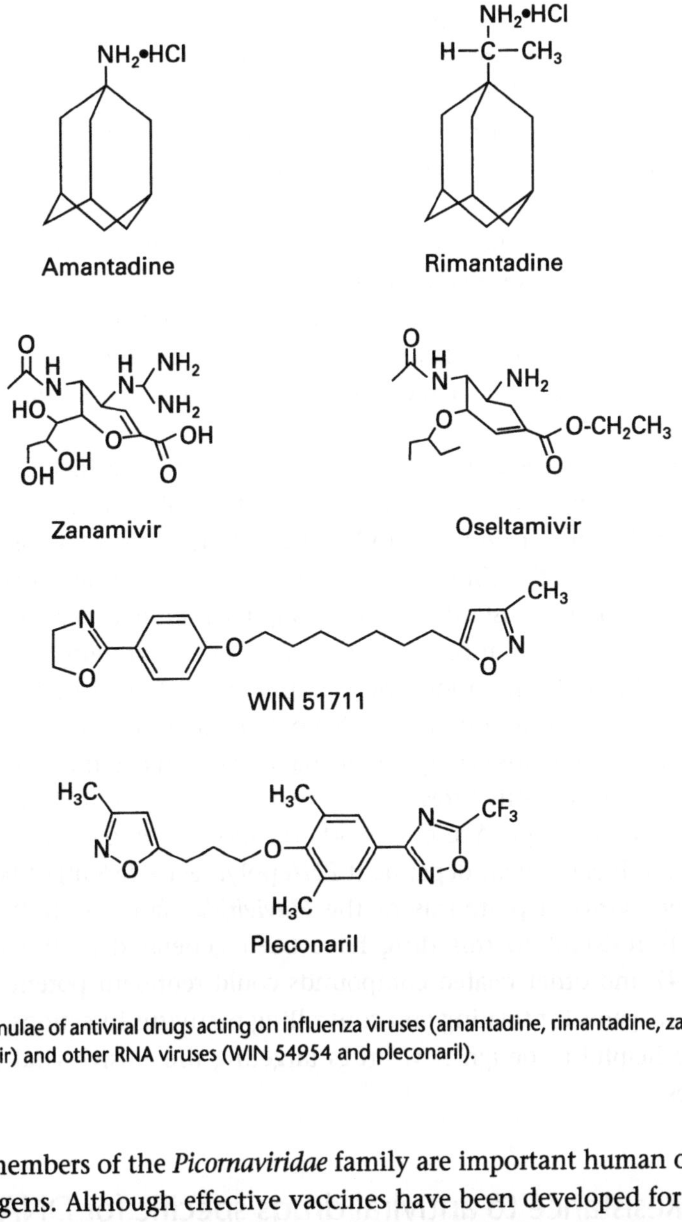

Fig. 3
Structural formulae of antiviral drugs acting on influenza viruses (amantadine, rimantadine, zanamivir and oseltamivir) and other RNA viruses (WIN 54954 and pleconaril).

Some members of the *Picornaviridae* family are important human or animal pathogens. Although effective vaccines have been developed for some of these viruses, such as the polio virus or hepatitis A virus, for other members of this group, the development of antiviral agents has become a priority (for a review see [150]). Structural analysis of the surface of the rhinovirus and enterovirus has revealed the presence of a hydrophobic pocket (usually referred as a 'canyon') which constitutes a target of antiviral compounds blocking viral uncoating and/or attachment. These compounds are collectively referred to as WIN compounds [151]; several drugs have been extensively studied, and resistance mutations to these drugs have been characterized (reviewed in [152]). One of the most promising agents acting on the capsid function is pleconaril, which is a metabolically stable WIN derivative (Fig. 3). This compound showed broad-spectrum and potent antiviral activity against the enterovirus and rhinovirus [153]. As previously noted for various anti-retroviral drugs, the development of resistance to pleconaril and other WIN derivatives leads to severely reduced infectivity and virulence or attenuated viral growth characteristics in cell culture ([154, 155]; reviewed in 152]).

Other antiviral agents targeting other viral functions include guanidine, a viral replication inhibitor effective against members of the *Picornaviridae* family (polio virus, rhinovirus and foot-and-mouth disease virus, which has not been used in the clinical setting due to its adverse side-effects and the rapid selection of resistant mutants [156]. Guanidine acts at the RNA synthesis step and resistance mutations map to the protein 2C, an ATPase involved in viral replication and encapsidation [157]. Despite significant efforts, efficient inhibitors of viral RNA polymerases, such as inhibitors of the polio virus or hepatitis C polymerase, have not been described, although the recently published structures of these two enzymes [158–161] may pave the way towards its design. A recent report described a new compound (VP32947) which inhibits the RNA-dependent RNA polymerase (NS5B) of bovine viral diarrhoea virus (a pestivirus of the *Flaviviridae* family) [162]. Although mutants resistant to this drug have been generated in the laboratory, VP32947 and other related compounds could represent potentially useful antiviral agents for treating and controlling pestivirus infections, and could also be helpful to design new drugs targeting the elusive viral RNA polymerases.

8 Resistance to antiviral drugs specific for DNA viruses

An important, still largely unanswered question is whether DNA viruses may participate in the high mutation frequencies and quasi-species dynamics which are typical of RNA viruses. The hepadnaviruses, which replicate *via* a

RT step catalyzed by a DNA polymerase devoid of a proofreading-repair activity, share high mutation frequencies with RNA viruses [163]. A strong case for quasi-species dynamics has been made for the geminivirus, a family of plant viruses with a circular, single-stranded DNA genome [164]. Other viruses with single-stranded DNA genomes of small size, such as the parvovirus, also display considerable heterogeneity and variations in host range [165]. For large DNA viruses, it has been suggested that loci-specific variations, for example, tandemly repeated sequences, will be far more likely than generalized high mutation frequencies at many loci (reviewed in [18]). Nevertheless, population heterogeneity and selection of inhibitor-resistant mutants may complicate the control of diseases associated with complex DNA viruses, as documented in the next section.

8.1 Inhibitors of viral replication of *Herpesviridae*

Approximately 90% of the human population is infected by at least one member of the herpes viruses. These viruses are responsible for genital and labial herpetic disease, chickenpox, retinitis, several tumors (lymphomas, sarcomas), etc. The most relevant infectious agents of this family are the herpes simplex virus types 1 and 2 (HSV-1 and -2), varicella zoster virus (VZV), cytomegalovirus (CMV), Epstein-Barr virus (EBV) and human herpes virus type 8 (HHV-8). The treatments currently in clinical use include nucleoside derivatives (acyclovir, vidarabine, famciclovir, valacyclovir, ganciclovir, trifluridine and cidofovir), pyrophosphate analogues (foscarnet), interferon α and an oligonucleotide of 21 nucleotides in length (fomivirsen) (for reviews see [166–169]).

Herpes virus isolates, whether from patients or adapted to cell culture, are heterogeneous populations. Data from a study of the molecular evolution of HSV-1 showed that its evolution *in vivo* is slower than for RNA viruses, with an estimated rate of evolution of 3.5×10^{-8} substitutions per site per year [170]. Despite the relatively low level of replication errors found in these viruses, drug-resistance mutations appear in the absence of antiviral drugs [171]. A drug-resistant mutant frequency of approximately one in 1500 plaque-forming viruses has been determined for HSV-1 populations that have never been exposed to selective pressure [172–174], and this rate could be 9- to 16-fold higher in the case of HSV-2 [175]. Once the treatment begins, the proportion of pre-existing treatment-resistant viruses would increase as a result of Darwinian positive selection. Therefore, prolonged antiviral treatments, often required for clinical management of herpes virus infections in immuno-compromised patients, favor the emergence of drug-resistant strains ([176, 177] and reviewed in [178]).

Nucleoside analogues (Fig. 4) must be converted into their tri-phosphorylated form in order to be biologically active. For acyclovir, famciclovir, valacyclovir and ganciclovir, the first phosphate is added by viral thymidine kinase (TK) in HSV or VZV, or by UL97 phosphotransferase in the case of CMV [179, 180], to obtain the monophosphate form of the inhibitor. Further phosphorylations are mediated by cellular kinases. The active triphosphate forms of these nucleosides competitively inhibit viral DNA polymerase and act as chain terminators. In general, the acquisition of resistance to nucleoside analogues in HSV and VZV appears to be mediated by mutations in the *tk* gene, usually rendering truncated or inactivated proteins [181–184], or alternatively through mutations leading to decreased TK activity. Examples of resistance associated with alterations in the viral TK have been reported for acyclovir [176, 178, 185, 186], famciclovir [187] and ganciclovir [178, 188, 189]. In addition, acyclovir, penciclovir (the oral prodrug of famciclovir), and cidofovir resistance-associated mutations have been found in the viral DNA polymerase-coding region, albeit less frequently than in the *tk* gene (for a review see [190]). For example, approximately 95 % of the clinical isolates resistant to acyclovir are TK mutants rather than DNA polymerase mutants [191, 192]. Polymerase mutations involve amino acid substitutions that either diminish inhibitor binding or its incorporation into the growing DNA chain [193-196].

Foscarnet is a pyrophosphate analogue (Fig. 4) and therefore is a prototype of a different class of inhibitors. It has a broad spectrum, being active against many DNA polymerases, including the ones from HSV-1 and -2, VZV, CMV, EBV, and HHV-6, apart from being also an inhibitor of HIV-1 RT and the hepatitis B virus DNA polymerase [197]. Foscarnet does not require intracellular metabolism for activation [198]. It is a non-competitive (or mixed-type) inhibitor that is not incorporated into the growing DNA [199]. It binds to the polymerase pyrophosphate-binding site blocking the pyrophosphate exchange during the catalytic cycle. As expected, the resistant phenotype has been related exclusively to mutations at the DNA polymerase level [178, 199, 200]. Foscarnet-resistant strains may remain susceptible to acyclovir and

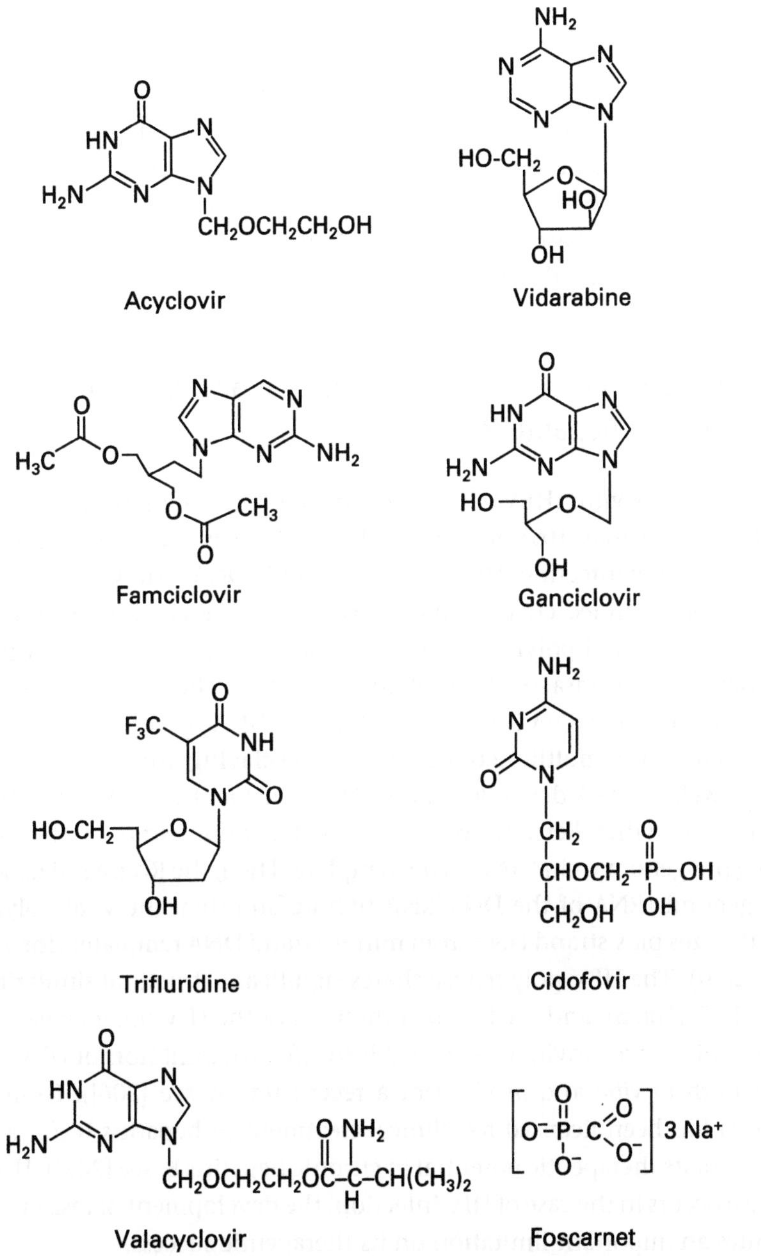

Fig. 4
Structural formulae of antiviral drugs targeting herpes virus replication.

ganciclovir [178], although dually resistant clinical isolates have been described [201].

There are other drugs in clinical development, such as herpes virus PR inhibitors (for a review see [202]) or compounds interfering with encapsidation [203], among others. Although development of resistance will probably be unavoidable, these new drugs will certainly be needed to design new alternative treatments based on drug combinations, and to inhibit strains resistant to acyclovir or other nucleoside drugs widely used in the clinical setting.

8.2 Inhibitors of reverse transcription as antiviral drugs for chronic hepatitis B

The hepatitis B virus (HBV) chronically infects 350 million people worldwide, and approximately 10% of these carriers will die as a direct consequence of persistent viral infection. HBV is a hepatotropic DNA virus with a 3.2-kb partial double-stranded circular genome with four overlapping reading frames encoding the viral polymerase, capsid, and surface proteins and a putative transcriptional transactivator protein termed "X". The HBV polymerase converts pre-genomic RNA into double-stranded DNA by reverse transcription. The viral RT is a multifunctional enzyme displaying protein priming activity, as well as DNA-dependent and RNA-dependent DNA polymerase, and RNase H activities. Retro-transcription involves minus-strand DNA synthesis using pre-genomic viral RNA as the template. Then, the RNase H degrades the pre-genomic RNA of the DNA/RNA hybrid, and then the viral polymerase synthesizes plus-strand DNA from minus-strand DNA templates (for a review see [204]). The HBV polymerase shares significant structural similarity with HIV-1 RT (Fig. 5), and nucleoside inhibitors of the HIV polymerase, such as lamivudine or adefovir, have turned into effective inhibitors of HBV replication both *in vitro* and *in vivo* (for a recent review see [206]). Lamivudine (Fig. 1) has been licensed for clinical treatment of hepatitis B (for a recent review of its therapeutic potential in chronic hepatitis B, see [207]). However, as also occurs in the case of HIV infection, the development of resistance constitutes an important limitation on its therapeutic success.

Resistance to lamivudine usually develops after 6 months of treatment and is associated with mutations in the highly conserved motif YMDD (Fig. 5). As in the case of HIV-1, the methionine residue found in this motif

Motif A

```
        423                 443
HBV      SNLSWLSLDVSAAFYHIPLHP
HIV-1    KKKSVTVLDVGDAYFSVPLDE
        102                 122
```

Motif B

```
        511                       537
HBV      VLGFRKIPMGVGLSPFLLAQFTSAICS
HIV-1    RYQYNVLPQGWKGSPAIFQSSMTKILE
        143                       169
```

Motif C

```
        547           561
HBV      LAFSYMDDVVLGAKS
HIV-1    VIYQYMDDLYVGSDL
        179           193
```

Motif D

```
        576           590
HBV      LLSLGIHLNPNKTKR
HIV-1    LLRWGLTTPDKKHQK
        209           223
```

Motif E

```
        592             608
HBV      GYSLNFMGYIIGSWGTL
HIV-1    EPPFLWMGYELHPDKWT
        224             240
```

Fig. 5
Alignments of conserved motifs within HBV polymerase and HIV-1 RT. Conserved residues are boxed. Sequences were taken from EMBL/GenBank accession files J02205 (HBV subtype adw2) and M15654 (isolate BH10), and the alignments were based on those given by Poch et al. [205].

is replaced by valine (M552V) or isoleucine (M552I) in lamivudine-resistant clinical isolates [208–211]. The resistance levels shown by isolates carrying the substitution M552I were significantly higher than those observed when the mutation M552V was present [209]. As in the case of HIV-1, the M552V polymerase variant showed reduced ability to synthesize viral DNA, indicating that the viral fitness would be compromised in the lamivudine-resistant mutants [212]. The M552V mutation is found *in vivo* always associated with an additional mutation, L528M, which is located in the conserved region B of HBV polymerase and HIV-1 RT. It has been shown that L528M in combination with M552V confers high-level resistance to lamivudine, although L528M alone has only a moderate impact on resistance [209]. The acquisition of lamivudine resistance appears to be associated with loss of viral fitness [213, 214]. In agreement with this proposal, it has been shown that in patients failing therapy (which occurred after 8 months of the initiation of lamivudine monotherapy), the resistant virus was quickly substituted by the wild-type HBV species after lamivudine withdrawal [215]. However, in some of these patients viral resistance reappeared sooner than with the initial course of treatment [215], suggesting that the resistant virus would persist, either inaccessible to the inhibitor or in the form of minority components of the viral quasi-species, constituting a sort of "molecular memory" ([41]; see also Section 1), that would result in a more efficient response to a selective constraint, such as the introduction of a previously administered drug.

No crystal structure is available for the HBV RT. However, amino acid sequence alignments indicate that the lamivudine-resistance mutations in HBV polymerase are the same as those observed in HIV-1 RT (i.e., M184V or M184I). In HIV-1 RT, the equivalent position of Leu-528 is occupied by Phe-160. This residue is highly conserved in HIV isolates, and non-conservative substitutions at this position lead to the loss of polymerase activity [216]. Phe-160 interacts with Tyr-115, and close to Met-184 [217]. If we assume a similar conformation at the nucleotide binding site of HBV polymerase, Phe-436, Leu-528, and Met-552 would be forming a cluster below the sugar moiety of the incoming nucleotide that would be critical for dNTP binding. Single mutants, such as M552I or M552V, and the double mutant L528M/M552V have shown to confer low-level or no resistance to other nucleoside inhibitors, such as lobucavir or adefovir [218, 219], which are under development to treat HBV infection. On the other hand, resistance to famciclovir (the oral form of penciclovir; Fig. 3) is acquired through the amino acid substitution L528M, in addition to other mutations whose relevance for drug resistance is still under investigation ([220–222] and references therein).

Mutations in the catalytic domain of the polymerase can also affect the amino acid sequence of the envelope protein (HBsAg) and *vice versa*. In particular, the genetic sequence for the neutralization domain of HBV known as the a determinant, which is located between residues 99 and 169 of HBsAg, overlaps with the major catalytic regions A and B of the polymerase. Although substitutions at motif C are likely to occur in the HbsAg region which is embedded in the lipid envelope [209], the lamivudine- and famciclovir-resistance mutation L528M is a potential neutralization escape mutant (for reviews see [223, 224]).

The estimated rate of evolution for HBV is approximately $< 2 \times 10^{-4}$ base substitutions/site/year [225], which is one to two orders of magnitude lower than the rate of evolution calculated for the positive- and negative-strand RNA viruses, including HIV. However, its half-life (24 h), the total daily production of virus (10^{11} virions), and its high viral load (2×10^{11}), together with the rate of cell death, with a half-life of infected hepatocytes of 10–100 days and a daily turnover of infected hepatocytes of 1–7%, reflect a highly dynamic process with a large production of the virus [226]. This situation parallels what we observed in the case of HIV infection, and suggests that many lessons learnt from drug-resistance management in HIV should also apply to HBV infection. However, emergence of resistance to lamivudine in HBV infection is slower and rarer than in HIV infection. The 10- to 100-day life of HBV-producing cells suggests that the generation time is 5 to 50 times longer in HBV than in HIV, and this could explain the slower adaptive response [227]. In the HIV field it is clear that therapeutic success implies prolonged effective therapy in order to achieve complete suppression of viral replication and, therefore, avoid the emergence of drug resistance. In order to improve the results of lamivudine monotherapy, studies on long-term therapy of combinations of lamivudine with interferon α or with other nucleoside analogues are certainly warranted.

9 Future directions: multiple-target antiviral therapy

Even though drug resistance seems inevitable, the development of new antiviral drugs fighting a resistant virus, as well as exploiting new targets, appears to be important to design more successful combination therapies, or to introduce treatments that would cope successfully with the genetic variation found in many viruses. For example, in the case of HIV-1, promising new drugs targeting viral entry or fusion and integration are in preclinical or clinical trials (for recent reviews see [228, 229]). The use of additional inhibitors could prolong suppression of viral replication, and should aim at treatments with diminished side-effects as compared with the combination therapies presently available.

One possibility for antiviral intervention that exploits the intrinsic nature of the viral quasi-species is the use of mutagens to increase viral mutation frequency. The mutation rate of many RNA viruses may approach the error threshold for viral population viability. Classical studies showed that chemical mutagenesis can cause a significant increase in mutation frequency in RNA viruses [230]. It has also been reported that chemical mutagenesis or X-ray irradiation of polio-virus-VSV-infected cells yielded a two-fold increase in viral mutation frequency together with a much larger decrease in viral replicative capacity [231]. More recently, Loeb and colleagues [232] showed that the sequential passage of HIV in cells grown in the presence of a mutagenic nucleoside (5-hydroxydeoxycytidine) resulted in the loss of viral replication. Viral extinction with a concomitant increase in the mutation frequency has been also reported for foot-and-mouth disease virus and polio virus, using 5-fluorouracil and ribavirin, respectively, as mutagenic nucleosides [233, 234]. Although the emergence of drug resistance could also be the Achilles's heel for therapies based on lethal mutagenesis, resistance to mutagenic analogues seems less likely to occur. Thus, the number of mutations required for drug resistance is expected to be relatively small in comparison with the number of nucleotide changes that would cause lethality, and in addition, it is unlikely that an immediate selective advantage for resistance to mutagenic nucleotides would arise, since the situation is different from what occurs with chain terminators, where resistance mutations afford an immediate selective growth advantage. Extinction (or lethal) mutagenesis appears as a promising new antiviral strategy, and research to develop this new approach is currently under way in several laboratories.

Acknowledgements

We thank José María Galán for help with the preparation of the figures. Support from the Commission for Cultural, Educational and Scientific Exchange between the United States of America and Spain (grant no. 99162), grants DGES PM 97-0060-C02-01, CAM no. 08.2/0046/2000, and an institutional grant of Fundación Ramón Areces are also acknowledged.

References

1 E. Domingo: Prog. Drug Res. *33*, 93 (1989).
2 E. Domingo, L. Menéndez-Arias, M.E. Quiñónez-Mateu, A. Holguín, M. Gutiérrez-Rivas, M.A. Martínez, J. Quer, I.S. Novella and J.J. Holland: Prog. Drug Res. *48*, 99 (1997).
3 I. Nájera, A. Holguín, M.E. Quiñónez-Mateu, M.A. Muñoz-Fernández, R. Nájera, C. López-Galíndez and E. Domingo: J. Virol. *69*, 23 (1995).
4 W.J. Lech, G. Wang, Y.L. Yang, Y. Chee, K. Dorman, D. McCrae, L.C. Lazzeroni, J.W. Erickson, J.S. Sinsheimer and A.H. Kaplan: J. Virol. *70*, 2038 (1996).
5 D.V. Havlir, S. Eastman, A. Gamst and D.D. Richman: J. Virol. *70*, 7894 (1996).
6 M.E. Quiñones-Mateu, A. Mas, T. Lain de Lera, V. Soriano, J. Alcamí, M.M. Lederman and E. Domingo: Virus Res. *57*, 11 (1998).
7 A. Weiner, A.L. Erickson, J. Kansopon, K. Crawford, E. Muchmore, A.L. Hughes, M. Houghton and C.M. Walker: Proc. Natl. Acad. Sci. USA *92*, 2755 (1995).
8 A.J. McMichael and R.E. Phillips: Annu. Rev. Immunol. *15*, 271 (1997).
9 P. Borrow and G.M. Shaw: Immunol. Rev. *164*, 37 (1998).
10 X. Forns, R.H. Purcell and J. Bukh: Trends in Microbiol. *7*, 402 (1999).
11 D.T. Evans, D.H. O'Connor, P. Jing, J.L. Dzuris, J. Sidney, J. da Silva, T.M. Allen, H. Horton, J.E. Venham, R.A. Rudersdorf et al.: Nat. Med. *5*, 1270 (1999).
12 A. Ciurea, P. Klenerman, L. Hunziker, E. Horvath, B.M. Senn, A.F. Ochsenbein, H. Hengartner and R.M. Zinkernagel: Proc. Natl. Acad. Sci. USA *97*, 2749 (2000).
13 R. Sousa: Trends Biochem. Sci. *21*, 186 (1996).
14 D.A. Steinhauer, E. Domingo and J. J. Holland: Gene *122*, 281 (1992).
15 J.W. Drake and J.J. Holland: Proc. Natl. Acad. Sci. USA *96*, 13910 (1999).
16 F. Gebauer, J.C. de la Torre, I. Gomes, M.G. Mateu, H. Barahona, B. Tiraboschi, I. Bergmann, P.A. de Mello and E. Domingo: J. Virol. *62*, 2041 (1988).
17 A. Arias, E. Lázaro, C. Escarmís and E. Domingo: J. Gen. Virol. *82*, 1049 (2001).
18 E. Domingo, C. Biebricher, M. Eigen and J.J. Holland: *Quasispecies and RNA virus evolution. Principles and consequences*, Landes Bioscience, Georgetown, Texas, USA 2001.
19 N. Sakamoto, N. Enomoto, H. Kurosaki, F. Marumo and C. Sato: J. Hepatol. *20*, 593 (1994).
20 J.W. Mellors, C.W. Rinaldo, Jr., P. Gupta, R.M. White, J.A. Todd and L.A. Kingsley: Science *272*, 1167 (1996).
21 D.D. Ho, A.U. Neumann, A.S. Perelson, W. Chen, J.M. Leonard and M. Markowitz: Nature 373, 123 (1995).

22 X. Wei, S.K. Ghosh, M.E. Taylor, V.A. Johnson, E.A. Emini, P. Deutsch, J.D. Lifson, S. Bonhoeffer, M.A. Nowak, B.H. Hahn et al.: Nature *373*: 117 (1995).
23 A.S. Perelson, A.U. Neumann, M. Markowitz, J.M. Leonard and D.D. Ho: Science *271*, 1582 (1996).
24 B.A. Larder, G. Darby and D.D. Richman: Science *243*, 1731 (1989).
25 J.H. Condra, W.A. Schleif, O.M. Blahy, L.J. Gabryelski, D.J. Graham, J.C. Quintero, A. Rhodes, H.L. Robbins, E. Roth, M. Shivaprakash et al.: Nature *374*, 569 (1995).
26 A.S. Perelson, P. Essunger, Y. Cao, M. Vesanen, A. Hurley, K. Saksela, M. Markowitz and D.D. Ho: Nature *387*, 188 (1997).
27 R.M. Gulick, J.W. Mellors, D. Havlir, J.J. Eron, C. Gonzalez, D. McMahon, D.D. Richman, F.T. Valentine, L. Jonas, A. Meibohm et al.: N. Engl. J. Med. *337*, 734 (1997).
28 S.M. Hammer, K.E. Squires, M.D. Hughes, J.M. Grimes, L.M. Demeter, J.S. Currier, J.J. Eron, Jr., J.E. Feinberg, H.H. Balfour, Jr., L.R. Deyton et al.: N. Engl. J. Med. *337*, 725 (1997).
29 E.A. Duarte, I.S. Novella, S.C. Weaver, E. Domingo, S. Wain-Hobson, D.K. Clarke, A. Moya, S.F. Elena, J.C. de la Torre and J.J. Holland: Infect. Agents Dis. *3*, 201 (1994).
30 I.S. Novella, E. Domingo and J.J. Holland: Mol. Med. Today 1, 248 (1995).
31 G. Weidt, W. Deppert, O. Utermohlen, J. Heukeshoven and F. Lehmann-Grube: J. Virol. *69*, 7147 (1995).
32 O. Taboga, C. Tami, E. Carrillo, J.I. Núñez, A. Rodríguez, J.C. Saíz, E. Blanco, M.L. Valero, X. Roig, J.A. Camarero et al.: J. Virol. *71*, 2606 (1997).
33 P.I. Marcus, L.L. Rodríguez and M.J. Sekellick: J. Virol. *72*, 542 (1998).
34 K. Morimoto, D.C. Hooper, H. Carbaugh, Z.F. Fu, H. Koprowski and B. Dietzschold: Proc. Natl. Acad. Sci. USA *95*, 3152 (1998).
35 Z. Chen, K. Li, R.R. Rowland, G.W. Anderson and P.G. Plagemann: J. Neurovirol. *4*, 560 (1998).
36 E.C. Hsu, F. Sarangi, C. Iorio, M.S. Sidhu, S.A. Udem, D.L. Dillehay, W. Xu, P.A. Rota, W.J. Bellini and C.D. Richardson: J. Virol. *72*, 2905 (1998).
37 C.L. Rowe, S.C. Baker, M.J. Nathan and J.O. Fleming: J. Virol. *71*, 2959 (1997).
38 P. Farci, A. Shimoda, A. Coiana, G. Diaz, G. Peddis, J.C. Melpolder, A. Strazzera, D.Y. Chien, S.J. Munoz, A. Balestrieri et al.: Science *288*, 339 (2000).
39 J.M. Pawlotsky, G. Germanidis, A.U. Neumann, M. Pellerin, P.O. Frainais and D. Dhumeaux: J. Virol. *72*, 2795 (1998).
40 J.M. Pawlotsky: Hepatology *32*, 889 (2000).
41 C.M. Ruiz-Jarabo, A. Arias, E. Baranowski, C. Escarmís and E. Domingo: J. Virol. *74*, 3543 (2000).
42 E. Domingo: Virology *270*, 251 (2000).
43 S.A. Frank, in: M.R. Rose and G.V. Landes: *Adaptation*, Academic Press, San Diego, California, USA 1996, 451.
44 M. Gell-Mann, in: G.A. Cowan, D. Pines and D. Meltzer (eds.): *Complexity metaphors, models and reality*, Addison-Wesley Publishing Co., Reading, Mass., USA 1994, 17.
45 B.D. Preston, B.J. Poiesz and L.A. Loeb: Science *242*, 1168 (1988).
46 J.D. Roberts, K. Bebenek and T.A. Kunkel: Science *242*, 1171 (1988).
47 V.K. Pathak and H.M. Temin: Proc. Natl. Acad. Sci USA *87*, 6019 (1990).
48 L. Mansky and H.M. Temin: J. Virol. *69*, 5087 (1995).
49 A.F. Labrijn and P.W.H.I. Parren, in: B. Korber, C. Brander, B. Haynes, J. Moore, R. Koup,

B. Walker and D. Watkins (eds.): *HIV Molecular Immunology Database*, part IV, Los Alamos National Laboratory, Los Alamos, New Mexico, USA 1999, 18.
50 L. Wu, N.P. Gerard, R. Wyatt, H. Choe, C. Parolin, N. Ruffing, A. Borsetti, A.A. Cardoso, E. Desjardin, W. Newman et al.: Nature *384*, 179 (1996).
51 A. Trkola, T. Dragic, J. Arthos, J.M. Binley, W.C. Olson, G.P. Allaway, C. Cheng-Mayer, J. Robinson, P.J. Maddon and J.P. Moore: Nature *384*, 184 (1996).
52 C.M. Hill, H. Deng, D. Unutmaz, V.N. Kewal-Ramani, L. Bastiani, M.K. Gorny, S. Zolla-Pazner and D.R. Littman: J. Virol. *71*, 6296 (1997).
53 J.P. Moore, Y. Cao, D.D. Ho and R.A. Koup: J. Virol. *68*, 5142 (1994).
54 C. Moog, H.J.A. Fleury, I. Pellegrin, A. Kirn and A.M. Aubertin: J. Virol. *71*, 3734 (1997).
55 J. Lewis, P. Balfe, C. Arnold, S. Kaye, R.S. Tedder and J.A. McKeating: J. Virol. *72*, 8943 (1998).
56 Y. Cao, L. Qin, L. Zhang, J.T. Safrit and D.D. Ho: N. Engl. J. Med. *332*, 201 (1995).
57 G. Pantaleo, S. Menzo, M. Vaccarezza, C. Graziosi, O.J. Cohen, J.F. Demarest, D. Montefiori, J.M. Orenstein, C. Fox, L.K. Schrager et al.: N. Engl. J. Med. *332*, 209 (1995).
58 D. Cecilia, C.A. Kleeberger, A. Munoz, J.V. Giorgi and S. Zolla-Pazner: J. Infect. Dis. *176*, 1365 (1999).
59 M.L. Tsang, L.A. Evans, P. McQueen, L. Hurren, C. Byrne, R. Penny, B. Tindall and D.A. Cooper: J. Infect. Dis. *170*, 1141 (1994).
60 T.C. VanCott, V.R. Polonis, L.D. Loomis, N.L. Michael, P.L. Nara and D.L. Birx: AIDS Res. Human Retrovir. *11*, 1379 (1995).
61 J.R. Mascola, S.W. Snyder, O.S. Weislow, S.M. Belay, R.B. Belshe, D.H. Schwartz, M.L. Clements, R. Dolin, B.S. Graham, G.J. Gorse et al: J. Infect. Dis. *173*, 340 (1996).
62 C. Spenlehauer, S. Saragosti, H.J. Fleury, A. Kirn, A.M. Aubertin and C. Moog: J. Virol. *72*, 9855 (1998).
63 T. Beaumont, A. van Nuenen, S. Broersen, W.A. Blattner, V.V. Lukashov and H. Schuitemaker: J. Virol. *75*, 2246 (2001).
64 A. McMichael: Cell *93*, 673 (1998).
65 S. Koenig, A.J. Conley, Y.A. Brewah, G.M. Jones, S. Leath, L.J. Boots, V. Davey, G. Pantaleo, J.F. Demarest, C. Carter et al.: Nat. Med. *1*, 330 (1995).
66 P. Borrow, H. Lewicki, X. Wei, M.S. Horwitz, N. Peffer, H. Meyers, J.A. Nelson, J.E. Gairin, B.H. Hahn, M.B.A. Oldstone et al.: Nat. Med. *3*, 205 (1997).
67 D.A. Price, P.J.R. Goulder, P. Klenerman, A.K. Sewell, P.J. Easterbrook, M. Troop, C.R.M. Bangham and R.E. Phillips: Proc. Natl. Acad. Sci. USA *94*, 1890 (1997).
68 P.J.R. Goulder, R.E. Phillips, R.A. Colbert, S. McAdam, G. Ogg, M.A. Nowak, P. Giangrande, G. Luzzi, B. Morgan, A. Edwards et al.: Nat. Med. *3*, 212 (1997).
69 T.M. Allen, D.H. O'Connor, P. Jing, J.L. Dzuris, B.R. Mothé, T.U. Vogel, E. Dunphy, M.E. Liebl, C. Emerson, N. Wilson et al.: Nature *407*, 386 (2000).
70 H. Mitsuya, K.J. Weinhold, P.A. Furman, M.H. St.Clair, S.N. Lehrman, R.C. Gallo, D. Bolognesi, D.W. Barry and S. Broder: Proc. Natl. Acad. Sci. USA *82*, 7096 (1985).
71 D. Finzi and R.F. Siliciano: Cell *93*, 665 (1998).
72 B. Young and D.R. Kuritzkes: AIDS *13* (suppl. 1), S11 (1999).
73 J.K. Wong, H.F. Günthard, D.V. Havlir, Z.-Q. Zhang, A.T. Haase, C.C. Ignacio, S. Kwok, E. Emini and D.D. Richman: Proc. Natl. Acad. Sci. USA *94*, 12574 (1997).
74 W. Cavert, D.W. Notermans, K. Staskus, S.W. Wietgrefe, M. Zupancic, K. Gebhard, K. Henry, S.-C. Zhang, R. Mills, H. McDade et al.: Science *276*, 960 (1997).

75 T.-W. Chun, D. Finzi, J. Margolick, K. Chadwick, D. Schwartz and R.F. Siliciano: Nat. Med. *1*, 1284 (1995).

76 T.-W. Chun, L. Carruth, D. Finzi, X. Shen, J.A. Digiuseppe, H. Taylor, M. Hermankova, K. Chadwick, J. Margolick, T.C. Quinn et al.: Nature *387*, 183 (1997).

77 T.-W. Chun, L. Stuyver, S.B. Mizell, L.A. Ehler, J.M. Mican, M. Baseler, A.L. Lloyd, M.A. Nowak and A.S. Fauci: Proc. Natl. Acad. Sci. USA *94*, 13193 (1997).

78 J.K. Wong, M. Hezareh, H.F. Günthard, D.V. Havlir, C.C. Ignacio, C.A. Spina and D.D. Richman: Science *278*, 1291 (1997).

79 D. Finzi, M. Hermankova, T. Pierson, L.M. Carruth, C. Buck, R.E. Chaisson, T.C. Quinn, K. Chadwick, J. Margolick, R. Brookmeyer et al.: Science *278*, 1295 (1997).

80 C.A. Michie, A. McLean, C. Alcock and P.C. Beverley: Nature *360*, 264 (1992).

81 T.-W. Chun, R.T. Davey, Jr., M. Ostrowski, J.S. Justement, D. Engel, J.I. Mullins and A.S. Fauci: Nat. Med. *6*, 757 (2000).

82 L. Zhang, B. Ramratnam, K. Tenner-Racz, Y. He, M. Vesanen, S. Lewin, A. Talal, P. Racz, A.S. Perelson, B.T. Korber et al.: New Engl. J. Med. *340*, 1605 (1999).

83 W.S. Hlavacek, N.I. Stilianakis, D.W. Notermans, S.A. Danner and A.S. Perelson: Proc. Natl. Acad. Sci. USA *97*, 10966 (2000).

84 L.K. Schrager and M.P. D'Souza: J. Amer. Med. Assoc. *280*, 67 (1998).

85 W. Cavert and A.T. Haase: Science *280*, 1865 (1998).

86 L. Menéndez-Arias and E. Domingo, in: B. Clotet, L. Menéndez-Arias, L. Ruiz, C. Tural, A. Vandamme, D. Burger, J. Schapiro, C. Boucher, R. D'Aquila and D. Richman (eds.): *Guide to Management of HIV Drug Resistance and Pharmacokinetics of Drug Therapy*, Taisa, Barcelona, Spain 2000, 31.

87 L. Menéndez-Arias and E. Domingo, in: B. Clotet, L. Menéndez-Arias, L. Ruiz, C. Tural, A. Vandamme, D. Burger, J. Schapiro, C. Boucher, R. D'Aquila and D. Richman (eds.): *Guide to Management of HIV Drug Resistance and Pharmacokinetics of Drug Therapy*, Taisa, Barcelona, Spain 2000, 55.

88 J. Hammond, C. Calef, B. Larder, R. Schinazi and J.W. Mellors, in: C.L. Kuiken, B. Foley, B. Hahn, B. Korber, F. McCutchan, P.A. Marx, J. Mellors, J.I. Mullins, J. Sodroski and S. Wolinsky (eds.): *Human Retroviruses and AIDS 1999: A compilation and analysis of nucleic acid and amino acid sequences*, Theoretical Biology and Biophysics Group, Los Alamos National Laboratory, Los Alamos, New Mexico, USA 1999, 542.

89 R.F. Schinazi, B.A. Larder and J.W. Mellors: Int. Antivir. News *8*, 65 (2000).

90 R. Schuurman, M. Nijhuis, R. van-Leeuwen, P. Schipper, D. de Jong, P. Collis, S.A. Danner, J. Mulder, C. Loveday and C. Christopherson: J. Infect. Dis. *171*, 1411 (1995).

91 R.M. Ribeiro and S. Bonhoeffer: Proc. Natl. Acad. Sci. USA *97*, 7681 (2000).

92 E. Domingo and J.J. Holland: Annu. Rev. Microbiol. *51*, 151 (1997).

93 E. Domingo, C. Escarmís, L. Menéndez-Arias and J.J. Holland, in: E. Domingo, R. Webster and J.J. Holland (eds.): *Origin and Evolution of Viruses*, Academic Press, San Diego, California, USA 1999, 141.

94 N.K.T. Back, M. Nijhuis, W. Keulen, C.A.B. Boucher, B.B. Oude Essink, A.B.P. van Kuilenburg, A.H. van Gennip and B. Berkhout: EMBO J. *15*, 4040 (1996).

95 W. Keulen, N.K.T. Back, A. van Wijk, C.A.B. Boucher and B. Berkhout: J. Virol. *71*, 3346 (1997).

96 M.D. Miller, K.E. Anton, A.S. Mulato, P.D. Lamy and J.M. Cherrington: J. Infect. Dis. *179*, 92 (1999).

97 K. Yoshimura, R. Feldman, E. Kodama, M.F. Kavlick, Y.-L. Qiu, J. Zemlicka and H. Mitsuya: Antimicrob. Agents Chemother. *43*, 2479 (1999).

98 P.R. Harrigan, C. Stone, P. Griffin, I. Nájera, S. Bloor, S. Kemp, M. Tisdale, B. Larder and the CNA2001 Investigative Group: J. Infect. Dis. *181*, 912 (2000).

99 R.W. Shafer, M.A. Winters, A.K.N. Iversen and T.C. Merigan: Antimicrob. Agents Chemother. *40*, 2887 (1996).

100 S.D.W. Frost, M. Nijhuis, R. Schuurman, C.A.B. Boucher and A.J. Leigh Brown: J. Virol. *74*, 6262 (2000).

101 P.R. Harrigan, S. Bloor and B.A. Larder: J. Virol. *72*, 3773 (1998).

102 B.A. Larder and S.D. Kemp: Science *246*, 1155 (1989).

103 P. Kellam, C.A. Boucher and B.A. Larder: Proc. Natl. Acad. Sci. USA *89*, 1934 (1992).

104 J. Goudsmit, A. de Ronde, E. de Rooij and R. de Boer: J. Virol. *71*, 4479 (1997).

105 A. de Ronde, M. van Dooren, L. van der Hoek, D. Bouwhuis, E. de Rooij, B. van Gemen, R. de Boer and J. Goudsmit: J. Virol. *75*, 595 (2001).

106 T. Shirasaka, M.F. Kavlick, T. Ueno, W.-Y. Gao, E. Kojima, M.L. Alcaide, S. Chokekijchai, B.M. Roy, E. Arnold, R. Yarchoan et al.: Proc. Natl. Acad. Sci. USA *92*, 2398 (1995).

107 A.K.N. Iversen, R.W. Shafer, K. Wehrly, M.A. Winters, J.I. Mullins, B. Chesebro and T.C. Merigan: J. Virol. *70*, 1086 (1996).

108 Y. Maeda, D.J. Venzon and H. Mitsuya: J. Infect. Dis. *177*, 1207 (1998).

109 P. Kosalaraksa, M.F. Kavlick, V. Maroun, R. Le and H. Mitsuya: J. Virol. *73*, 5356 (1999).

110 R.W. Shafer, A.K. Iversen, M.A. Winters, E. Aguiniga, D.A. Katzenstein and T.C. Merigan: J. Infect. Dis. *172*, 70 (1995).

111 M.F. Kavlick, K. Wyvill, R. Yarchoan and H. Mitsuya: J. Infect. Dis. *98*, 1506 (1998).

112 J.-C. Schmit, K. van Laethem, L. Ruiz, P. Hermans, S. Sprecher, A. Sonnerborg, M. Leal, T. Harrer, B. Clotet, V. Arendt et al.: AIDS *12*, 2007 (1998).

113 J.G. García-Lerma, P.J. Gerrish, A.C. Wright, S.H. Qari and W. Heneine: J. Virol. *74*, 9339 (2000).

114 A. De Antoni, A. Foli, J. Lisziewicz and F. Lori: J. Infect. Dis. *176*, 899 (1997).

115 C. Tamalet, J. Izopet, N. Koch, J. Fantini and N. Yahi: AIDS *12*, F161 (1998).

116 M.A. Winters, K.L. Coolley, Y.A. Girard, D.J. Levee, H. Hamdan, R.W. Shafer, D.A. Katzenstein and T.C. Merigan: J. Clin. Invest. *102*, 1769 (1998).

117 J.J. de Jong, J. Goudsmit, V.V. Lukashov, M.E. Hillebrand, E. Baan, R. Huismans, S.A. Danner, J.H. ten Veen, F. de Wolf and S. Jurriaans: AIDS *13*, 75 (1999).

118 B.A. Larder, S. Bloor, S.D. Kemp, K. Hertogs, R.L. Desmet, V. Miller, M. Sturmer, S. Staszewski, J. Ren, D.K. Stammers et al.: Antimicrob. Agents Chemother. *43*, 1961 (1999).

119 C. Briones, A. Mas, G. Gómez-Mariano, C. Altisent, L. Menéndez-Arias, V. Soriano and E. Domingo: Virus Res. *66*, 13 (2000).

120 C. Tamalet, N. Yahi, C. Tourrès, P. Colson, A.-M. Quinson, I. Poizot-Martin, C. Dhiver and J. Fantini: Virology *270*, 310 (2000).

121 A. Mas, M. Parera, C. Briones, V. Soriano, M.A. Martínez, E. Domingo and L. Menéndez-Arias: EMBO J. *19*, 5752 (2000).

122 K. van Vaerenbergh, K. van Laethem, J. Albert, C.A.B. Boucher, B. Clotet, M. Floridia, J. Gerstoft, B. Hejdeman, C. Nielsen, C. Pannecouque et al.: Antimicrob. Agents Chemother. 44, 2109 (2000).

123 M.A. Winters, K.L. Coolley, P. Cheng, Y.A. Girard, H. Hamdan, L.C. Kovari and T.C. Merigan: J. Virol. *74*, 10707 (2000).

124 T. Imamichi, T. Sinha, H. Imamichi, Y.-M. Zhang, J.A. Metcalf, J. Falloon and H.C. Lane: J. Virol. *74*, 1023 (2000).
125 T. Imamichi, S.C. Berg, H. Imamichi, J.C. López, J.A. Metcalf, J. Falloon and H.C. Lane: J. Virol. *74*, 10958 (2000).
126 T. Imamichi, M.A. Murphy, H. Imamichi and H.C. Lane: J. Virol. *75*, 3988 (2001).
127 Z. Chen, Y. Li, H.B. Schock, D. Hall, E. Chen and L.C. Kuo: J. Biol. Chem. *270*, 21433 (1995).
128 H.B. Schock, V.M. Garsky and L.C. Kuo: J. Biol. Chem. *271*, 31957 (1996).
129 H. Jacobsen, K. Yasargil, D.L. Winslow, J.C. Craig, A. Kröhn, I.B. Duncan and J. Mous: Virology *206*, 527 (1995).
130 K.E. Potts, M.L. Smidt, S.P. Tucker, T.R. Stiebel, Jr., J.J. McDonald, W.C. Stallings and M.L. Bryant: Antivir. Chem. Chemother. *8*, 447 (1997).
131 P.S. Eastman, J. Mittler, R. Kelso, C. Gee, E. Boyer, J. Kolberg, M. Urdea, J.M. Leonard, D.W. Norbeck, H. Mo et al.: J. Virol. *72*, 5154 (1998).
132 J. Martínez-Picado, A.V. Savara, L. Sutton and R.T. D'Aquila: J. Virol. *73*, 3744 (1999).
133 M. Nijhuis, R. Schuurman, D. de Jong, J. Erickson, E. Gustchina, J. Albert, P. Schipper, S. Gulnik and C.A.B. Boucher: AIDS *13*, 2349 (1999).
134 J. Martínez-Picado, A.V. Savara, L. Shi, L. Sutton and R.T. D'Aquila: Virology *275*, 318 (2000).
135 Y.M. Zhang, H. Imamichi, T. Imamichi, H.C. Lane, J. Falloon, M.B. Vasudevachari and N.P. Salzman: J. Virol. *71*, 6662 (1997).
136 L. Doyon, G. Croteau, D. Thibeault, F. Poulin, L. Pilote and D. Lamarre: J. Virol. *70*, 3763 (1996).
137 L. Doyon, C. Payant, L. Brakier-Gingras and D. Lamarre: J. Virol. *72*, 6146 (1998).
138 L. Moutouh, J. Corbeil and D.D. Richman: Proc. Natl. Acad. Sci. USA *93*, 6106 (1996).
139 J.-C. Schmit, J. Cogniaux, P. Hermans, C. van Vaeck, S. Sprecher, B. van Remoortel, M. Witvrouw, J. Balzarini, J. Desmyter, E. de Clercq et al.: J. Infect. Dis. *174*, 962 (1996).
140 R. Webster, in: E. Domingo, R. Webster and J.J. Holland (eds.): *Origin and Evolution of Viruses*, Academic Press, San Diego, California, USA 1999, 377.
141 R.B. Couch: N Engl J Med *343*, 1778 (2000).
142 L.R. Forrest, A. Kukol, I.T. Arkin, D.P. Tieleman and M.S. Sansom: Biophys. J. *78*, 55 (2000).
143 D. Salom, B.R. Hill, J.D. Lear and W.F. DeGrado: Biochemistry *39*, 14160 (2000).
144 H. Masuda, H. Suzuki, H. Oshitani, R. Saito, S. Kawasaki, M. Nishikawa and H. Satoh: Microbiol. Immunol. *44*, 833 (2000).
145 D.M. Fleming: Lancet *353*, 668 (1999).
146 L.V. Gubareva, L. Kaiser and F.G. Hayden: Lancet *355*, 827 (2000).
147 T.J. Blick, A. Sahasrabudhe, M. McDonald, I.J. Owens, P.J. Morley, R.J. Fenton and J.L. McKimm-Breschkin: Virology *246*, 95 (1998).
148 J.M. Barnett, A. Cadman, F.M. Burrell, S.H. Madar, A.P. Lewis, M. Tisdale and R. Bethell: Virology *265*, 286 (1999).
149 C.A. Silagy: Lancet *353*, 669 (1999).
150 L. Carrasco: Pharmacol. Ther. *64*, 215 (1994).
151 M.A. McKinlay, D.C. Pevear and M.G. Rossmann: Annu. Rev. Microbiol. *46*, 635 (1992).
152 H.A. Rotbart: Antivir. Chem. Chemother. *11*, 261 (2000).
153 G.L. Kearns, S.M. Abdel-Rahman, L.P. James, D.L. Blowey, J.D. Marshall, T.G. Wells and R.F. Jacobs: Antimicrob. Agents Chemother. *43*, 634 (1999).

154 S.R. Yasin, W. Al-Nakib and D.A. Tyrrell: Antimicrob. Agents Chemother. *34*, 963 (1990).
155 D.C. Pevear, T.M. Tull, M.E. Seipel and J.M. Groarke: Antimicrob. Agents Chemother. *43*, 2109 (1999).
156 R.M. Friedman: J. Virol. *6*, 628 (1970).
157 T. Pfister and E. Wimmer: J. Biol. Chem. *274*, 6992 (1999).
158 J.L. Hansen, A.M. Long and S.C. Schultz: Structure *5*, 1109 (1997).
159 H. Ago, T. Adachi, A. Yoshida, M. Yamamoto, N. Habuka, K. Yatsunami and M. Miyano: Structure *7*, 1417 (1999).
160 S. Bressanelli, L. Tomei, A. Roussel, I. Incitti, R.L. Vitale, M. Mathieu, R. De Francesco and F.A. Rey : Proc. Natl. Acad. Sci. USA *96*, 13034 (1999).
161 C.A. Lesburg, M.B. Cable, E. Ferrari, Z. Hong, A.F. Mannarino and P.C. Weber: Nat. Struct. Biol. *6*, 937 (1999).
162 S.G. Baginski, D.C. Pevear, M. Seipel, S.C. Sun, C.A. Benetatos, S.K. Chunduru, C.M. Rice, and M.S. Collett: Proc. Natl. Acad. Sci. USA *97*, 7981 (2000).
163 J.I. Esteban, M. Martell, W.F. Carman and J. Gómez, in: E. Domingo, R. Webster and J.J. Holland (eds.): *Origin and Evolution of Viruses*, Academic Press, San Diego, California, USA 1999, 345.
164 M. Isnard, M. Granier, R. Frutos, B. Reynaud and M. Peterschmitt: J. Gen. Virol. *79*, 3091 (1998).
165 C.R. Parrish and U. Truyen, in: E. Domingo, R. Webster and J.J. Holland (eds.): *Origin and Evolution of Viruses*, Academic Press, San Diego, California, USA 1999, 421.
166 R. Snoeck, G. Andrei and E. De Clercq: Drugs *57*, 187 (1999).
167 R. Snoeck: Int. J. Antimicrob. Agents *16*, 157 (2000).
168 C. J. Harrison: Adv. Pediatrics *47*, 335 (2001).
169 T. J. Brown, M. Vander Straten and S. K. Tyring: Dermatol. Clin. *19*, 23 (2001).
170 H. Sakaoka, K. Kurita, Y. Iida, S. Takada, K. Umene, Y.T. Kim, C.S. Ren and A.J. Nahmias: J. Gen. Virol. *75*, 513 (1994).
171 J. D. Hall and R. E. Almy: Virology *116*, 535 (1982).
172 U. B. Dasgupta and W. C. Summers: Proc. Natl. Acad. Sci. USA *75*, 2378 (1978).
173 J. D. Hall, D. M. Coen, B. L. Fisher, M. Weisslitz, S. Randall, R. E. Almy, P. T. Gelep and P. A. Schaffer: Virology *132*, 26 (1984).
174 C.C. Hwang and H.H. Chen: Gene *152*, 191 (1995).
175 R.T. Sarisky, T.T. Nguyen, K.E. Duffy, R.J. Wittrock and J.J. Leary: Antimicrob. Agents Chemother. *44*, 1524 (2000).
176 G. Darby, H. J. Field and S. A. Salisbury: Nature *289*, 81 (1981).
177 H.H. Balfour, Jr., C. Benson, J. Braun, B. Cassens, A. Erice, A. Friedman-Kien, T. Klein, B. Polsky and S. Safrin: J. Acquir. Immune Defic. Syndr. *7*, 254 (1994).
178 P. Reusser : J Hosp. Infect. *33*, 235 (1996).
179 D.J. Tenney, G. Yamanaka, S.M. Voss, C.W. Cianci, A.V. Tuomari, A.K. Sheaffer, M. Alam and R.J. Colonno: Antimicrob. Agents Chemother. *41*, 2680 (1997).
180 C.L. Talarico, T.C. Burnette, W.H. Miller, S.L. Smith, M.G. Davis, S.C. Stanat, T.I. Ng, Z. He, D.M. Coen, B. Roizman et al.: Antimicrob. Agents Chemother. *43*, 1941 (1999).
181 R. T. Sarisky, M. R. Quail, P. E. Clark, T. T. Nguyen, W. S. Halsey, R. J. Wittrock, J. O. Bartus, M. M. Van Horn, G. M. Sathe, S. Van Horn et al.: J. Virol. *75*, 1761 (2001).
182 C. McLaren, M. S. Chen, I. Ghazzouli, R. Saral and W. H. Burns: Antimicrob. Agents Chemother. *28*, 740 (1985).
183 P. A. Chatis and C. S. Crumpacker: Virology *180*, 793 (1991).

184 E. L. Hill, G. A. Hunter and M. N. Ellis: Antimicrob. Agents Chemother. *35*, 2322 (1991).
185 C. L. Talarico, W. C. Phelps and K. K. Biron: J. Virol. *67*, 1024 (1993).
186 G. Boivin, C. K. Edelman, L. Pedneault, C. L. Talarico, K. K. Biron and H. H. Balfour: J. Infect. Dis. *170*, 68 (1994).
187 M. R. Boyd, S. Safrin and E. R. Kern: Antivir. Chem. Chemother. *4*, 3 (1993).
188 A. Erice, S. Chou, K. K. Biron, S. C. Stanat, H. H. Balfour and M. C. Jordan : N. Engl. J. Med. *320*, 4139 (1989).
189 A. P. Limaye, L. Corey, D. M. Koelle, C. L. Davis and M. Boeckh: Lancet *356*, 645 (2000).
190 D.M. Coen: Antivir. Res. *15*, 287 (1991).
191 J.C. Pottage and H.A. Kessler: Infect. Agents Dis. *4*, 115 (1995).
192 J. Christophers, J. Clayton, J. Craske, R. Ward, P. Collins, M. Trowbridge and G. Darby: Antimicrob. Agents Chemother. *42*, 868 (1998).
193 J.S. Gibbs, H.C. Chiou, K.F. Bastow, Y.-C. Cheng and D.M. Coen: Proc. Natl. Acad. Sci. USA *85*, 6672 (1988).
194 C.B.C. Hwang, K.L. Ruffner and D.M. Coen: J. Virol. *66*, 1774 (1992).
195 L. Huang, K.K. Ishii, H. Zuccola, A.M. Gehring, C.B.C. Hwang, J. Hogle and D.M. Coen: Proc. Natl. Acad. Sci. USA *96*, 447 (1999).
196 G. Andrei, R. Snoeck, E. De Clercq, R. Esnouf, P. Fiten and G. Opdenakker : J. Gen. Virol. *81*, 639 (2000).
197 B. Eriksson, B. Öberg and B. Wahren: Biochim. Biophys. Acta *696*, 115 (1982).
198 S. Safrin, C. Crumpacker, P. Chatis, R. Davis, R. Hafner, J. Rush, H.A. Kessler, B. Landry and J. Mills: N. Engl. J. Med. *325*, 551 (1991).
199 D. Derse, K. F. Bastow and Y-C. Cheng: J. Biol. Chem. *10*, 10251 (1982).
200 B. Visse, B. Dumont, J. M. Huraux and A. M. Fillet : J. Infect. Dis. *178*, S55 (1998).
201 S. Safrin, S. Kemmerly, B. Plotkin, T. Smith, N. Weissbach, D. De Veranez, L. D. Phan and D. Cohn: J. Infect. Dis. *169*, 193 (1994).
202 L. Waxman and P.L. Darke: Antivir. Chem. Chemother. *11*, 1 (2000).
203 M. van Zeijl, J. Fairhurst, T.R. Jones, S.K. Vernon, J. Morin, J. LaRocque, B. Feld, B. O'Hara, J.D. Bloom and S.V. Johann: J. Virol. *74*, 9054 (2000).
204 F. Zoulim and C. Trépo: J. Hepatol. *29*, 151 (1998).
205 O. Poch, I. Sauvaget, M. Delarue and N. Tordo: EMBO J. *8*, 3867 (1989).
206 J. Torresi and S. Locarnini: Gastroenterology *118*, S83 (2000).
207 B. Jarvis and D. Faulds: Drugs *58*, 101 (1999).
208 R. Ling, D. Mutimer, M. Ahmed, E.H. Boxall, E. Elias, G.M. Dusheiko and T.J. Harrison: Hepatology *24*, 711 (1996).
209 M.I. Allen, M. Deslauriers, C.W. Andrews, G.A. Tipples, K.-A. Walters, D.L.J. Tyrrell, N. Brown for the Lamivudine Clinical Investigation Group, and L.D. Condreay: Hepatology *27*, 1670 (1998).
210 Y. Benhamou, M. Bochet, V. Thibault, V. Di Martino, E. Caumes, F. Bricaire, P. Opolon, C. Katlama and T. Poynard: Hepatology *30*, 1302 (1999).
211 K.S. Gutfreund, M. Williams, R. George, V.G. Bain, M.M. Ma, E.M. Yoshida, J.-P. Villeneuve, K.P. Fischer and D.L.J. Tyrrell: J. Hepatol. *33*, 469 (2000).
212 S.K. Ladner, T.J. Miller and R.W. King: Antimicrob. Agents Chemother. 42, 2128 (1998).
213 M. Melegari, P.P. Scaglioni and J.R. Wands: Hepatology *27*, 68 (1998).
214 S.K. Ono, N. Kato, Y. Shiratori, J. Kato, T. Goto, R.F. Schinazi, F.J. Carrilho and M. Omata: J. Clin. Invest. *107*, 449 (2001).

215 D.T.-Y. Lau, M.F. Khokhar, E. Doo, M.G. Ghany, D. Herion, Y. Park, D.E. Kleiner, P. Schmid, L.D. Condreay, J. Gauthier et al.: Hepatology *32*, 828 (2000).
216 M. Gutiérrez-Rivas, A. Ibáñez, M.A. Martínez, E. Domingo and L. Menéndez-Arias: J. Mol. Biol. *290*, 615 (1999).
217 H. Huang, R. Chopra, G.L. Verdine and S.C. Harrison: Science *282*, 1669 (1998).
218 X. Xiong, C. Flores, H. Yang, J.J. Toole and C.S. Gibbs: Hepatology *28*, 1669 (1998).
219 S.K. Ono-Nita, N. Kato, Y. Shiratori, K.-H. Lan, H. Yoshida, F.J. Carrilho and M. Omata: J. Clin. Invest. *103*, 1635 (1999).
220 T.T. Aye, A. Bartholomeusz, T. Shaw, S. Bowden, A. Breschkin, J. McMillan, P. Angus and S.A. Locarnini: J. Hepatol. *26*, 1148 (1997).
221 Bartholomeusz, L.C. Groenen and S.A. Locarnini: Intervirology *40*, 337 (1997).
222 Seignères, C. Pichoud, S.S. Ahmed, O. Hantz, C. Trépo and F. Zoulim: J. Infect. Dis. *181*, 1221 (2000).
223 W. Carman, H. Thomas and E. Domingo: Lancet *341*, 349 (1993).
224 S.A. Locarnini. Hepatology *27*, 294 (1998).
225 R. Girones and R.H. Miller: Virology *170*, 595 (1989).
226 M. Nowak, S. Bonhoeffer, A. Hill, R. Boehme, H. Thomas and H. McDade: Proc. Natl. Acad. Sci. USA *93*, 4398 (1996).
227 S. Bonhoeffer, R.M. May, G.M. Shaw and M.A. Nowak: Proc. Natl. Acad. Sci. USA *94*, 6971 (1997).
228 E. de Clercq: Rev. Med. Virol. *10*, 255 (2000).
229 J.P. Moore and M. Stevenson: Nature Rev. Mol Cell. Biol. *1*, 40 (2000).
230 K.W. Mundry and A. Gierer: Z. Vererbungsl. *89*, 614 (1958).
231 J.J. Holland, E. Domingo, J.C. de la Torre and D.A. Steinhauer: J. Virol. *64*, 3960 (1990).
232 L.A. Loeb, J.M. Essigmann, F. Kazazi, J. Zhang, K.D. Rose and J.I. Mullins: Proc. Natl. Acad. Sci. USA *96*, 1492 (1999).
233 S. Sierra, M. Dávila, P.R. Lowenstein and E. Domingo: J. Virol. *74*, 8316 (2000).
234 S. Crotty, D. Maag, J.J. Arnold, W. Zhong, J.Y.N. Lau, Z. Hong, R. Andino and C.E. Cameron: Nat. Med. *6*, 1375 (2000).

Progress in Drug Research, Vol. 57 (E. Jucker, Ed.)

Applications of yeast in drug discovery

By Doreen Ma

Lilly Research Laboratories
Eli Lilly and Company
Indianapolis, IN 46285, USA
<ma_doreen@lilly.com>

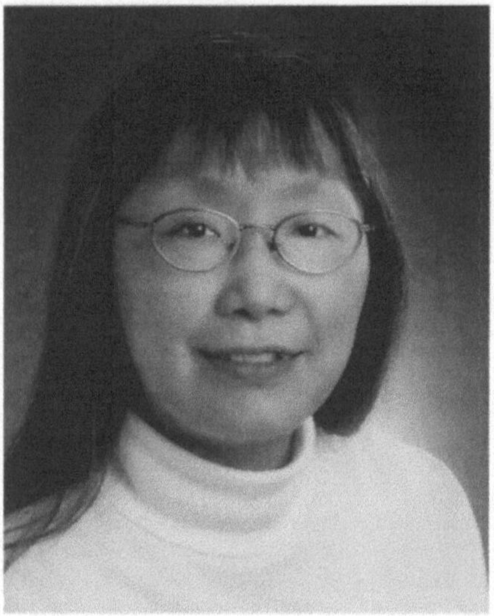

Doreen Ma

graduated from the California Institute of Technology with a Ph. D. in Biochemistry. As a post-doctoral fellow of the American Cancer Society, she studied the role of MAP kinases in the yeast pheromone response pathway at the University of California, Berkeley. In 1992, she joined the Biomolecular Screening Department at Eli Lilly and Company. She is currently a senior scientist in the Infectious Diseases Division and focuses her research on discovery of new antifungal therapeutics.

Summary

The yeast *Saccharomyces cerevisiae* is perhaps the best-studied eukaryotic organism. Its experimental tractability, combined with the remarkable conservation of gene function throughout evolution, makes yeast the ideal model genetic organism. Yeast is a non-pathogenic model of fungal pathogens used to identify antifungal targets suitable for drug development and to elucidate mechanisms of action of antifungal agents. As a model of fundamental cellular processes and metabolic pathways of the human, yeast has improved our understanding and facilitated the molecular analysis of many disease genes. The completion of the Saccharomyces genome sequence helped launch the post-genomic era, focusing on functional analyses of whole genomes. Yeast paved the way for the systematic analysis of large and complex genomes by serving as a test bed for novel experimental approaches and technologies, tools that are fast becoming the standard in drug discovery research

Contents

1	Introduction	120
2	*Saccharomyces cerevisiae* as a model system for human diseases	122
2.1	The cell cycle and cancer	123
2.2	Sterol metabolism	127
3	*Saccharomyces cerevisiae* as a model system for pathogenic fungi	129
3.1	Sterol biosynthesis pathway and antifungal drug resistance	131
3.2	Sordarins and their molecular target, elongation factor 2 (EF2)	134
4	Genomics and functional genomics	136
4.1	Bioinformatics and specialized databases for genomic scale projects	137
4.2	Systematic functional genomics – the EUROFAN model	139
4.3	Genome-wide transcript profiling	139
4.3.1	DNA microarrays	141
4.4	Proteomics	145
4.4.1	2D-PAGE and mass spectrometry	146
4.4.2	Transposon-tagged mutagenesis	147
4.4.3	Biochemical genomics – GST-fusion proteins	149
4.4.4	Protein microarrays	150
4.4.5	Yeast two-hybrid analysis – global network of protein-protein interactions	152
4.5	Metabolome	154
5	Conclusion	156
	References	157

Keywords

Saccharomyces cerevisiae, cell cycle, checkpoint control, sterol metabolism, *Candida albicans*, ergosterol biosynthesis, elongation factor 2, antifungals, genomics, functional genomics, transcription profiling, DNA microarray, haploinsufficiency, protein microarray, mass spectrometry, 2D-PAGE, transposon mutagenesis, yeast two-hybrid, transcriptome, proteome, metabolome.

Glossary of abbreviations

aa, amino acid; *A. fumigatus, Aspergillus fumigatus*; BLAST, basic local alignment search tool; bp, base pair; *C. albicans, Candida albicans*; *C. elegans, Caenorhabditis elegans*; *C. glabrata, Candida glabrata*; *C. krusei, Candida krusei*; *C. parapsilosis, Candida parapsilosis*; *C. neoformans, Cryptococcus neoformans*; CYP, Cytochrome P-450; cDNA, complementary DNA; DNA, deoxyribonucleic acid; *D. melanogaster, Drosophila melanogaster*; *E. coli, Escherichia coli*; EF, elongation factor; EST, expressed sequence tag; EUROFAN, European functional analysis network; FDA, Food and Drug

Administration; GFP, green fluorescent protein; GPCR, heterotrimeric GTP-binding protein-coupled receptor; GRM™, genome reporter matrix; kDa, kilodalton; Mb, megabase; HMG-CoA, 3-hydroxyl-3-methylglutaryl coenzyme A; MIPS, Martinsried Institute for Protein Sciences; mRNA, messenger RNA; MOA, mechanism of action; NORF, non-annotated ORF; ORF, open reading frame; PAGE, polyacrylamide gel electrophoresis; PDR, pleiotropic drug resistance; RNA, ribonucleic acid; SAGE, serial analysis of gene expression; SAR, structure activity relationship; *S. cerevisiae*, *Saccharomyces cerevisiae*; *S. pombe*, *Schizosaccharomyces pombe*; SGD, *Saccharomyces* genome database; tRNA, transfer RNA; YPD™, Yeast proteome database.

1 Introduction

Saccharomyces cerevisiae, budding yeast, has a history of being used as a model eukaryote. Because yeast can exist in both haploid and diploid stages, its life cycle is uniquely suited for genetic manipulation. As a unicellular organism, its growth rate is comparable to bacterial species and so provides data in a shorter time period than other eukaryotic model systems. Furthermore, the ability to transform yeast with plasmid or DNA fragments enables precise alteration of the genetic make-up of this organism to examine the consequences of such mutations. Yeast geneticists and cell biologists have relied on these sophisticated tools for decades to understand the functions of genes and have applied this knowledge to elucidate gene functions in higher eukaryotes including humans. The vast knowledge base accumulated through independent investigations was further assisted with the publication of the complete genome sequence of *S. cerevisiae* in early 1996 [1, 2]. The publication was the first for a eukaryotic genome and it established the utility of *S. cerevisiae* as a model eukaryote. Independent researchers have observed in many cases that pathways are conserved from yeast to human. The ability of human genes to complement the deficiency of a yeast homolog, or *vice versa*, further confirmed the functional conservation. Mushegian et al. [3] surveyed a sample of 70 positionally cloned human disease genes and found that 29 genes were cloned through functional complementation of their yeast homologs. Additional evidence has come with the publications of three eukaryotic genomes, *C. elegans*, *D. melanogaster* and humans.

The publication of the *C. elegans* 97 Mb genome made possible the first comprehensive comparison of two eukaryotic genomes, yeast, a unicellular microorganism, and worm, a multicellular animal [4, 5]. Proteins involved in core biological processes, such as DNA and RNA metabolism, protein synthesis, protein folding and protein degradation, intermediary metabolism, transport and secretion, are highly conserved between the two species. In addition, numerous shared domains and motifs are identified that function similarly in the two organisms, making inference of protein functions possible with knowledge of the counterpart. The publication of the genome sequence of *D. melanogaster* in 2000 [6] further enhanced the value of *S. cerevisiae* as a model genetic organism.

It is remarkable that a complex organism, such as the fruit fly, has only 13,000 genes, only double that of the yeast genome, a unicellular eukaryote. With three complete or essentially complete eukaryotic genomes, Rubin et al. performed a comparative analysis of the three genomes and their proteomes [7]. This analysis underscored the comparison of worm and yeast genomes, and demonstrated that a core proteome exists to perform biological processes common to all organisms. Significantly, when all protein domains are searched against the three genomes, 744 out of a total of 1,400 are present in all three organisms. This finding further substantiates the fact that there are universal concepts of life that are highly conserved through evolution. Additionally, Rubin et al. [7] assembled a panel of 289 genes that are affected in a variety of human diseases and asked if homologs exist in the 3 completed genomes surveyed. Based on BLAST scores, over 46 genes have a clear match in yeast (E values $< 1 \times 10^{-40}$). An additional 70-plus genes have E values in the range of 1×10^{-6} and 1×10^{-40}, indicating significant homology perhaps within the conserved protein domains. Together these genes represent opportunities for research in yeast to contribute towards a detailed understanding of complex human diseases. In this article, I will provide examples that illustrate how *S. cerevisiae* has been used as a eukaryote model for the human and also as a non-pathogenic model for human fungal pathogens.

The advent of genomics in the past decade has transformed the approach of practicing researchers. Instead of focusing on one gene, one protein, one pathway at a time, we look on the level of the entire genome. This comprehensive view requires development of new and systematic tools that can quickly and accurately yield information with or without hypotheses. Large volumes of information must then be catalogued and analyzed to facilitate interpretation. Advances in areas such as DNA sequencing, bioinformatics and functional genomics have been tremendous and the *S. cerevisiae* genome has been applied to each of these pioneering areas to validate the technology. In addition, results from these studies in yeast identified limitations of each technology and led to the improvement or invention of entirely new tools for the analysis of larger genomes. I will present a general view of available genomic tools, how these have been applied to answer questions in yeast and how the learning can be applied to the functional analysis of the Human genome.

One utility of yeast in drug discovery outside the scope of this review is the expression and production of heterologous proteins for research and other purposes. In recent years, non-conventional yeasts, such as *Pichia pastoris*, *Yarrowia lipolytica* and *Kluyveromyces lactis*, have been added to the repertoire of this application. A vast literature exists on this topic and I refer readers to several thorough reviews for such information [8–13]. One notable exception is the expression of orphan GPCRs in yeast to elucidate function and to screen for potential agonists and antagonists. Numerous studies were conducted in *Saccharomyces* on a variety of receptors [9–14] that revealed ligand specificity, receptor/G-protein interactions and also the identification of novel components of the G-protein signaling pathway [14–20].

2 *Saccharomyces cerevisiae* as a model system for human diseases

The comparative analysis between the *S. cerevisiae*, *C. elegans* and *D. melanogaster* proteomes [7] showed great promise that we may reliably infer possible functions of human proteins from study of the cognate proteins in these model organisms. Indeed, with the Human genome publication in February 2001 by two different groups [21, 22], the concept of evolutionary conservation of core biological processes is borne out. Primary cell functions, such as basic metabolism, DNA replication, transcription of DNA into RNA and translation of RNA into protein, are all highly conserved from yeast to human. The biggest difference between humans and flies, or humans and yeast, is the complexity of proteins and gene expression. The fact that the human genome is estimated at 30,000 genes, a mere five-fold that of a unicellular eukaryote, *S. cerevisiae*, suggests that biological sophistication does not depend on the number of genes but rather upon the intricate regulation of gene expression. The basic modules of gene regulation present in every eukaryote are combined in novel ways to generate a considerably more complex network in the human. Similarly, when the *S. cerevisiae* and human proteomes were compared, the human has more multi-domain proteins with combinations of domains not previously seen in *S. cerevisiae* or other organisms. Conservation is well maintained in functional categories such as rho GTPase signaling, protein-protein interaction and nuclear interaction domains. Conspicuously missing in the yeast genome are genes involved in cell-cell communication, developmental and homeostatic regulation, and acquired immunity. However, over the entire proteome, apparent homologs could be identified in the Human genome that correspond to 46% of the yeast proteome [21, 22]. Therefore, approaches in yeast that ignored the complexity and focused primarily on component parts would most likely yield useful information that is applicable to the human counterparts.

Yeast has been applied as a model system to study numerous diseases in the human. The positional cloning of the gene responsible for cystic fibrosis (CFTR) [23] took many years of research. After the gene was cloned and sequenced, homology to yeast *YCF1* (yeast cadmium factor) was immediately recognized and CFTR inferred to function as a transmembrane ion transporter. Yeast prion research has facilitated understanding of human diseases like Creutzfeldt-Jakob disease (CJD). Recent investigation of yeast prion protein Sup35 in *S. cerevisiae* and *C. albicans* led to a hypothesis of how particular prion diseases cross the species line, an important aspect in understanding how mad cow disease spreads to the human but why scrapie does not [24]. A recent review of congenital disorders of glycosylation (CDG) also pointed to yeast as the model system to elucidate molecular defects in the pathway leading to N-linked glycosylation that are responsible for CDG [25]. Study of yeast *SGS1* (slow growth suppressor), a DNA helicase involved in premature aging of yeast mother cells, helped unravel the molecular basis of genetic instability disorders in the human, such as Werner's syndrome, Bloom syndrome and Rothmund-Thomson syndrome [26–28]. In the sections below, I will review more extensively two areas of yeast research that have contributed significantly to the understanding of human diseases, cell cycle research and sterol metabolism.

2.1 The cell cycle and cancer

The cell cycle is one of the most conserved processes in eukaryotes. Murray and Marks conducted a search for new components of the cell cycle in the

Human genome based on current knowledge in model organisms and, surprisingly, found very few novel cyclins, no new cyclin-dependent kinases or components of the spindle checkpoint [29]. With the machinery that is involved in cell cycle regulation being so well conserved from yeast to human, Murray and Marks suggest that the majority of components necessary for the cell cycle have been identified through extensive studies in the cell cycling process of model systems like *S. cerevisiae* and *S. pombe*.

An extensive review by Nurse looked back at the history of cell cycle research over the last century and provided many examples demonstrating the power of combining yeast genetics and molecular biology [30]. The early existence of a set of cell division cycle (cdc) mutants [31] and the ease of genetic manipulation in yeast propelled the understanding of the cell cycle from a cellular process of copying and partitioning hereditary materials to the molecular details of cell cycle machinery and control [30]. The concept of checkpoint control also originated based on the many yeast mutants that have defects at specific stages of the cell cycle [32]. The phenotypes of the mutants suggested that the specific stages are ordered into interdependent pathways. To progress from one stage to next, the cells "check" to ensure that the previous stage has been executed correctly. Various checkpoint mechanisms have been elucidated. The DNA damage and replication checkpoint blocks mitosis when DNA damage occurs or when DNA replication is incomplete. The spindle checkpoint likewise prevents exit from mitosis if the spindle is not assembled or if the chromosomes are not aligned and attached to the spindle. Mounting evidence shows that interfering with the activity of checkpoint proteins results in uncontrolled proliferation and, ultimately, genomic instability. Ever since the identification of checkpoint control mutants in *S. cerevisiae*, it has been hypothesized that checkpoint control in the human plays a similar role in maintaining genome stability. I refer the readers to excellent reviews detailing the connection of checkpoint control with cancer development [33, 34] and I provide a few recent publications below as examples of how yeast homologs have helped to elucidate the role checkpoint proteins play in different types of cancers.

The spindle checkpoint defect was originally defined in budding yeast by mutants that fail to arrest in the cell cycle on treatment with microtubule depolymerizing drugs. One of the proteins involved in spindle checkpoint control in *S. cerevisiae* is *BUB1* (budding uninhibited by benzimidazole). Mutant *bub1* fails to properly arrest mitosis in response to the loss of microtubule function induced by treatment with benzimidazole [35]. *BUB1*, together with *MPS1* (monopolar spindle), *MAD1-3* (mitotic arrest defective) and *BUB3* in yeast, ensures that all chromosomes are attached to the mitotic spindle and aligned at the metaphase plate. Deletion mutants of any of the spindle checkpoint proteins have a higher rate of chromosome loss when exposed to low doses of microtubule depolymerizing drugs such as nocodazole and benomyl [35]. The observation that in most colorectal cancers, chromosomal instability leads to aneuploidy similar to the genomic instability caused by defects in spindle checkpoint mutants in yeast, led Cahill et al. to evaluate the role of the human homolog of *BUB1*, *hBUB1*, in colorectal cancer cell lines [36]. The human *BUB1* was isolated by searching the EST database for clones similar to *S. cerevisiae* and murine *BUB1* genes [36]. This group sequenced *hBUB1* in 19 colorectal cancer cell lines to search for mutations that may account for the chromosomal instability phenotype. One deletion mutation was identified that corresponds to removal of a highly conserved domain 1 essential for kinetochore localization in *S. cerevisiae* [37]. Another missense mutation caused the substitution of a conserved serine to tyrosine. Both mutations were heterozygous but exhibited a dominant-negative effect when overexpressed. Furthermore, by adopting a similar strategy for *hBUB1* cloning, Cahill et al. identified another homolog in the human, *hBUBR1* [36]. One mutation identified in *hBUBR1* is located in the conserved domain 2 necessary for the protein kinase activity to phosphorylate another checkpoint protein, *BUB3* [38]. These results demonstrated that correlation exists between the loss of spindle checkpoint and chromosome instability phenotype in colorectal cancer cell lines [36]. Similarly, mutant forms of Bub1p were identified in tumors from Brca2-deficient animals, indicating that mutations in mitotic checkpoint genes are also involved in the pathogenesis of inherited breast cancer [39].

Another spindle checkpoint component in *S. cerevisiae* is *MAD2* (mitotic arrest defective) that functions in the same regulatory pathway as *BUB1* to monitor spindle defects. Michel et al. recently demonstrated that haploinsufficiency at the *hMAD2* (human *MAD2*) locus is associated with a high rate of aneuploidy in human cancer cells and murine primary embryonic fibroblasts [40]. In addition, mice with one intact copy of *hMAD2* developed papillary lung adenocarcinomas at a high frequency with long latency [40]. The results from studies of *hBUB1* and *hMAD2* suggest that loss of spindle checkpoint function is involved in the progression of tumorigenesis.

Questions remain as to whether interfering with the mitotic checkpoint can affect the outcome of the disease. Study of *S. cerevisiae* spindle checkpoint components, especially on the genomic scale, may help to address this issue. Simon et al. performed transcription profiling on 23 FDA-approved cytotoxic anticancer agents applied to a panel of isogenic yeast strains, of which each was defective in a particular DNA repair or cell cycle gene function [41]. The panel of isogenic yeast strains included genes involved in various DNA damage repair pathways, such as nucleotide excision repair, mismatch repair, base excision repair, and cell cycle checkpoint. For the majority of the profiles, the various mutants involved in a particular pathway showed similar sensitivity, indicating that the observed response is pathway-specific rather than mutant-specific. In general, the authors observed 3 types of profiles based on the mode of chemotherapeutic action [41]. One class of agents has selective toxicity targeting a specific pathway and thus offers the potential to improve selectivity for killing cancer cells over that of normal cells. The second class of agents shows toxicity in many pathway defects, indicating the introduction of multiple types of DNA damage. The study showed that results in yeast are predictive of human cell responses to DNA damaging agents. The third class of agents lacks selectivity between the mutants because cell killing is not likely to be due to DNA damage. Through analysis of how sensitive mutated yeast strains are responding to these chemotherapeutic agents and by extrapolation to their human counterparts, we may one day be able to predict the outcome of a particular chemotherapeutic regimen. Alternatively, we may understand how these chemotherapeutic agents differentially affect the cancer cells and help minimize the serious side-effects that are associated with current chemotherapy.

In conclusion, cell cycle research in yeast has greatly aided our understanding of the human cell cycle and of cell cycle regulators in cancer development. In addition to checkpoint controls, yeast research has also furthered our understanding of cyclins and cyclin-dependent kinases and their involvement in cancer [42]. Detailed molecular and mechanistic dissection is easier in yeast and identification of other components involved in the same pathway using synthetic lethal screening is yet another advantage of the yeast system [43]. Furthermore, anticancer drugs could be evaluated using a strategy similar to Simon et al. [41] to discover therapeutic agents with selective killing properties. In 1997, Hartwell et al. [44] proposed how yeast genetics could be used to streamline anticancer drug discovery. With the examples described, this approach is certainly a fruitful endeavor and the completion of the Human Genome Project will undoubtedly further accelerate the process of identifying mutations in human orthologs of proteins demonstrated to be crucial components of the cell cycle pathway. A detailed molecular description of cancers and an anticancer drug targeted to the molecular defect seems to be in our near future.

2.2 Sterol metabolism

Extensive knowledge exists for the fungal ergosterol biosynthesis and metabolism pathway. The human counterpart of ergosterol is cholesterol, structurally different from ergosterol but synthesized and regulated in a similar manner. The conservation of eukaryotic sterol homeostasis has allowed a detailed molecular approach to be applied to the human pathway using yeast genetics. In fact, the search for targets suitable for developing drugs for the human hypercholesterolemia has driven an intense effort since the 1980s to identify the molecular components of this pathway.

The most prominent molecular target in the human sterol pathway is HMG-CoA reductase, an enzyme that catalyzes the conversion of HMG-CoA to mevalonate and the rate-limiting enzyme of sterol biosynthesis. Many blockbuster cholesterol-lowering drugs, such as lovastatin, fluvastatin, and atorvastatin, all target this crucial enzyme [45]. Rine et al. succeeded in isolating the yeast genes encoding HMG-CoA reductase by applying a new concept at the time, the gene dosage effect [46]. The authors surmised that by selective amplification of target genes, a concomitant increase in gene products might be able to confer resistance to certain metabolic inhibitors. In this case, they utilized compactin, a hypocholesterolemic agent that is known to inhibit HMG-CoA reductase. Exposing yeast cells to high concentrations of compactin causes lethality. The genetic screen demands that the specific yeast strain(s) harboring a plasmid that contains the gene encoding HMG-CoA reductase be able to suppress the lethality due to the overproduction of the reductase. Two genes, *HMG1* and *HMG2*, were identified in this novel screen [46] and DNA sequence analysis revealed a high degree of conservation in the catalytic domain between yeast and human HMG-CoA reductase [47]. Expression of human HMG-CoA reductase could compensate for the loss of both *HMG1* and *HMG2 in vivo*, one of the first examples of functional conservation from yeast to human [47]. A recent review by Sturley summarized many years of yeast research in this area and how the cumulative knowledge was applied to current efforts in understanding not only the cholesterol biosynthesis pathway but also sterol homeostasis [48].

Based on the high conservation of the sterol metabolism pathway between yeast and man, various expression-profiling studies were conducted in yeast to evaluate the transcriptional response to drug exposure. Dimster-Denk and colleagues utilized a panel of 864 isogenic yeast strains, a subset of the yeast genome, each containing a different reporter gene fusion, to evaluate the expression profiles of eight compounds that target four different enzymatic steps of the sterol biosynthesis pathway [49]. They observed very specific feedback regulation for inhibition of HMG-CoA synthase. Only 34 genes out of the 864-strain array had two-fold or more changes in expression. Half of the genes are known to be involved in ergosterol biosynthesis and have mammalian homologs. Many of the remaining 17 genes are of unknown function and investigations may well lead to identification of new components in this pathway. Genes induced or repressed by at least two-fold range from ten to twenty percent for the statins to almost forty percent for sulconazole. These gene expression patterns may reflect the specificity of these drugs [49], providing valuable information in the process of drug discovery to minimize serious side-effects.

The most revealing aspect of the Dimster-Denk et al. study is the induced expression of a subset of genes encoding enzymes of sterol biosynthesis (*ERG2*, *ERG8*, *ERG9*, *ERG12* and *ERG19*) by all eight drugs examined [49]. These genes could be used as biomarkers for identifying mutations or compounds that affect the sterol biosynthesis pathway. An expression-profiling study based on the entire yeast genome has already demonstrated the utility of this approach [50]. In total, Hughes et al. generated 300 expression profiles, mainly for deletion mutants, but also for 13 well-characterized compounds. These profiles were then subjected to two-dimensional hierarchical clustering that revealed groups of coregulated transcripts as well as functional groupings. One of the coregulated transcript clusters is the "ergosterol cluster" containing many known components of the ergosterol biosynthetic pathway, a finding confirming the work of Dimster-Denk et al. [49]. Results showed that the transcript profile of yeast cells exposed to lovastatin, an HMG-CoA reductase inhibitor, closely mimics the profile of yeast cells with reduced expression of *HMG2*, the gene encoding HMG-CoA reductase. Such pattern matching between expression profiles from yeast cells exposed to a compound with unknown MOA and a comprehensive panel of mutant profiles may therefore identify the compound's MOA.

Identification of novel drug targets is yet another utility demonstrated by this comprehensive gene profiling study. Hughes et al. identified *ERG28* to be involved in ergosterol biosynthesis, based on the close resemblance of expression profiles between an *erg28* deletion strain and other mutants of the pathway [50]. Subsequent study showed that *ERG28* is involved in sterol C-4 demethylation along with *ERG26* and *ERG27* [51]. All three *ERG* genes have significant homologs in the human and for *ERG28, hERG28* show functional conservation by restoring wild-type growth to a yeast *erg28* deletion mutant [50]. Although *ERG28* is not essential for survival, deletion of either *ERG26* or *ERG27* is a lethal event [52]. Thus a novel component of the ergosterol and, most likely, the cholesterol biosynthesis pathway in the human was identified using yeast gene expression profiling.

In summary, similar to cell cycle research, yeast sterol metabolism pathway research has yielded many opportunities for drug discovery in the human sterol metabolism pathway. Applications range from identification of novel molecular components as potential drug targets and evaluation of drug specificity, to elucidation of molecular target(s) of compounds known to inhibit this essential process.

3 *Saccharomyces cerevisiae* as a model system for pathogenic fungi

Invasive fungal infections are more prevalent than ever. Recent statistics showed that *Candida* species are now the fourth most common cause of nosocomial bloodstream infection and fungal infections accounted for 12% of all nosocomial bloodstream infections in ICU settings [53, 54]. Large populations of immunocompromised and neutropenic patients, combined with the widespread use of implanted devices, all contribute to the increased incidence of fungal infections. Unfortunately, the number of antifungal therapeutics available for clinical use is very limited and each has its shortcomings. Amphotericin B, widely accepted as the gold standard of antifungal treatment, has a dose-limiting nephrotoxicity issue, whereas emerging resistance and a narrow spectrum of activity have limited the efficacy of triazoles.

The unmet medical need for treatment of fungal infections is apparent in light of the high mortality rate in neutropenic patients caused by fungal infections [55, 56]. The ideal antifungal agent should have a broad spectrum of activity, be administered either orally or parenterally, be fungicidal instead of fungistatic to avoid resistance, and be safe at the efficacious dose. Development of antifungal agents is complicated by the conservation of essential biological processes from fungi to humans. The most desirable targets are those that maintain a high degree of similarity across fungal species but that diverge considerably from their homologs in humans. Putative targets should also be essential for survival of the pathogen. At present, it is still very difficult to identify an antifungal drug target unique to fungi with no counterparts present in the human [57]. When a complete genomic sequence of various fungal species becomes available, researchers could then select antifungal targets based on *in silico* comparison of the fungal and Human genomes to maximize both the therapeutic index and the spectrum of activities.

With the recent publication of the Human genome [21, 22], the urgent task for antifungal drug discovery is to obtain the complete sequence of major fungal pathogens such as *C. albicans*, *A. fumigatus* and *C. neoformans*. At the time of writing of this review, whole-genome shotgun and cosmid sequencing of the *C. albicans* genome has already achieved a 10.4X genome coverage and the assembly of the sequences yielded more than 9000 ORFs encoding proteins with 100 amino acids or greater. The assembly and all ORFs are available at the Stanford Sequencing Center website, http://www-sequence.stanford.edu/group/candida. A major hindrance in studying *C. albicans* is the lack of molecular genetics tools applicable to this genome, in contrast to *S. cerevisiae* [58]. By using *S. cerevisiae* as a model system, researchers hope to circumvent this problem. Two published studies compared the *C. albicans* and *S. cerevisiae* genomes to investigate the extent of gene order conservation [59] and the existence of an intact sexual cycle in *C. albicans* [60]. More comparative analyses between these genomes will undoubtedly be made to elucidate common biological processes engaged by these two organisms.

In addition to the *C. albicans* genome, sequencing projects for two other human fungal pathogens, *A. fumigatus* and *C. neoformans*, have begun. Information on the progress of these sequencing projects can be accessed at http://www.aspergillus.man.ac.uk/sequence_info/sequence and http://www.sequence.stanford.edu/group/cryptococcus, respectively. The availability of molecular genetics tools for *S. cerevisiae* continues to facilitate the validation of chosen targets because functional analysis in the pathogenic fungi remains a challenge. In the next two sections, I will discuss examples of how investigations in *S. cerevisiae* have led to elucidation of mechanisms of action and/or mechanisms of resistance for two classes of antifungals, the azoles and the sordarins.

3.1 Sterol biosynthesis pathway and antifungal drug resistance

Sterols are essential lipid components of eukaryotic membranes and sterol biosynthesis is a process targeted by multiple antifungal drugs, including azoles, allylamines and morpholines [61]. All key enzymes of the sterol biosynthesis pathway in *S. cerevisiae* have been identified and characterized [61]. Squalene epoxidase, encoded by *ERG1* (ergosterol), is the target of the allylamine class of antifungals, including terbinafine [62]. Both *ERG24*, encoding sterol C-14 reductase, and *ERG2*, encoding sterol C-8 desaturase, are targets of the morpholine antifungals [63]. Lanosterol 14α-demethylase, the product of the *ERG11* gene, is a CYP-dependent enzyme and the target of azole antifungals. In all instances, studies of MoA and resistance were greatly enhanced by the knowledge of the *S. cerevisiae* sterol biosynthesis pathway, facilitated by the availability of molecular genetic tools. The study of azole drug resistance described below illustrates various applications of yeast in the elucidation of this alarming phenomenon.

The introduction of azoles in the 1980s and the subsequent widespread prophylactic use of fluconazole in the 1990s have given rise to azole resistance. In the past two decades, a substantial shift took place in the epidemiology of candidemia due to different *Candida* species: Candidal infection due to non-albicans species overtook that of *C. albicans* [64, 65]. Selection of azole non-susceptible species such as *Candida krusei* and induction of resistant organisms are thought to have contributed to this shift. As mentioned above, azoles target lanosterol 14α-demethylase, a crucial enzyme in the sterol biosynthesis pathway. Many biochemical studies have shown that multiple mechanisms are involved in resistance to azoles, including uptake and efflux [66, 67], changes in membrane fluidity [68], alteration of membrane sterol components [69, 70] and, finally, modification at the target site. Investigations in yeast have furthered our understanding of the resistance phenomenon at the molecular level.

Studies on *S. cerevisiae* identified a single form of CYP during purification of microsomal fractions of vegetatively growing yeast. This CYP was later associated with the gene *ERG11* cloned and demonstrated to possess lanosterol 14α-demethylase activity [71]. Kirsch et al. [72] utilized the presumed homology between the *S. cerevisiae* and *C. albicans* enzymes and low-stringency hybridization to isolate the DNA encoding the *C. albicans* enzyme. They demonstrated that the cloned sequence rescued a deletion mutant of *ERG11* in *S. cerevisiae*, showing a conserved function of the *C. albicans* enzyme similar to that of *S. cerevisiae*. Similar strategies were adopted to clone the human ortholog of the demethylase. The deduced amino acid sequence has approximately 40% amino acid identity between human and *S. cerevisiae* counterparts [73]. Heterologous expression of the *C. albicans* enzyme in *S. cerevisiae* and its ability to substitute for the lack of *S. cerevisiae* Erg11p makes the molecular genetics study of pathogen genes in *S. cerevisiae* possible. To probe the structure of the demethylase, Lamb et al. [74] conducted site-directed mutagenesis of the *C. albicans* sterol 14α-demethylase and heterologously expressed these mutants in *S. cerevisiae*. They concluded that a specific mutant, T315A, showed fluconazole resistance through reduced affinity to Erg11p, accompanied by a significant drop in enzymatic activity. For the first time, a single base mutation in the *ERG11* sequence was directly linked to altered drug binding affinity. Recently, additional mutations in the *C. albicans ERG11* gene were sequenced and introduced into *S. cerevisiae* (Y132H and I471T) [75]. Kakeya et al. demonstrated that either mutation was sufficient to confer azole resistance, but that enhanced resistance was observed when both mutations were present in the same organism [75]. These findings support that resistance to azole is the result of multiple mutations.

The heterologous expression of orthologs was applied to the human cytochrome CYP3A4, the major drug-metabolizing enzyme within the liver [76]. The study compared the potency of several azoles against the human CYP3A4 and the *C. albicans* Erg11p expressed in yeast. The approximately thirty-fold differential between the IC_{50} values of these two enzymes *versus* several azoles was interpreted as being sufficient to provide an acceptable therapeutic index in a clinical setting. Interestingly, Lamb et al. also showed that both enzymes favor the same enantiomeric configuration of the azole compounds diclobutrazol and SCH39304, providing further insight into the drug interaction model [76].

The complete genome sequence of *S. cerevisiae* also facilitated the search for paralogs of enzymes in the sterol biosynthetic pathway. *ERG5* was discovered during the yeast genome project when chromosome XIII was sequenced. *ERG5* is not essential under laboratory conditions and may represent the product of a gene duplication event. *S. cerevisiae ERG11* and *ERG5* have 24% amino acid identity and 41% homology. Kelly et al. determined that Erg5p has similar affinity to azole drugs as Erg11p and thus may be a factor in drug susceptibility [77].

ERG3 encodes the C-5 desaturase and has been reported to contribute to azole resistance in *S. cerevisiae* [70, 78]. Again, by homology to *S. cerevisiae ERG3*, *C. albicans ERG3* was cloned and showed to complement the absence of the *S. cerevisiae* ortholog [79]. By introducing mutant *erg3* alleles from a clinical *C. albicans* strain (the Darlington strain), Miyazaki et al. deduced the importance of two particular amino acid residues that are conserved in three fungal and one plant species [79]. Another approach commonly practiced in yeast molecular genetics, transposon-mediated mutagenesis [80], was applied to screen for mutants affected by azoles [81]. Mutants of *erg3* were isolated that confer resistance to fluconazole, another line of evidence supporting the significant role *ERG3* plays in azole resistance. This study also yielded mutants of *ERG11* and *PDR5* (pleiotropic drug resistance) that confer hypersensitivity to azoles when disrupted. Three genes previously not known to be involved in azole sensitivity were also identified, *SWI7*, *SPT7* and *YMR034c*. The latter is a putative sterol transporter whose disruption caused hypersensitivity to fluconazole. *SWI7* (mating type switching) and *SPT7* (suppressor of Ty) are part of the *in vivo* transcription activation machinery in yeast. The author surmised that these factors might be involved in the regulation of drug transporters such as *PDR5*, which has been shown in multiple studies to be responsible for azole drug efflux [81, 82].

S. cerevisiae is a model system for the study of drug efflux effects on azole resistance in *C. albicans*. *C. albicans* orthologs cloned based on homology with *S. cerevisiae* counterparts are numerous and their effects on drug resistance are also similar [83]. The dissection of how many transporters are responsible for the efflux of azoles is complicated by the existence of approximately 200 transporters within the *S. cerevisiae* genome. It is highly likely that a comparable number of transporters are present in the *C. albicans* genome. Some transporters have been characterized but many have no associated function. DeRisi et al. conducted a transcript profiling study of *pdr1* and *pdr3* mutants to delineate the network of transporters involved in pleiotropic drug resistance [84]. One of the groups of genes up-regulated by the activated mutants is the well-recognized ABC transporter (ATP-binding cassette) which contains *PDR5*. However, other groups, including permeases responsible for transport of hydrophobic substrates and lipids, genes related to cell wall metabolism, and stress response are also regulated by *PDR1* and *PDR3*. Thus *PDR1/3*-mediated resistance to chemicals like azoles may involve modulation of membrane and cell wall components as well as active efflux, a significant finding in light of the molecular target of the azoles. Investigation of pleiotropic drug resistance in *S. cerevisiae* serves as a framework for a similar study of whether a pathogenic fungus such as *C. albicans* utilizes the same mechanism for defense against noxious chemicals. Finally, the systematic disruption of all yeast genes has been completed and researchers are now able to characterize each of the disrupted transporter genes with regard to substrates and sensitivity to various chemicals. Such systematic analysis will give rise to a comprehensive view of the diverse classes of transporters in yeast and provide insights into drug resistance mechanisms.

3.2 Sordarins and their molecular target, elongation factor 2 (EF2)

The elucidation of MOA for a potential class of antifungal agent, the sordarins has generated considerable interest around the molecules. This class of compounds was first described as antifungal agents in 1970 [85, 86] and was rediscovered in a screen designed to isolate fungal-specific protein synthesis inhibitors [87]. Previous to Kinsman et al. [87], the mode of action of this class of antifungals had not been examined. No derivatives of sordarins are on the market yet but some sordarin derivatives, such as GM 222712 and GM 237354, show excellent *in vitro* activities against a diverse set of pathogenic fungi, including *Candida* spp., *C. neoformans*, *Pneumocystis carinii* and some filamentous fungi [88]. The lack of activity against human protein synthesis [88] is surprising considering the high degree of conservation of protein synthesis within the eukaryotic kingdom. By assaying chromatographic fractions for their ability to bind to tritiated sordarins, Domínguez and Martín identified elongation factor 2 (EF2) as the molecular target of this class of molecule [89]. EF2 is one of the soluble factors required for the elongation phase of translation. Together with EF1α and EF3, this soluble elongation factor catalyzes the translocation of ribosome along mRNA. Both EF1α and EF2 belong to the GTPase superfamily and are required for translation in all eukaryotes, while EF3 is unique to fungi and essential for fungal protein synthesis [90]. EF2 is a highly conserved protein with 66% amino acid identity and 85% homology to its human ortholog [91]. Considering these facts together, it is intriguing that a highly selective inhibitor could be discovered against this cellular target.

Great progress has been made on understanding how sordarins inhibit protein synthesis in fungi, using *S. cerevisiae* as a model system. Classical genetics was engaged to isolate and characterize sordarin-resistant mutants in yeast, resulting in two complementation groups [92]. A genomic library was constructed from one of the dominant sordarin-resistant mutants and transformed into wild-type yeasts to select for plasmid-conferred resistance. *EFT2*, encoding EF2, was found to be the gene conferring resistance to sordarins, consistent with the biochemical approach described above [89]. All mutants from this major complementation group were sequenced and most mutations clustered on a 50-amino acid segment of EF2, the same region the authors defined as a sordarins binding pocket using a modeling exercise. In addition, all mutants displayed negligible binding to sordarins, corroborating that this 50-amino acid region is involved in drug binding. An independent study conducted by Justice et al. [93] also isolated mutants with mutations clustering around the same 50-amino acid region. Sequence alignment between *S. cerevisiae* EF2 and its prokaryotic counterpart EF-G demonstrates that mutations in EF2 conferring resistance to sordarins are located close to mutations in EF-G that lead to fusidic acid resistance.

Analysis of the second complementation group by Capa et al. [92] identified the ribosomal stalk protein rpP0 (also known as L10e, the eukaryotic counterpart of L10 in prokaryotes) encoded by *RPL10* (ribosomal protein L10) as the mutated locus [94]. Similarly, Justice et al. [95] reported that mutations in L10e confer resistance to sordarins. Protein rpP0 has been localized to the base of the stalk structure conserved in large ribosomal subunits and mutational analysis has shown it to be essential [96]. Furthermore, rpP0 is one of the proteins reported to be cross-linked to EF2 in 80S ribosomes by bifunctional reagents [97]. Recent data from cryo-electron microscopy also demonstrated substantial interaction between EF2 and the stalk region of the 80S ribosomes [98]. Both genetic studies [94, 95] observed the requirement of ribosomes for high-affinity binding of sordarins to EF2, suggesting that sordarins are interfering with the interactions between EF2 and rpP0 within the ribosome. The authors indicate that the involvement of multiple elements in the translation machinery could explain the large selectivity of sordarins, even though individual components are highly conserved [94, 95].

To investigate further the activity and selectivity of sordarins, Domínguez et al. [99] evaluated a panel of sordarin derivatives for their ability to inhibit cell-free translation from five different pathogenic fungi (*C. albicans*, *C. glabrata*, *C. krusei*, *C. parapsilosis* and *C. neoformans*). The ability to inhibit protein synthesis in these organisms correlated well with inhibition of fungal growth and suggests that resistance to sordarins in specific organisms is due to intrinsic differences in the molecular target. Shastry et al. [100] isolated and expressed EF2s from various *Candida* species, including those sensitive and intrinsically resistant to sordarins, in *S. cerevisiae*. Results from *in vitro* translation and growth inhibition assays showed that residues in an 8-amino acid region (517–524), in particular residues 521, 523 and 524, within EF2 are responsible for the selectivity of this class of compounds [100]. The difference between *S. cerevisiae* and the human in the corresponding residues likewise accounts for the insensitivity of the human protein to sordarins, a conclusion that could not have been reached without the precise molecular details afforded by *S. cerevisiae*.

Investigations in *S. cerevisiae* have provided a deeper understanding of how two classes of antifungals exert their action and how fungi develop resistance against these agents. It is hoped that this information will help researchers develop novel antifungal therapeutics with a broader spectrum and higher selectivity. As more complete fungal genomes become available, *S. cerevisiae* is likely to serve as a useful model system because of the many experimental advantages associated with this well-studied organism.

4 Genomics and functional genomics

Discussions of the Human Genome Project started more than a decade ago and, in the beginning, the value of such a large-scale sequencing project was highly controversial. At the time, DNA sequencing technology and throughput were not advanced enough to support this seemingly enormous effort. Ultimately, a compromise plan was made to initiate pilot projects on the relatively small genomes of model organisms such as *E. coli* and *S. cerevisiae*, together with building comprehensive genetic and physical maps of the Human genome [101]. It was surmised that by performing similar processes on a scale smaller than that of the Human genome, the technology necessary for automated sequencing and computational analysis of genome information would either be refined or invented outright. The publication of the Human genome in early 2001 [22] is a testimony to the success of this approach. Sequencing technology advanced rapidly to the point that current automatic sequencing machines can easily generate up to a half million bases per day. Furthermore, the explosion of genomic sequences (over 40 complete bacterial, archaeal and eukaryotic genomes) has necessitated the accelerated development of new algorithms and software. Eventually, by performing systematic analyses on the genes and proteins in these model organisms, researchers intend to translate this information to the homologous human genes and proteins. Integration of sequence and functional data is the biggest barrier faced by scientists today and whole genome approaches are being devised to reduce this integration gap. *S. cerevisiae*, the first eukaryotic organism to be sequenced completely, was a milestone for the Human Genome Project and has continued to serve as a test bed for new genomics and functional genomics tools. In this review, I will discuss various tools and technologies spawned by the availability of the complete *Saccharomyces* sequence.

4.1 Bioinformatics and specialized databases for genomic scale projects

The complete 12 Mb-genome of *S. cerevisiae* defines around 6000 ORFs, of which an estimated one-third to one-half has no homology to known proteins. These "orphan" genes are incentives for developing new technologies to elucidate gene and protein functions. In order to accommodate and analyze the large number and volume of datasets generated from these systematic analyses, new algorithms and software are continually being developed. Numerous excellent reviews have addressed the development of bioinformatics tools for functional genomics and drug discovery that stemmed from yeast genomic research [102–105]. Specialized databases, such as both SGD [106, 107] and MIPS [108], provide access to the sequences as well as annotation and bioinformatics tools for analysis. Without these organized databases, it would be difficult to utilize this sequence resource for systematic functional analysis. In addition, YPD™, a curated proteome database for *S. cerevisiae*, is also an invaluable resource to the yeast research community [109].

MIPS served as the informatics center for the European yeast sequencing effort. Much information on the function of this well-studied organism has accumulated through decades of research on yeast genetics and cell biology, including codon adaptation bias, phenotypes of disruptants and motifs. Application of the classification scheme developed by Riley [110] to the yeast genome placed all ORFs into seven major and 173 minor classes [2]. The structural characteristics of all yeast ORFs are based on the comparison of sequences with known 3D structures. Secondary structure and transmembrane domain predictions were based on a computational algorithm [2]. These data sets are continuously updated with either new information or improved analysis tools. Recently, MIPS also incorporated data from systematic functional analysis projects such as EUROFAN, described in section 4.2 below.

The SGD provides access to the vast knowledge available for *Saccharomyces*, similarly to MIPS, and aims to disseminate this knowledge so researchers can efficiently exploit this information. SGD also serves as the yeast community's repository for gene nomenclature [107]. In the last two years, SGD extended its reach to protein structure and catalogued the comparison between the first two eukaryotic genomes sequenced, *S. cerevisiae* and *C. elegans* [5, 111]. Both the SGD and MIPS yeast databases were created around *S. cerevisiae*, but the software development and organization of these specialized databases have served as a model for similar databases for the metazoans.

The YPD™ is a curated proteome database for *S. cerevisiae* and consists of roughly 6000 protein reports, one for each predicted ORF with detailed descriptions of characterized proteins. All annotations in YPD™ are mined from the literature by trained curators who are yeast researchers [109] and YPD™ too has recently added systematic functional analysis data from various sources, transcriptional profiling and protein-protein interactions [112]. Furthermore, this database is also a model for the organization and presentation of comprehensive protein information. Proteome, Inc. followed YPD™ with PombePD™ and WormPD™ to provide the same kind of information on *S. pombe* and *C. elegans* [113]. There are plans to expand this database to encompass all fungi, including important fungal pathogens such as *C. albicans* and *A. fumigatus* to constitute the Fungal BioKnowledge™ Library [114].

4.2 Systematic functional genomics – the EUROFAN model

EUROFAN aims to elucidate the function of all novel genes contained in the Saccharomyces genome [115]. This network of laboratories evolved from the European sequencing consortium that contributed more than 60% of the yeast genomic sequence. The network is composed of research consortia that develop and perform genome-wide analysis, and of functional analysis nodes that conduct studies on specific areas of yeast biology based on the phenotype of the deletion strain [115]. MIPS coordinates and acts as the central database for all results. The network also has a genetic archive and stock center as a central depository for all molecular biology tools and yeast strains. In contrast to the European yeast community, no such coordinated effort of systematic analysis was made in North America. However, both sides of the Atlantic agreed that having a complete set of disruptants would be a valuable resource for the yeast research community [115, 116]. In August 2000, the international deletion consortium announced the completion of specific deletion strains for over 95% of the yeast ORFs and this resource is now available commercially through either Research Genetics or ATCC (American Type Culture Collection). Phenotypes of deletion strains are part of the information now available at MIPS [117]. Deletion strains have been mentioned numerous times before in this review, underscoring the importance of this resource not only to yeast researchers but also to those who use yeast as a model system for their studies. This set of deletion strains is also required for the haploinsufficiency analysis described in section 4.3.1 below.

4.3 Genome-wide transcript profiling

The completion of the genomic sequences of *S. cerevisiae* made available for the first time a comprehensive blueprint of a eukaryote. Even after decades of intensive study of this unicellular organism, on publication of the genome in 1996, functions for only a third to half of the genes were either previously characterized or derived from putative sequence homology. In order to explore the functions of the entire genome, new and systematic analyses need to be conducted. The genome-wide survey of gene expression pattern or function is one of the approaches that has been applied in the post-genomic age to fill the gap between gene and function. Numerous techniques were employed to evaluate gene expression on a genomic scale, including DNA microarrays, SAGE and GRM™.

SAGE has been applied to evaluate global gene expression during normal growth and cell cycle progression [118]. The technique and principles of SAGE were described in detail [119]. Briefly, SAGE requires the isolation of unique sequence tags from individual transcripts. DNA sequencing of the concatenated tags reveals the identity of individual tags and allows for identification and quantification of cellular transcripts. Importantly, the SAGE approach is not dependent on annotated ORFs, an advantage that led to a significant finding, the discovery of NORFs (nonannotated open reading frames). Because the yeast genome has been annotated for all ORFs larger than 300 bp, genes encoding proteins below this cutoff are not annotated, yet SAGE data suggested that there are approximately 160 NORF genes transcribed at a detectable level in the yeast genome. NORF genes might also be underrepresented in classical mutagenesis studies due to their small target size. The existence of NORFs has prompted yeast researchers to retune their sensitivity to small proteins and redesign DNA microarrays to include intergenic regions where potential NORF genes are located.

The GRM™ was previously mentioned in Section 2.2 as being utilized to evaluate the transcriptional response to inhibitors of sterol metabolism [49]. Based on gene expression patterns of mutants in the sterol metabolism pathway, results derived from GRM™ analysis are qualitatively comparable to those of the DNA microarray. The major difference between DNA microarrays and GRM™ is the construction of 6000-plus GFP-gene fusions for each of the ORFs in the yeast genome. These reporters are maintained in individual strains in a 96-well format. To obtain a gene expression profile for any compound, these arrays were exposed to the compound incorporated in a solid growth medium. After a defined period of growth, the arrays were scanned and the level of fluorescence from GFP is the measure of gene expression. One advantage of GRM™ over DNA microarrays is the minimal manual handling required that is conducive to high-throughput automation. On the other hand, to compare a mutant profile to that of the wild-type, the 6000-plus reporters will need to be introduced in the mutant strain for evaluation. Efficient transformation in *S. cerevisiae* can overcome this barrier easily though it is more challenging to apply this technology to other eukaryotic genomes. However, different innovative approaches that target the same problem are essential in the validation of any technology. Results are corroborated and limitations detected, helping researchers to make an educated choice on which tool to select for a specific biological question. The DNA microarray has emerged in the past few years from a variety of tools as the researchers' choice to initiate systematic functional genomics studies.

4.3.1 DNA microarrays

The basis of DNA microarrays is the universal and specific rules of nucleic acid base pairing. Membrane-supported arrays of nucleic acids, based on Southern's discovery, have been used for many years for biological experiments [120]. Recent technological advances have allowed miniaturization of nucleic acid arrays and much higher data throughput. Two basic DNA microarrays are commonly employed: the high-density arrays of oligonucleotides or complementary DNAs. The focus below is to illustrate the utility of DNA microarrays. For principles behind the construction of the two types of arrays, please refer to existing extensive reviews [121, 122].

The main advantage of DNA microarrays is their ability to measure every gene of the genome simultaneously, obviating the need for hypothesis-driven investigation. More often than not, analysis of microarray experimental results yielded discoveries that could not have been predicted from current knowledge. Many yeast DNA microarray studies focused on cellular processes that were heavily investigated in the past, including diauxic shift [123], transcription [124], mitotic cell cycle [125], sporulation [126], phosphate uptake [127] and responses to environmental stimuli [128]. Transcriptional changes occur in as many as 10–20% of all genes and only a fraction of these alterations have been characterized before.

Perhaps not surprisingly, the genes that respond dramatically to a given condition (i.e., with large changes in gene expression), are likely to be genes already linked to that specific process. Molecular geneticists focus their studies on genes with characteristically large and easily reproduced effects. More subtle gene expression changes are less detectable using conventional molecular genetics tools such as mutagenesis, and thus likely to be missed in these analyses resulting in incomplete understanding of any given process. Previous to the genome-wide survey of gene expression during sporulation, fifty genes were linked to or characterized as being involved in this important process. This number has now increased 10-fold with many new, uncharacterized genes that are potentially involved in the sporulation process. The temporal pattern of gene expression during sporulation is also delineated [126]. About one-third of the genes induced during sporulation peaked between 2 and 5 h after transfer into the sporulation medium, corresponding to the transition between two major stages of sporulation controlled by the transcription factor Ndt80p. The authors suggested that this transition may be governed by a recombination checkpoint to ensure that the meiotic prophase is complete before progressing to the next stage [126]. They also noted the similarity between yeast sporulation and human gametogenesis and predicted that many genes discovered in their analysis may have significant human homologs that could play similar roles in human gametogenesis.

Information harnessed from the DNA microarray study frequently generates hypotheses for further investigations needed to corroborate the microarray observations. Another example to demonstrate how DNA microarrays help elucidate the role of a protein with a hitherto unknown function is *SRB5* (suppressor of RNA polymerase B). A study designed to evaluate the requirement of key components in the transcriptional machinery revealed that deletion of *SRB5* adversely affected numerous genes in the pheromone response pathway, including those responsible for pheromone production and maturation, and the signal transduction circuitry [124]. On further investigation, *SRB5* was found to be necessary for mating in yeast, though *srb5* deletion mutants still mate at a low level, another surprise for a well-dissected pathway. Again subtle phenotypes seem to be missed in mutant hunts widely acknowledged to have achieved saturation. In another investigation of the phosphate uptake system in yeast, Ogawa et al. [127] identified 13 novel genes involved in this cellular process. They went on to demonstrate that five of these genes are involved in polyphosphate metabolism.

DNA microarrays are also useful in the identification of cis-regulatory elements or promoters required for transcriptional regulation. Promoters act as transducers, receiving signals from internal and external sources and responding by changing the level of transcription. Genes required in any given cellular process are transcribed in a coordinate manner by activating promoters upstream of the ORF and promoters of co-regulated genes often contain specific sequence motifs that correlate well with the gene expression pattern. The study of the mitotic cell cycle in yeast showed that those genes whose transcription peaks in the G1 phase of the cell cycle have an MCB (Mlu cell-cycle box) within 500 bp of their translational start site [125]. Similarly, Chu et al. [126] were able to identify MSE (middle gene sporulation element) sites in the immediate upstream regions of 70% of the genes whose induction peaks at the end of the meiotic prophase. The availability of complete genome sequences and large numbers of gene expression profiles, together with development of computational methodology, will accelerate the identification of novel regulatory elements not only in yeast but also in higher eukaryotes [129, 130].

Transcript profiling can also be considered as a phenotype in a genetics sense. In multiple yeast studies, profiles of mutant strains often differ from the wild-type strain and the differences are usually indicative of the mutant defect. Similarly, when yeast cells respond to external stimuli, such as a change in environment or exposure to drugs, specific gene expression changes occur that can be considered as transcriptional "fingerprints". If the gene expression pattern of a mutant correlates with that of a response to an external stimulus, the mutation and the external stimulus are likely to affect the same pathway. Extending this idea to drug discovery, if a drug specifically interacts with and inactivates a cellular target, the gene expression pattern of cells exposed to the drug should coincide with the profile of a mutant in which the specific target is inactivated. Furthermore, information on off-target effects, additional gene expression changes that are inconsistent with target inactivation, can be applied to improve drug specificity in an SAR. Recall the utility of the yeast expression profile study in identifying additional targets in the sterol metabolism pathway from section 2.2 [50]. Hughes et al. is cited here to demonstrate the power of the compendium in identifying drug targets [50].

The compendium is comprised of profiles from yeast deletion mutants and profiles of 13 well-characterized compounds. All profiles were performed under standard conditions to allow direct comparisons and to draw inferences with increased statistical confidence. The experimental design included 63 negative controls in which 2 untreated isogenic wild-type cultures were compared to each other. Data derived from the controls were used to delimit the "biological noise" of the study [50]. Hierarchical clustering was then conducted on all profiles to correlate clusters of profiles and transcripts with cellular functions. One of the compounds evaluated was dyclonine, a commonly used topical anaesthetic. The expression profile of dyclonine most closely resembled profiles resulting from perturbation of the ergosterol pathway, especially that of the *erg2* deletion mutant [50]. The authors also showed that a heterozygous yeast strain with one functional copy of *ERG2* (encoding sterol C-8 isomerase) is hypersensitive to dyclonine, whereas overexpression of *ERG2* confers resistance, indicating that *ERG2* is the cellular target of dyclonine. Based on sequence similarity between yeast *ERG2* and the human sigma receptor, the authors suggested that dyclonine binds the sigma receptor and inhibits nerve conductance by reducing potassium current, an interesting hypothesis that remains to be tested.

The approach can be extrapolated to examine drug specificity, namely whether pathways unrelated to the drug target were affected or not on challenge with the drug. Such an example occurred in the study conducted by Marton et al. [131] in which FK506, a clinically used immunosuppressant, was found to have secondary effects unrelated to its binding to immunophilins. Importantly, both these studies helped establish that genetic and pharmacological inhibition of gene function can result in extremely similar changes in gene expression, paving the way for similar studies to be conducted using arrays of human DNA. In fact, this type of experiment is anticipated in the near future with the recent publication of the first array of the entire Human genome [132].

The study by Hughes et al. [50] also demonstrated the power of the gene dosage effect in yeast. The dyclonine hypersensitivity of a strain having only one copy of the target gene renders this strain less fit to survive, compared to its wild-type counterpart, in the presence of the drug [50]. Giaever et al. took advantage of this haploinsufficiency phenotype and applied the method to identify MOAs for drugs [133]. At the point that the study was performed, systematic construction of heterozygous deletion strains in yeast was at its infancy. However, using 233 heterozygous strains, the Giaever study demonstrated the feasibility of this approach to encompass all 6000-plus strains when the strain construction is complete. Each of the 233 strains was uniquely tagged with a 20-base oligonucleotide "barcode", incorporated when the deletion strain was generated [134]. These unique barcodes allowed quantitative analysis of the relative abundance of each strain in the pool by hybridization of the amplified DNA tags to an oligonucleotide array. All 233 heterozygous strains were pooled and exposed to tunicamycin, a compound known to inhibit glycosylation in yeast. Over the course of 15 generations, three strains showed a significant decrease in population within the pool [133]. The three heterozygous strains had deletions of the known target of tunicamycin *ALG7* (asparagine-linked glycosylation), as well as two uncharacterized ORFs, *YMR266w* and *YMR007w*. *YMR266w* encodes a 953-aa protein with homology to the multi-facilitator superfamily that probably functions as a permease to export tunicamycin. *YMR007w* encodes a 126-aa protein of unknown function. Strains containing homozygous deletion of both *YMR007w* and *YMR266w* were still sensitive to tunicamycin, indicating that these genes are not the cellular targets of this drug. Again no prior knowledge of the target is required for the haploinsufficiency approach and only those targets that affect the fitness of the organism in the presence of the drug will be identified [133]. Off-target effects of the drugs would also be identified, similarly to the gene expression profile studies. In August 2000, the international consortium that generates deletion strains for all annotated yeast genes announced the completion of this effort at the Yeast Genetics and Molecular Biology Meeting. Description of the construction of deletion mutants was detailed in Winzeler et al. [135]. It is now possible to use all heterozygous yeast strains in a drug-induced haploinsufficeincy experiment.

DNA microarrays have been utilized to answer many different biological questions and new applications will undoubtedly be found. Applying the complete yeast genome as a test for this new technology provides validation of the tool and valuable information on yeast biology that is transferable to higher eukaryotes. Numerous examples in this section also showed that yeast could be used as a tool for classification of drugs and their mode of action.

4.4 Proteomics

Proteomics, the large-scale analysis of proteins, is a natural extension of large-scale sequencing and genomic scale transcript profiling. The avalanche of DNA sequences on hand does not translate to an understanding of the biological functions encoded by the sequences. Sequence homology is helpful in suggesting a function of a protein for which the homolog's role is characterized but assignments are usually limited to the molecular function and homology is usually insufficient to predict the cellular context in which the protein exerts its action. Moreover, one gene could encode multiple gene products arising from alternative splicing and post-translational modifications. Thus the proteome of an organism may have little linear relationship to its genome. Since proteins mediate most cellular processes that in turn ensure survival of the organism, the systematic study of proteins is an important key to unlocking the mystery of life. This is also important from a drug discovery viewpoint since most marketed drugs target proteins and their associated activities. New computational methods have been devised to provide a functional linkage of proteins [136]. Simultaneously, different technologies have been attempted to analyze proteins in a high-throughput fashion.

4.4.1 2D-PAGE and mass spectrometry

Historically, two-dimensional (2D) polyacrylamide gels have been used to display large numbers of proteins since the 1970s. The barriers to a systematic analysis of the proteome using 2D gels are lack of gel reproducibility and lack of rapid and sensitive techniques to analyze the resolved spots. In the last decade, biological mass spectrometry emerged as a powerful analytical tool for the high-throughput analysis of proteins and has eliminated some of the limitations of the 2D-PAGE. Futcher et al. examined the yeast proteome using 2D-PAGE and evaluated the abundance of 1400 visual spots [137]. They concluded that protein abundance has a broad dynamic range and admitted that with the technology available, they could only observe the most abundant proteins due to resolution limits of the 2D-PAGE. Gygi et al. confirmed the limitations of the 2D-PAGE technique in an extensive study to identify low abundance proteins [138]. They analyzed 50 spots migrating within a 4 cm^2 area and showed that the proteins all have codon bias values > 0.1. It is known that highly expressed proteins have large codon bias values, usually > 0.2. In the area of the gel that was analyzed, 57 proteins were predicted to be present based on sequence analysis (isoelectric point). Only 14 proteins were detected, none with a codon bias value < 0.1, even though more than one-half of yeast genes fall in this category. Through silver staining, the authors were also able to establish a lower visualization limit of 1000 copies of protein/cell. 2D-PAGE coupled with mass spectrometry identification is unsuited for analysis of low abundance proteins and its application in systematic proteomic analysis is likewise limited [138]. Recognizing the limitations of 2D-

PAGE, other technologies were developed to resolve proteins that directly feed into mass spectrometry for analysis.

Link et al. [139] coupled multidimensional chromatography and tandem mass spectrometry to analyze proteolytically digested purified yeast 80S ribosomes. The identities of the fragmented peptides were deduced by comparing the mass of peptides to the predicted masses of peptides generated from *in silico* digestions applied to genomic database sequences. The power of this approach was demonstrated in that it identified 75 of 78 predicted ribosomal proteins. The advantages of the direct mass spectrometry method are higher throughput due to automation, increased sensitivity for low abundance protein, and the availability of vastly expanded databases.

In a publication that expanded the use of this technology to the entire yeast genome, Washburn et al. demonstrated that this approach is appropriate for large-scale analysis of the proteome [140]. The yeast proteome was fractionated into 3 preparations (soluble, lightly washed insoluble and heavily washed insoluble) and analyzed as described above. Some 1484 proteins were detected and identified, including integral and peripheral membrane proteins. Closer scrutiny of the proteins revealed that the distribution of high and low abundance proteins so detected approximates that of the entire yeast genome. In addition, proteins with molecular weight > 180 kDa or isoelectric point > 10 were also detected and identified. As encouraging as the results are, the authors point out that this technology is not yet quantitative, an key attribute vital to drug discovery research. By applying these emerging proteomics technologies to the yeast proteome, we comprehend the limitations and advantages of each method and the need for improvement to tackle a much larger and complicated proteome like that of the human.

4.4.2 Transposon-tagged mutagenesis

In a pioneering publication before the complete yeast genome sequence was published, Burns et al. [80] demonstrated the power of utilizing transposon-mediated insertion mutagenesis to characterize the functions of yeast genes. The approach does not require prior knowledge of DNA sequence or annotated ORFs. Since the publication of the yeast genome in 1996, an improved and larger-scale analysis based on the same technique was detailed in Ross-Macdonald et al. [141]. To understand the rich information that could be derived from this technique, we need to discuss the various features of the mini-transposon and the phenotypes they exhibit when integrated into the genome.

The transposon contains a *lacZ* reporter gene that will result in β-galactosidase production in yeast only when the insertion is in-frame with the coding region of an expressed gene. Flanked by recombination sites, the transposon can be excised from the yeast gene, leaving behind a full-length, haemagglutinin (HA) epitope-tagged protein for immunolocalization with anti-HA antibodies. Unique DNA sequences present in the transposon were used to design primers for identifying the point of insertion in the yeast genome. The transposon also has *URA3* and *tet*^{R} genes as selection markers in yeast and bacteria, respectively.

Using high-throughput methods, Ross-Macdonald et al. generated over 11,000 strains that expressed the β-galactosidase reporter gene and, for 6,358 of these strains, the exact insertion sites were determined. More than 85% of the insertions occurred within annotated ORFs affecting 1,917 ORFs distributed over all 16 chromosomes of the yeast genome. Additionally, insertions were also detected in NORFs, some with repeated insertions. A mutant phenotype and a distinct localization pattern of disruption within NORFs verified the importance of NORFs in normal cellular functions. To analyze phenotypes on a genomic scale, the authors transformed over 7,000 insertion alleles into a haploid yeast strain and found that most gene disruptions due to the insertions were non-lethal. These mutants were then put through multiple phenotypic microarrays to look for growth phenotypes under different conditions. Application of the clustering algorithm to the data gathered from phenotypic analysis allowed the mutants to be classified into 21 groups. Not surprisingly, mutants involved in the same cellular process tended to cluster together. The function of an uncharacterized protein could thus be inferred from proteins belonging to the same cluster, similarly to the strategy adopted in large-scale DNA microarray analysis (Section 4.3.1). Further, immunolocalizations were carried out for 1,340 strains that have in-frame HA tags fused to the intact full-length protein. Discrete cellular localization was observed for 201 strains and an additional 214 strains showed cytoplasmic staining. Such data of a previously uncharacterized protein are again useful in generating a hypothesis for its biological role since co-localization is required for proteins to function as a unit in cells. In comparison to published DNA microarray data on sporulation [126], Ross-Macdonald et al. [141] observed that 14 out of 31 meiotic genes identified by the study indicated little or no induction in the microarray study. Evidence was given in the paper that two genes were indeed verified as being involved in meiosis.

One major obstacle to achieving saturation mutagenesis with this technique is the sheer number of insertions needed to cover the entire yeast genome, especially with small genes. It was estimated that 30,000 additional insertions in yeast ORFs would be required to mutagenize 90% of the yeast genome. This number is certainly within reach for a relatively small genome like yeast, but would be difficult to attain for the Human genome if similar technology were to be implemented. For yeast researchers, however, information derived from the Ross-Macdonald et al. study has given many investigators a jump-start for their favorite proteins and cellular pathways.

4.4.3 Biochemical genomics – GST-fusion proteins

Systematic functional analysis of proteins requires not only the identity of the polypeptides to be known, but also the association of biochemical activity with the proteins in a cellular context. Frequently, encoded activity detected by sensitive biochemical assays cannot be purified in sufficient quantity for detailed genetics or biochemical study. Martzen et al. came up with a new genomic strategy to identify yeast genes encoding any biochemical activity [142]. Briefly, the authors constructed an array of 6,144 individual yeast strains, each carrying a plasmid expressing a different GST-ORF fusion under control of a copper-inducible promoter. The array was then organized into 64 pools each containing 96 gene fusions. Fusion proteins were then purified from each of the 64 pools to be assayed for the desired biochemical activity. Deconvolution of the active pool was performed to identify the strain and the ORF responsible for the desired activity. In this manner, Martzen et al. were able to identify three previously unknown genes, a cytrochrome c methyltransferase, a cyclic phosphodiesterase and an uncharacterized processing activity involved in tRNA splicing [142]. Conventional purification of the cyclic phosphodiesterase from wild-type cells was carried out to confirm that the biochemical activity indeed associates with the ORF identified (*YGR247w*). Follow-up investigation of the cytochrome c methyltransferase activity also confirmed that *YHR109w* is responsible for the detected activity [143]. This method is both rapid (ORF-associated activity could be identified in 2 weeks time) and sensitive (highly expressed GST fusions with activities well above the intrinsic cellular level). On the other hand, limitations also exist for this technology. First, the GST fusions must be functional. The literature showed that in many instances N-terminal GST-fusions have a high probability of functionally complementing the corresponding genetic mutations. Second, overexpression of the GST-ORF must not be toxic to the cell, a condition frequently encountered with tightly regulated genes. Third, if other polypeptides are required for biochemical activity, such factors must have sufficient affinity to the GST-ORF to stay intact as a complex during the purification procedures. Fourth, this strategy relies on the comprehensive information on yeast ORFs. Unless a NORF is demonstrated to have some function through other analyses, the non-annotated ORFs will not be included in the array. In addition to the demonstrated application of this approach, the authors also suggested two other uses for this array, to identify potential protein substrates for any protein modification enzymes and to identify genes encoding proteins that bind any drug, ligand or macromolecule. The GST-fusion could also act as a handle for capturing protein complexes for subsequent mass spectrometry analysis to decipher protein-protein interactions.

As this array is being employed to solve biological questions in yeast, we will continue to learn from the successes and failures of this strategy in studying the proteome. The implementation of this strategy in systematic analysis of the human proteome is not likely to be limited by the number of GST-ORFs required to cover the genome (estimated at 30,000 from the recent publications) [21, 22] but rather by the ability of bioinformatics to generate a well-annotated set of ORFs [144].

4.4.4 Protein microarrays

Analogous to DNA microarrays, protein microarrays aim to facilitate the study of protein function by enabling the simultaneous processing of thousands of proteins. Two studies were published in late 2000 that describe the manufacture of high-density protein microarrays and their application for high throughput screening of protein biochemical activity [145, 146].

MacBeath and Schreiber immobilized proteins on chemically derivatized glass slides and showed that the proteins retained their functional capability through three different applications [145]. Protein-protein interaction was demonstrated between three pairs of proteins that are known to interact with each other. Protein kinases also showed the ability to specifically phosphorylate their cognate substrates and small molecules were found to bind their respective receptors with predicted affinities. Zhu et al. focused on the application of identifying protein substrates for predicted yeast protein kinases [146]. Out of the 122 potential protein kinases derived from the yeast genome, 119 were overexpressed and analyzed in this study. Instead of glass slides, proteins were covalently arrayed in microwells made of disposable silicone elastomer, poly(dimethylsiloxane) through the use of a crosslinker. The 119 protein kinases were assayed against 17 different polypeptide substrates, including the protein kinase itself, to look for autophosphorylation. Most kinases were able to phosphorylate at least one substrate but a few were not. Lack of activator in the purified fraction may contribute to the lack of *in vitro* kinase activity. One example given was Cdc28p, a cyclin-dependent kinase, which was not active in the assay, presumably due to the insufficient amount of activating cyclins. In another example, Hog1p was only found to be active in the assays after treatment of the cells with high salt before purification. Hog1p is the protein kinase involved in regulating osmolarity in yeast. One surprising finding of Zhu et al. is the ability of 27 protein kinases to phosphorylate a tyrosine-glutamate polymer *in vitro*. All protein kinases in yeast are classified as serine/threonine protein kinases, with the exception of two that are members of the histidine kinase family. Interestingly, in this study, the authors identified 27 potential tyrosine kinases. An independent study [147] confirmed that one of the putative tyrosine kinases identified, Rim11p, is indeed a bona fide tyrosine kinase phosphorylating a tyrosine residue on its *in vivo* substrate. The remaining kinases will require similar detailed studies to confirm that *in vitro* tyrosine kinase activity exhibited by these kinases is relevant for their functions *in vivo*.

Early development of protein microarrays has been slow primarily because proteins are easily denatured when placed on solid surfaces. This barrier seems to be removed in the studies described above. Undoubtedly, the technology will be applied to answer biological questions on a genomic scale, as DNA microarrays have come of age in the past few years.

4.4.5 Yeast two-hybrid analysis – global network of protein-protein interactions

Most biological functions arise from interactions among many components and proteins are no exception to this general principle. In order to understand the cellular processes, biologists have traditionally isolated and purified large protein complexes and analyzed them in detail. New technology such as mass spectrometry analysis helps in this effort considerably, as described above in the analysis of components in the 80S ribosome [139]. Many inferences could be made for an uncharacterized protein if it were to associate with characterized protein complexes. To complement this approach of reducing a complex to its constituents, the two-hybrid system is designed to identify protein partners, a pair at a time, to build up a complex network of protein-protein interactions.

The concept of yeast two-hybrid analysis was based on the fact that the functional DNA-binding domain (DB) and the transcription-activation domain (AD) need not be covalently attached for efficient activation of the promoter [148]. In the standard 2-hybrid analysis, the coding sequences of the DB and AD are cloned into separate vector molecules. The coding sequence of a candidate protein whose partners are sought (known as "bait") is fused in-frame with DB. A library of coding sequences for proteins that are potential partners with the bait (called "prey") is fused in-frame with AD. Bait and prey are maintained in yeast strains of opposite sexes and conjugation between these strains results in a diploid strain containing both bait and prey [149, 150]. The mating strategy facilitates high-throughput analysis using the 2-hybrid system. If the bait and the prey physically interact, DB and AD are brought in close proximity and the reconstituted transcription activator can turn on the reporter genes. Indirect interaction between bait and prey mediated by another cellular protein could also turn reporter genes on [151]. Recent improvements of the 2-hybrid system have increased the specificity of the assay by scoring phenotypes conferred by three different reporter genes in the same cell to eliminate promoter context-dependent false positives [151–153].

The advantages of the yeast 2-hybrid system are similar to other yeast-based techniques, namely powerful genetic selection coupled with the ability to screen a large number of sequences. The assay is performed in yeast cells and is thus not limited by artificial conditions imposed on an *in vitro* system. Since the assay is based on physical binding, it allows a wide variety of protein-protein interactions to be detected and characterized. One inherent requirement of the system is that neither the bait nor the prey may activate transcription on its own. The problem of membrane-anchored proteins being transported to and properly folded in the nucleus has also been noted. Another potential limitation is the failure of yeast cells to undergo various post-translational modifications required for particular interactions in higher organisms. Further details of the yeast 2-hybrid system and early examples of its application were reviewed by Vidal & Legrain [154].

The yeast 2-hybrid system has recently been applied to generate protein interaction maps for *S. cerevisiae* and *C. elegans* [155–157]. Ito et al. [155] cloned each of the yeast ORFs as both DB and AD fusions. These fusions were then pooled with 96 fusions per pool and 430 mating reactions between different pools were conducted representing ~ 10% of the total permutations possible. From this vast experiment, 866 positives resulted, of which 750 pairs yielded DNA sequence data to determine the identities of the fusion protein. The authors eliminated proteins that interacted with more than 3 unrelated partners and were left with 183 independent interactions. Only 12 of these interactions were previously known according to the annotations in YPD™ and an additional 32 were homotypic interactions, suggesting dimerization or oligomerization of these polypeptides. The authors suggested that among the remaining unknown interactions, 26 seem to be biologically relevant and thus likely to be interacting. The rest of the interactions were classified as novel, among them uncharacterized proteins interacting with proteins of known function, a starting point to generate testable hypotheses. More interestingly, the authors utilized the interaction data to construct interaction schemes and elaborated on the possibilities of deriving protein functions from such clusters with yeast vesicular transport as an example [155]. They cautioned researchers that interaction data should only be viewed as hypotheses until data from expression profiles, subcellular localization, genetics and other approaches corroborate or validate the inference.

Similarly, Uetz et al. [156] conducted an extensive screen of the yeast proteome and detected 957 putative interactions encompassing 1,004 yeast proteins. The authors likewise hypothesized the function of uncharacterized proteins based on their interaction partners and the cellular pathways these known proteins participate in, commonly known as the principle of guilt-by-association. An extension of this work incorporated all published interactions from the entire yeast community in addition to the two genomic scale datasets to comprise 2,709 putative interactions involving 2,039 proteins [158]. Their goal was to construct comprehensive interaction maps from the data. Surprisingly, only one large network of protein interactions was obtained, representing 2,358 links among 1,548 individual proteins. An additional 203 networks were derived and the majority had four or fewer proteins. The authors observed the presence of clusters within the large network that are related to the cellular roles of the proteins in a particular cluster. This observation again illustrates the power of guilt-by-association in assigning potential cellular roles to hitherto uncharacterized ORFs. Authors from all three studies [155, 156, 158] expressed both optimism and caution in the challenge ahead to scale up the 2-hybrid system for analysis of the human proteome. Uetz et al. [156] called for further comparison of datasets across species to identify conserved protein-protein interactions in an effort to decipher the large volume of interaction data anticipated by the research community.

Walhout et al. [159], in a review of the *C. elegans* interaction mapping effort, estimated that 45% of protein-protein interactions were not detected in their 2-hybrid system, suggesting that large-scale 2-hybrid analyses may only provide partial coverage of the protein-protein interactions within a given proteome. More comprehensive understanding of a given proteome appears likely to require the development, implementation and integration of data from several complementary approaches.

4.5 Metabolome

The last topic for review is the concept of the metabolome. In the last decade, the research community has moved from large-scale systematic analysis of the genome and transcriptome to the proteome, and now to the metabolome. The metabolome is defined as the complete set of metabolites (low-molecular-weight intermediates) in a cell, tissue or organ [160]. Transcription analysis was revolutionized by the availability of DNA microarrays screening large numbers of genes for mRNA abundance. The current state of proteomics is admittedly at an early stage of development because of the technical challenge presented by proteins, a much more diverse set of structures compared to DNA and mRNA. The metabolome, proteome and transcriptome are context-dependent such that the total complement of transcripts, proteins or metabolites varies according to changes in physiology and environment. In addition, both metabolites and proteins are functional entities within the cell. There are less than 600 metabolites, a number much lower than the 6000-or-so genes and proteins present in yeast. Thus there is no direct correlation between metabolite and gene in a way that there is for mRNAs and proteins.

Metabolomics, as a new field of functional genomics, is needed to elucidate roles of uncharacterized genes which, when mutated, failed to register an observable phenotype (a silent mutation). Raamsdonk et al. [161] reasoned that if the silent mutation is in a gene involved in metabolism, the cell must be able to bypass the block and utilize other pathways to compensate leaving no obvious change in overall flux through the system. However, changes in the use of metabolic pathways should result in measurable changes in intracellular metabolites. By comparing alterations in metabolite concentrations between the wild-type and the mutant, the authors hope to detect a phenotype for the mutation. They demonstrated the feasibility of this approach with a mutant strain containing a mutation in one of the genes encoding 6-phosphofructo-2-kinase (6PF-2-K). Deletion of either gene confers no detectable growth defect, but analysis of metabolites in the glycolysis pathway showed a clear increase in the intracellular concentration of the substrate, fructose-6-phosphate, a phenotype tying the mutant and the gene to a cellular role. Raamsdonk et al. has coined this approach FANCY, for functional analysis by co-responses in yeast. Three different physical methods were applied in FANCY and the integrated data resulted in an overall profile of the metabolites in the cell. Profiles of mutants containing defective genes involved in similar pathways are closely related and thus clustered as a group when compared to each other. As long as a gene with a known function is part of a cluster, functions of other genes may be inferred. Ideally, to elucidate the function of an uncharacterized gene, the metabolite profile of a mutant would be compared to a library of such profiles generated by individually deleting genes of known function. This library does not yet exist but with the availability of all single-ORF deletion mutants available, the feasibility of this approach could be determined in the near future. This technology provides much potential in assigning cellular roles to the vast number of genes that have no known homologs.

5 Conclusion

From the days of classical genetics to the present genomic and post-genomic age, *Saccharomyces cerevisiae* has served the role of a model organism with amazing resilience. Interest in this organism has not waned, making it one of the most investigated organisms. In the past thirty years, many techniques were developed to understand how yeast cells function on a molecular level. Novel concepts and information derived from these studies have not only aided our understanding of this eukaryote but also helped establish a framework for drug discovery research on fungal pathogens and higher eukaryotes.

Budding yeast also has the distinction of being the first eukaryote to have its complete genome sequenced, reinforcing the biological importance placed on this unicellular eukaryote. Mobilization and coordination of laboratories worldwide were required to accomplish this feat and eventually the concept of the sequencing consortium was applied to many large-scale sequencing projects, including the Human Genome Project. The availability of the complete genome sequence led to another explosion of research on this simple organism aimed at systematically deciphering the roles of all genes within the genome. This lofty goal is a powerful incentive for yeast researchers and technologists alike to cooperate in search of new and high-throughput tools, essential tools for efficient and economical drug discovery.

Within the last five years, tremendous effort has resulted in the invention of tools such as novel algorithms and software for analyzing and visualizing genomic data, DNA microarrays, protein arrays and many more. By virtue of the relatively small genome size and the availability of a vast array of conventional validation tools, yeast continues to be the organism of choice to validate new technologies. In some instances, validations conducted using the yeast genome have indicated limitations of the technology, requiring significant retooling. Recognition of severe limitations also led to development of new tools to either complement shortcomings or to replace existing tools. Such knowledge is essential to scale up the effort required to tackle the much larger Human genome. Intensive research in this area will continue to provide yeast researchers with an ever increasing number of avenues to explore this simple organism in hopes that, one day, they can describe in molecular detail the mystery of life not only for *S. cerevisiae* but for the human as well. Understanding the complex molecular circuitry required for correct execution of cellular processes will aid the pharmaceutical industry in selecting the most appropriate targets for the amelioration of disease. Additionally, the holistic view of humans generated through genomic approaches will increase our awareness of potential off-target effects and may help to minimize side-effects associated with a given therapeutic agent.

References

1 A. Goffeau, B.G. Barrell, H. Bussey, R.W. Davis, B. Dujon, H. Feldmann, F. Galibert, J.D. Hoheisel, C. Jacq, M. Johnston et al.: Science *274*, 546 (1996).

2 H.W. Mewes, K. Albermann, M. Bahr, D. Frishman, A. Gleissner, J. Hani, K. Heumann, K. Kleine, A. Maierl, S.G. Oliver et al.: Nature *387* (suppl), 7 (1997).

3 A.R. Mushegian, D.E. Bassett Jr., M.S. Boguski, P. Bork and E.V. Koonin: Proc. Natl. Acad. Sci. USA *94*, 5831 (1997).

4 The *C. elegans* Sequencing Consortium: Science *282*, 2012 (1998).

5 S.A. Chervitz, L. Aravind, G. Sherlock, C.A. Ball, E.V. Koonin, S.S. Dwight, M.A. Harris, K S. Dolinski, S. Mohr, T. Smith et al.: Science *282*, 2022 (1998).

6 M.D. Adams, S.E. Celniker, R.A. Holt, C.A. Evans, J.D. Gocayne, P.G. Amanatides, S.E. Scherer, P.W. Li, R.A. Hoskins, R.F. Galle et al.: Science *287*, 2185 (2000).

7 G.M. Rubin, M.D. Yandell, J.R. Wortman, G.L.G. Miklos, C.R. Nelson, I.K. Hariharan, M.E. Fortini, P.W. Li, R. Apweiler, W. Fleischmann et al.: Science *287*, 2204 (2000).

8 M.C. Hensing, R.J. Rouwenhorst, J.J. Heijnen, J.P. van Dijken and J.T. Pronk: Antonie Van Leeuwenhoek *67*, 261 (1995).

9 G. Gellissen and C.P. Hollenberg: Gene *190*, 87 (1997).

10 A. Dominguez, E. Ferminan, M. Sanchez, F.J. Gonzalez, F.M. Perez-Campo, S. Garcia, A.B. Herrero, A. San Vicente, J. Cabello, M. Prado et al.: Int. Microbiol. *1*, 131 (1998).

11 G.P.L. Cereghino and J.M. Cregg: Curr. Opin. Biotechnol. *10*, 422 (1999).

12 J.L. Cereghino and J.M. Cregg: FEMS Microbiol. Rev. *24*, 45 (2000).

13 S. Ostergaard, L. Olsson and J. Nielsen: Microbiol. Mol. Biol. Rev. *64*, 34 (2000).

14 K. King, H.G. Dohlman, J. Thorner, M.G. Caron and R.J. Lefkowitz: Science *250*, 121 (1990).

15 L.A. Price, E.M. Kajkowski, J.R. Hadcock, B.A. Ozenberger and M.H. Pausch: Mol. Cell. Biol. *15*, 6188 (1995).

16 J.R. Broach and J. Thorner: Nature *384* (Suppl.), 14 (1996).

17 E.M. Kajkowski, L.A. Price, M.H. Pausch, K.H. Young and B.A. Ozenberger: J Receptor & Signal Transduction Res. *171*, 293 (1997).

18 J.R. Erickson, J.J. Wu, J.G. Goddard, G. Tigy, K. Kawanishi, L.D. Tomei and M.C. Kiefer: J. Biol. Chem. *273*, 1506 (1998).

19 C. Klein, J.I. Paul, K. Sauve, M.M. Schmidt, L. Arcangeli, J. Ransom, J. Trueheart, J.P. Manfredi, J.R. Broach and A.J. Murphy: Nat. Biotechnol. *16*, 1334 (1998).

20 M.J. Cismowski, A. Takesono, C. Ma, J.S. Lizano, X. Xie, H. Fuernkranz, S.M. Lanier and E. Duzic: Nat. Biotechnol. *17*, 878 (1999).

21 J.C. Venter, M.D. Adams, E.W. Myers, P.W. Li, R.J. Mural, G.G. Sutton, H.O. Smith, M. Yandell, C.A. Evans, R.A. Holt et al.: Science *291*, 1304 (2001).

22 International Human Genome Sequencing Consortium (IHGSC): Nature *409*, 860 (2001).
23 J.R. Riordan, J.M. Rommens, B. Kerrem, N. Alon, R. Rozmahel, Z. Grzelczak, J. Zielenski, S. Lok, N. Plavsic, J.L. Chou et al.: Science *245*, 1066 (1989).
24 P. Chien and J.S. Weissman: Nature *410*, 223 (2001).
25 M. Aebl and T. Hennet: Trends Cell Biol. *11*, 136 (2001).
26 D.A. Sinclair, K. Mills and L. Guarente: Science *277*, 1313 (1997).
27 H. Cohen and D.A. Sinclair: Proc. Natl. Acad. Sci. USA *98*, 3174 (2001).
28 W.M. Fricke, V. Kaliraman and S.J. Brill: J. Biol. Chem. *276*, 8848 (2001).
29 A.W. Murray and D. Marks: Nature *409*, 844 (2001).
30 P. Nurse: Cell *100*, 71 (2000).
31 L.H. Hartwell, R.K. Mortimer, J. Culotti and M. Culotti: Genetics *74*, 267 (1973).
32 L.H. Hartwell and T. Weinert: Science *246*, 629 (1989).
33 K. Wassmann and R. Benezra: Curr. Opin. Genet. Dev. *11*, 83 (2001).
34 R.D. Gardner and D.J. Burke: Trends Cell Biol. *10*, 154 (2000).
35 M.A. Hoyt, L. Totis and B.T. Roberts: Cell *66*, 507 (1991).
36 D.P. Cahill, C. Lengauer, J. Yu, G.J. Riggins, J.K.V. Willson, S.D. Markowitz, K.W. Kinzler and B. Vogelstein: Nature *392*, 300 (1998).
37 S.S. Taylor and F. McKeon: Cell *89*, 727 (1997).
38 B.T. Roberts, K.A. Farr and M.A. Hoyt: Mol. Cell Biol. *14*, 8282 (1994).
39 H. Lee, A.H. Trainer, L.S. Friedman, F.C. Thistlethwaite, M.J. Evans, B.A.J. Ponder and A.R. Venkitaraman: Mol. Cell *4*, 1 (1999).
40 L.S. Michel, V. Liberal, A. Chatterjee, R. Kirchwegger, B. Pasche, W. Gerald, M. Dobles, P.K. Sorger, V.V.V.S. Murty and R. Benezra: Nature *409*, 355 (2001).
41 J.A. Simon, P. Szankasi, D.K. Nguyen, C. Ludlow, H.M. Dunstan, C.J. Roberts, E.L. Jensen, L.H. Hartwell and S.H. Friend: Cancer Res. *60*, 328 (2000).
42 F. Cross, M. Yuste-Rojas, S. Gray and M. Jacobson: Mol. Cell *4*, 11 (1999).
43 V. Doye and E.C. Hurt: Trends Genet *11*, 235 (1995).
44 L.H. Hartwell, P. Szankasi, C.J. Roberts, A.W. Murray and S.H. Friend: Science *278*, 1064 (1997).
45 A.W. Alberts, J. Chen, G. Kuron, V. Hunt, J. Huff, C. Hoffman, J. Rothrock, M. Lopez, H. Joshua, E. Harris et al.: Proc. Natl. Acad. Sci. USA *77*, 3957 (1980).
46 J. Rine, W. Hansen, E. Hardeman and R.W. Davis: Proc. Natl. Acad. Sci. USA *80*, 6750 (1983).
47 M.E. Basson, M. Thorsness, J. Finer-Moore, R.M. Stroud and J. Rine: Mol. Cell Biol. *8*, 3797 (1988).
48 S.L. Sturley: Biochim. Biophys. Acta *1529*, 155 (2000).
49 D. Dimster-Denk, J. Rine, J. Phillips, S. Scherer, P. Cundiff, K. DeBord, D. Gilliland, S. Hickman, A. Jarvis, L. Tong and M. Ashby: J. Lipid Res. *40*, 850 (1999).
50 T.R. Hughes, M.J. Marton, A.R. Jones, C.J. Roberts, R. Stoughton, C.D. Armour, H.A. Bennett, E. Coffey, H. Dai, Y.D. He et al.: Cell *102*, 109 (2000).
51 D. Gachotte, J. Eckstein, R. Barbuch, T. Hughes, C. Roberts and M. Bard: J. Lipid Res. *42*, 150 (2001).
52 D. Gachotte, R. Barbuch, J. Gaylor, E. Nickel and M. Bard: Proc. Natl. Acad. Sci. USA *95*, 13794 (1998).
53 M.B. Edmond, S.E. Wallace, D.K. McClish, M.A. Pfaller, R.N. Jones and R.P. Wenzel: Clin. Infect. Dis. *29*, 239 (1999).

54 M.J. Richards, J.R. Edward, D.H. Culver and R.P. Gaynes: Crit. Care Med. *27*, 887 (1999).
55 J.M. Wallace, R. Lim, B.L. Browdy, P.C. Hopewell, J. Glassroth, M.J. Rosen, L.B. Reichman and P.A. Kvale: Chest *114*, 131 (1998).
56 C. Viscoli, C. Girmenia, A. Marinus, L. Collette, P. Martino, B. Vandercam, C. Doyen, B. Lebeau, D. Spence, V. Krcmery et al.: Clin. Infect. Dis. *28*, 1071 (1999).
57 E.A. Wills, M.R. Redinbo, J.R. Perfect and M. Del Poeta: Emerg. Ther. Targets *4*, 1 (2000).
58 M.D. De Backer, P.T. Magee and J. Pla: Annu. Rev. Microbiol. *54*, 463 (2000).
59 C. Seoighe, N. Federspiel, T. Jones, N. Hansen, V. Bivolarovic, R. Surzycki, R. Tamse, C. Komp, L. Huizar, R.W. Davis et al.: Proc. Natl. Acad. Sci. USA *97*, 14433 (2000).
60 K.W. Tzung, R.M. Williams, S. Scherer, N. Federspiel, T. Jones, N. Hansen, V. Bivolarevic, L. Huizar, C. Komp, R. Surzycki et al.: Proc. Natl. Acad. Sci. USA *98*, 3249 (2001).
61 G. Daum, N.D. Lees, M. Bard and R.T. Dickson: Yeast *14*, 1471 (1998).
62 N.S. Ryder: Biochem. Soc. Trans. *19*, 774 (1991).
63 R.I. Baloch and E.I. Mercer: Phytochemistry *26*, 663 (1987).
64 D. Abi-Said, E. Anaissie, O. Uzon, I. Raad, H. Pinzcowski and S. Vartivarian: Clin. Infect. Dis. *24*, 1122 (1997).
65 M.F. Price, M.T. LaRocco and L.O. Gentry: Antimicrob. Agents Chemother. *38*, 1422 (1994).
66 D. Sanglard, K. Kuchler, F. Ischer, J.L. Pagani, M. Monod and J. Bille: Antimicrob. Agents Chemother. *39*, 2378 (1995).
67 K. Venkateswarlu, D.W. Denning, N.J. Manning and S.L. Kelly: FEMS Microbiol. Lett. *131*, 337 (1995).
68 N.D. Lees, F.W. Kleinhans, M.C. Broughton, D.E. Pennington, V.A. Ricker and M. Bard: Steroids *53*, 567 (1989).
69 C.A. Hitchcock, K.J. Barrett-Bee and N.J. Russell: J. Med. Vet. Mycol. *25*, 329 (1987).
70 P.F. Watson, M.E. Rose, S.W. Ellis, H. England and S.L. Kelly: Biochem. Biophys. Res. Commun. *164*, 1170 (1989).
71 V.F. Kalb, C.W. Woods, T.G. Turi, C.R. Dey, T.R. Sutter and J.C. Loper: DNA 6, 529 (1987).
72 D.R. Kirsch, M.H. Lai and J. O'Sullivan: Gene *68*, 229 (1988).
73 M. Stromstedt, D. Rozman and M.R. Waterman: Arch. Biochem. Biophys. *329*, 73 (1996).
74 D.C. Lamb, D.E. Kelly, W.H. Schunck, A.Z. Shyadehi, M. Akhtar, D.J. Lowe, B.C. Baldwin and S.L. Kelly: J. Biol. Chem. *272*, 5682 (1997).
75 H. Kakeya, Y. Miyazaki, H. Miyazaki, K. Nyswaner, B. Grimberg and J.E. Bennett: Antimicrob. Agents Chemother. *44*, 2985 (2000).
76 D.C. Lamb, D.E. Kelly, B.C. Baldwin and S.L. Kelly: Chem. Biol. Interact. *125*, 165 (2000).
77 S.L. Kelly, D.C. Lamb, B.C. Baldwin, A.J. Corran and D.E. Kelly: J. Biol. Chem. 15, 9986 (1997).
78 P.F. Watson, M.E. Rose and S.L. Kelly: J. Med. Vet. Mycol. *26*, 153 (1988).
79 Y. Miyazaki, A. Gerber, H. Miyazaki, D. Falconer, T. Parkinson, C. Hitchcock, B. Grimberg, K. Nyswaner and J.E. Bennett: Gene *236*, 43 (1999).
80 N.B. Burns, P.B. Grimwade, E.Y. Ross-Macdonald, K. Choi, K. Finbery, G.S. Roeder and M. Snyder: Genes Dev. *8*, 1087 (1994).
81 D.P. Kontoyiannis: Antimicrob. Agents Chemother. *43*, 2731 (1999).
82 E. Balzi, M. Wang, S. Leterme, L. Van Dyck and A. Goffeau: J. Biol. Chem. *269*, 2206 (1994).
83 A. Kolaczkowska and A. Goffeau: Drug Resistance Update *2*, 403 (1999).

84 J. DeRisi, B. van den Hazel, P. Marc, E. Balzi, P. Brown, C. Jacq and A. Goffeau: FEBS Lett. *470*, 156 (2000).
85 D. Hauser and H.P. Sigg: Helv. Chim. Acta *54*, 1178 (1971).
86 S.J. Coval, M.S. Puar, D.W. Phife, J.S. Terracciano and M. Patel: J. Antibiot. (Toyko) *48*, 1171 (1995).
87 O.S. Kinsman, P.A. Chalk, H.C. Jackson, R.F. Middleton, A. Shuttleworth, B.A.M. Rudd, C.A. Jones, H.M. Noble, H.G. Wildman, M.J. Dawson et al.: J. Antibiot. (Tokyo) *51*, 41 (1998).
88 E. Herreros, C.M. Martinez, M.J. Almela, M.S. Marriott, F. Gómez de las Heras and D. Gargallo-Viola: Antimicrob. Agents Chemother. *42*, 2863 (1998).
89 J.M. Domínguez and J. J. Martín: Antimicrob. Agents Chemother. 42, 2279 (1998).
90 G.P. Belfield and M.F. Tuite: Mol. Microbiol. *9*, 411 (1993).
91 J.P. Parenthesis, L.D. Phan, W.R. Gleason, D.C. LaPorte, D.M. Livingston and J.W. Bodley: J. Biol. Chem. *267*, 1190 (1992).
92 L. Capa, A. Mendoza, J.L. Lavandera, F. Gómez de las Heras and J.F. García-Bustos: Antimicrob. Agents Chemother. *42*, 2694 (1998).
93 M.C. Justice, M.J. Hsu, B. Tse, T. Ku, J. Balkovec, D. Schmatz and J. Nielsen: J. Biol. Chem. *273*, 3148 (1998).
94 M.G. Gómez-Lorenzo and J.F. García-Bustos: J. Biol. Chem. *273*, 25041 (1998).
95 M.C. Justice, T. Ku, M.J. Hsu, K. Carniol, D. Schmatz and J. Nielsen: J. Biol. Chem. *274*, 4869 (1999).
96 M. Remacha, A. Jimenez-Diaz, C. Santos, E. Briones, R. Zambrano, M.A. Rodriguez-Gabriel, E. Guarinos and J.P.G. Ballesta: Biochem. Cell Biol. *73*, 959 (1995).
97 T. Uchiumi, M. Kikuchi and K. Ogata: J. Biol. Chem. *261*, 9663 (1986).
98 M.G. Gómez-Lorenzo, C.M.T. Spahn, R.K. Agrawal, R.A. Grassucci, P. Penczek, K. Chakraburtty, J.P.G. Ballesta, J.L. Lavandera, J.F. García-Bustos and J. Frank: EMBO J. *19*, 2710 (2000).
99 J.M. Domínguez, V.A. Kelly, O.S. Kinsman, M.S. Marriott, F. Gómez de las Heras and J.J. Martín: Antimicrob. Agents Chemother. *42*, 2274 (1998).
100 M. Shastry, J.Nielsen, T. Ku, M.J. Hsu, P. Liberator, J. Anderson, D. Schmatz and M.C. Justice: Microbiology *147*, 383 (2001).
101 B.M. Alberts, D. Botstein, S. Brenner, C.R. Cantor, R.F. Doolittle, L. Hood, V.A. McKusick, D. Nathans, M.V. Olson, S. Orkin et al.: Report of the Committee on Mapping and Sequencing the Human Genome, National Academy Press, Washington D.C. 1988.
102 D.B. Searls: Drug Discovery Today *5*, 135 (2000).
103 P.D. Karp, M. Krummenacker, S. Paley and J. Wagg: Trends Biotechnol. *17*, 275 (1999).
104 E.V. Koonin, L. Aravind and A.S. Kondrashov: Cell *101*, 573 (2000).
105 M.Y. Galperin and E.V. Koonin: Nature Biotechnol. *18*, 609 (2000).
106 K. Dolinski, C.A. Ball, S.A. Chervitz, S.S. Dwight, M.A. Harris, S. Roberts, T. Roe, J.M. Cherry and D. Botstein: Yeast *14*, 1453 (1998).
107 J.M. Cherry, C. Adler, C. Ball, S.A. Chervitz, S.S. Dwight, E.T. Hester, Y. Jia, G. Juvik, T. Roe, M. Schroeder et al.: Nucl. Acids Res. *26*, 73 (1998).
108 H.W. Mewes, K. Albermann, K. Heumann, S. Liebl and F. Pfeiffer: Nucl. Acids Res. *25*, 28 (1997)
109 P.E. Hodges, W.E. Payne and J.I. Garrels: Nucl. Acids Res. *26*, 68 (1998).
110 M. Riley: Microbiol. Rev. *57D*, 862 (1993).

111 S.A. Chervitz, E.T. Hester, C.A. Ball, K. Dolinski, S.S. Dwight, M.A. Harris, G. Juvik, A. Malekian, S. Roberts, T. Roe et al.: Nucl. Acids Res. *27*, 74 (1999).

112 P.E. Hodges, A.H. McKee, B.P. Davis, W.E. Payne and J.I. Garrels: Nucl. Acids Res. *27*, 69 (1999).

113 M.C. Constanzo, J.D. Hogan, M.E. Cusick, B.P. Davis, A.M. Fancher, P.E. Hodges, P. Kondu, C. Lengieza, J.E. Lew-Smith, C. Lingner et al.: Nucl. Acids Res. *28*, 73 (2000).

114 M.C. Constanzo, M.E. Crawford, J.E. Hirschman, J.E. Kranz, P, Olsen, L.S. Robertson, M.S. Skrzypek, B.R. Braun, K.L. Hopkins, P. Kondu et al.: Nucl. Acids Res. *29*, 75 (2001).

115 S. Oliver: Trends Genet. *12*, 241 (1996).

116 M. Johnston: Trends Genet. *12*, 242 (1996).

117 H.W. Mewes, D. Frishman, C. Gruber, B. Geier, D. Haase, A. Kaps, K. Lemcke, G. Mannhaupt, F. Pfeiffer, C. Schüller et al.: Nucl. Acids Res. *28*, 37 (2000).

118 V.E. Velculescu, L. Zhang, W. Zhou, J. Vogelstein, M.A. Basrai, D.E. Bassett Jr., P. Hieter, B. Vogelstein and K.W. Kinzler: Cell *88*, 243 (1997).

119 V.E. Velculescu, L. Zhang, B. Vogelstein and K.W. Kinzler: Science *270*, 484 (1995).

120 E.M. Southern: J. Mol. Biol. *98*, 503 (1975).

121 D.J. Lockhart and E.A. Winzeler: Nature *405*, 827 (2000).

122 P.O. Brown and D. Botstein: Nature Genet. *21* (Suppl.), 33 (1999).

123 J.L. DeRisi, V.R. Iyer and P.O. Brown: Science *278*, 680 (1997).

124 F.C.P. Holstege, E.G. Jennings, J.J. Wyrick, T.I. Lee, C.J. Hengartner, M. R. Green, T.R. Golub, E.S. Lander and R.A. Young: Cell *95*, 717 (1998).

125 R.J. Cho, M.J. Campbell, E.A. Winzeler, L. Steinmetz, A. Conway, L. Wodicka, T.G. Wolfsberg, A.E. Gabrielian, D. Landsman, D.J. Lockhart et al.: Mol. Cell *2*, 65 (1998).

126 S. Chu, J. DeRisi, M. Eisen, J. Mullholland, D. Botstein, P.O. Brown and I. Herskowitz: Science *282*, 699 (1998).

127 N. Ogawa, J. DeRisi and P.O. Brown: Mol. Biol. Cell *11*, 4309 (2000).

128 A.P. Gasch, P.T. Spellman, C.M. Kao, O. Carmel-Harel, M.B. Eisen, G. Storz, D. Botstein and P.O. Brown: Mol. Biol. Cell *11*, 4241 (2000).

129 J.W. Fickett and W.W. Wasserman: Curr. Opin. Biotechnol. *11*, 19 (2000).

130 P. Bucher: Curr. Opin. Struct. Biol. *9*, 400 (1999).

131 M.J. Marton, J.L. DeRisi, H.A. Bennett, V. R. Iyer, M.R. Meyer, C.J. Roberts, R. Stoughton, J. Burchard, D. Slade, H. Dai et al.: Nature Med. *4*, 1293 (1998).

132 D.D. Shoemaker, E.E. Schadt, C.D. Armour, Y.D. He, P. Garrett-Engele, P.D. McDonagh, P.M. Loerch, A. Leonardson, P.Y. Lum, G. Cavet et al.: Nature *409*, 922 (2001).

133 G. Giaever, D.D. Shoemaker, T.W. Jones, H. Liang, E.A. Winzeler, A. Astromoff and R.W. Davis: Nature Genet. *21*, 278 (1999).

134 D.D. Shoemaker, D.A. Lashkari, D. Morris, M. Mittmann and R.W. Davis: Nature Genet. *14*, 450 (1996).

135 E. A. Winzeler, D.D. Shoemaker, A. Astromoff, H. Liang, K. Anderson, B. Andre, R. Bangham, R. Benito, J.D. Boeke, H. Bussey et al.: Science *285*, 901 (1999).

136 D. Eisenberg, E.M. Marcotte, I. Xenarios and T.O. Yeates: Nature *405*, 823 (2000)

137 B. Futcher, G.I. Latter, P. Monardo, C.S. McLaughlin and J.I. Garrels: Mol. Cell Biol. *19*, 7357 (1999).

138 S.P. Gygi, G.L. Corthals, Y. Zhang, Y. Rochon and R. Aebersold: Proc. Natl. Acad. Sci. USA *97*, 9390 (2000).

139 A.J. Link, J. Eng, D.M. Schietz, E. Carmack, G.J. Mize, D.R. Morris, B.M. Garvik and J.R. Yates, III: Nature Biotechnol. *17*, 676 (1999).

140 M.P. Washburn, D. Wolters, J.R. Yates, III: Nature Biotechnol. *19*, 242 (2001).
141 P. Ross-Macdonald, P.S.R. Coelho, T. Roemer, S. Agarwal, A. Kumar, R. Jansen, K.H. Cheung, A. Sheehan, D. Symoniatis, L. Umansky et al.: Nature *402*, 413 (1999).
142 M.R. Martzen, S.M. McCraith, S.L. Spinelli, F.M. Torres, S. Fields, E.J. Grayhack and E.M. Phizicky: Science *286*, 1153 (2000).
143 B. Polevoda, M.R. Martzen, B. Das, E.M. Phizicky and F. Sherman: J. Biol. Chem. *275*, 20508 (2000).
144 E. Birney, A. Bateman, M.E. Clamp and T.J. Hubbard: Nature *409*, 827 (2001).
145 G. MacBeath and S.L. Schreiber: Science *289*, 1760 (2000).
146 H. Zhu, J.F. Klemic, S. Chang, P. Bertone, A. Casamayor, K.G. Klemic, D. Smith, M. Gerstein, M.A. Reed and M. Snyder: Nature Genet. *26*, 283 (2000).
147 K. Malathi, Y. Xiao and A.P Mitchell: Genetics *153*, 1145 (1999).
148 S. Fields and O. Song: Nature *340*, 245 (1989).
149 C. Bendixen, S. Gangloff and R. Rothstein: Nucl. Acids Res. *22*, 1778 (1994).
150 M. Fromont-Racine, J.C. Rain and P. Legrain: Nature Genet. *16*, 277 (1997).
151 P. Bartel C.T. Chien, R. Sternglanz and S. Fields: BioTechniques *14*, 920 (1993).
152 M. Vidal, in: P.L. Bartel and S. Fields (eds): The Yeast Two-Hybrid System, Oxford University Press, New York, NY 1997, 109.
153 P. James, J. Halladay and E.A. Craig: Genetics *144*, 1425 (1996).
154 M. Vidal and P. Legrain: Nucl. Acids Res. *27*, 919 (1999).
155 T. Ito, K. Tashiro, S. Muta, R. Ozawa, T. Chiba, M. Nishizawa, K. Yamamoto, S. Kuhara and Y. Sakaki: Proc. Natl. Acad. Sci. USA *97*, 1143 (2000).
156 P. Uetz, L. Giot, G. Cagney, T.A. Mansfield, R.S. Judson, J.R. Knight, D. Lockshon, V. Narayan, M. Srinivasan, P. Pochart et al.: Nature *403*, 623 (2000).
157 A.J.M. Walhout, R. Sordella, X. Lu, J.L. Hartley, G.F. Temple, M.A. Brasch, N. Thierry-Mieg and M. Vidal: Science *287*, 116 (2000).
158 B. Schwikowski, P. Uetz and S. Fields: Nature Biotechnol. *18*, 1257 (2000).
159 A.J.M. Walhout, S.J. Boulton and M. Vidal: Yeast *17*, 88 (2000).
160 S.G. Oliver, M.K. Winson, D.B. Kell and F. Baganz: Trends Biotechnol. *16*, 373 (1998).
161 L.M. Raamsdonk, B. Teusink, D. Broadhurst, N. Zhang, A. Hayes, M.C. Walsh, J.A. Berden, K.M. Brindle, D.B. Kell, J.J. Rowland et al.: Nat. Biotechnol. *19*, 45 (2001).

Progress in Drug Research, Vol. 57 (E. Jucker, Ed.)

Sympathetic nervous system and experimental diabetes: role of adrenal medullary hormones

By Chaman Lal Kaul
and Poduri Ramarao

Department of Pharmacology & Toxicology
National Institute of Pharmaceutical Education and Research
S.A.S. Nagar (Mohali)
Punjab 160 062, India

<kaulniper@yahoo.com>

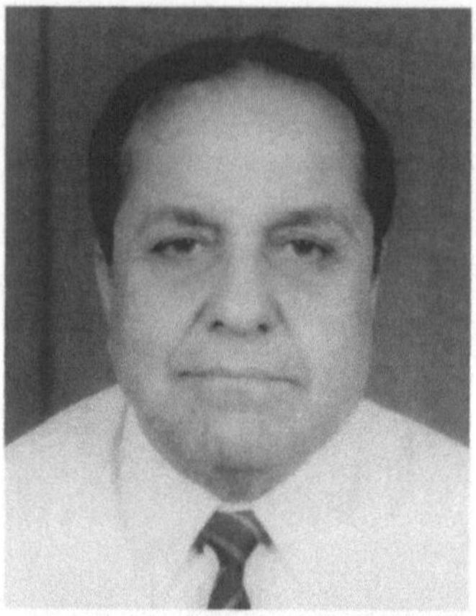

Chaman Lal Kaul

is First Director of the National Institute of Pharmaceutical Education and Research (NIPER), after his position as Director of Research & Development of Boots Pharmaceutical Ltd., Bombay. He was also Group Leader of Pharmacology at the Ciba-Geigy Research Centre, Bombay. Dr. Kaul worked as a Research Associate at the Chelsea College of Science and Technology, University of London, and went on to earn his Ph.D. in 1964 from the University of Glasgow (U.K.). He was employed at several research centers in the U.K. and Switzerland. His research has centered on development and preclinical studies of new drugs, stability, bioavailability, pharmaceutical formulations and quality control.

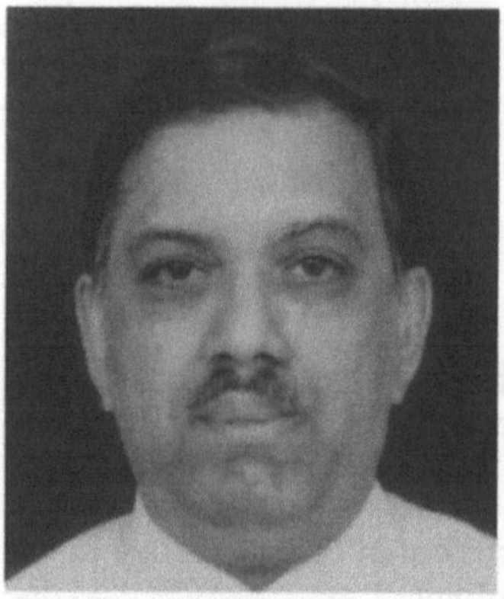

Poduri Ramarao

is Professor of Pharmacology at NIPER and was a Reader and Lecturer of Pharmacology at the Department of Pharmaceutics, BHU, in Varanasi, India. He worked as a Research Associate at the College of Pharmacy, University of Illinois at Chicago and Beth Israel Hospital, Harvard Medical School in Boston, between 1987 and 1990. His research focusses on receptor mechanisms in hypertension, diabetes and opioid tolerance and dependence.

Summary

The sympathetic nervous system is of major importance in the regulation of various physiological functions. The present review discusses the mechanisms which control glucose homeostasis and the role of the sympathetic nervous system in experimental diabetes with special emphasis on the role of adrenal medullary hormones, over-activity of the sympathetic nervous system and its relationship to hypertension in the diabetic state and the effect of stress. The chapter also reviews the ability of various drugs and pharmacological agents to produce hyperglycemia in experimental animals and how this information can be used in screening new chemical entities and in differentiating the mode of action of these agents.

Contents

1	Introduction	165
2	Role of the sympathetic nervous system	166
3	Role of the adrenal medulla	167
4	Effect of adrenalectomy and chemical sympathectomy	169
5	Effect of various agents on hyperglycemic response of streptozotocin (STZ)	169
5.1	α- and β-adrenoceptor blocking drugs	169
5.2	GO 8288 and diazoxide	171
5.3	6-amino-nicotinamide (6-AN)	172
5.4	Prostaglandins	173
5.5	Chlorpromazine	174
5.6	Glucagon	174
5.7	Angiotensin II	174
5.8	Histamine	175
5.9	Dopamine derivatives	175
5.10	Clonidine	176
6	Stress and hyperglycemia	176
7	Conclusions	178
	References	178

Keywords

Sympathetic nervous system, hyperglycemia, streptozotocin, diabetes, stress.

Glossary of abbreviations

GTT, glucose tolerance test; 6-AN, 6-amino-nicotinamide; 6-OHD, 6-hydroxydopamine; ICV, intracerebroventricular; NE, norepinephrine; PPS, pentose phosphate shunt; SNS, sympathetic nervous system; STZ, streptozotocin.

1 Introduction

The circulating concentration of glucose prevailing in the blood is the result of a number of mechanisms operating in the body, e.g., the breakdown of glycogen from the liver, conversion of amino acids to glucose by the liver, glucose uptake into tissues and clearance from the body by the kidneys. There is some disagreement at present as to whether the stress-induced increase in blood glucose is mediated by neural stimulation of the liver or by hormonal factors. It has been suggested that the changes in the blood sugar level which occur during an emergency like stress are mediated by multi-synaptic, hypothalamic-hepatic connections, whereas for the long term, regulation of blood-glucose levels are maintained by hormonal factors, e.g., the adrenal medulla, hypothalamic-pituitary-pancreas connection [1–3]. Furthermore, it has been suggested that in stress, the hypothalamic noradrenaline system initiates an increase in blood sugar by activating the hypothalamic-hepatic neural pathway [1, 4].

The present review will summarize the precise role of the sympathetic nervous system in experimental diabetes, the effect of α- and β-adrenoceptor blockers, chemical sympathectomy and the role of the adrenal medulla. The review will also summarize the mode of action of a variety of drugs and pharmacological agents which produce hyperglycemia in experimental animals and how this information may be useful in screening new pharmacological agents and in differentiating the mode of action of these agents.

2 Role of the sympathetic nervous system

The sympathetic nervous system is of major importance in the regulation of numerous physiological functions. There are no consistent reports regarding changes in the catecholamine levels in diabetes. Circulating noradrenaline levels are increased in poorly controlled diabetes and decreased in those with evidence of neuropathy [5–7]. Using the indirect method of estimation of noradrenaline, Christlieb [8] reported no changes in noradrenaline stores in rats made diabetic with alloxan. No significant difference in the catecholamine levels in the brain and heart of streptozotocin (STZ) diabetes rats has been reported 14 weeks after STZ administration [9–10]. A decrease in the levels of noradrenaline has been reported in carotid arteries of alloxan-treated rabbits [11].

Although there are no consistent reports on the endogenous catecholamine stores, the urinary excretion of catecholamines and its metabolite is markedly increased in the STZ diabetic rat. This increase is seen as early as three days after STZ administration, indicating increased sympathetic activity [9, 12].

The increased sympathetic activity is further manifested by the increased disappearance of [^{3}H]-NE from the rat heart in both age and weight match controls. This is further supported by a significant difference seen in the ratio of [^{3}H]-NE at 1 to 3 h and a decrease in the ratio of [^{3}H]-NE to total radioactivity at 3 h [9, 10].

The increased sympathetic activity seen in these diabetic animals is in line with the reports that hypertension may have an important relationship with diabetes [8, 13]. In fact, these STZ-treated diabetic animals develop hypertension early, as compared to controls when their renal arteries are bilaterally clamped [14]. These results are further supported by the observation of Kawashima et al. [15] that STZ induces not only diabetes but also chronic hypertension in rats. Increased sympathetic activity in untreated diabetes has been reported [6]. Increased sympathetic activity in the insulin-resistance state in Wistar rats has also been reported and this may be related to the hypertension associated with diabetes mellitus in the clinic [16].

There are, however, some reports where decreased turnover of noradrenaline in the STZ diabetic animals [17] and in spontaneously diabetic mice has been reported [18]. Amongst the various possible mechanisms which will reduce the sympathetic nerve activity is the possibility that the lack of regeneration properties in the nerves was caused by diabetes. However, experiments reported with 6-hydroxydopamine (6-OHD) did not show any significant difference in the restoration of noradrenaline tissue levels between diabetes and non-diabetes, indicating thereby that experimental diabetes does not influence the regeneration of nerves damaged by toxic substances [18].

3 Role of the adrenal medulla

The adrenal medulla of rats and humans contains two distinct types of adrenal medullary chromaffin cells in the ratio of 4:1 for adrenaline and noradrenaline, respectively [19]. The amount of neurotransmitter released is dependent on the preganglionic neurons whose activity is controlled by tracts of neurons descending to the spinal cord from supraspinal centers [20]. Depending upon the physiological and pharmacological stimuli, the neural input of the adrenal medulla is adjusted, with the result that adrenaline and noradrenaline are secreted in the blood and these circulating amines help in the restoration of homeostasis. One of the good examples of neurally mediated stimulation of catecholamine release is the response to hypoglycemia. It has been reported that, during hypoglycemia, adrenaline populations of chromaffin cells are preferentially stimulated as compared to noradrenaline-containing cells [21–23]. This hypothesis has been supported by the fact that the circulating adrenaline levels are distinctly higher as compared to noradrenaline, even when the ratio of adrenaline and noradrenaline content of the adrenal medulla is taken into consideration [23, 24]. The differential release of adrenaline and noradrenaline following various stimuli has not been clearly established to date because of the limitations of the methodologies available. Furthermore, the blood concentrations of noradrenaline levels are constituted partly by the adrenal medulla and partly by the sympathetic neurons, which makes the interpretation difficult. However, recent studies by Vollmer and his co-workers, using an intra-adrenal microdialysis technique in conscious rats, have shown selective stimulation of adrenaline-containing chromaffin cells following hypoglycemia produced by insulin [25].

It has been reported that sympathochromaffin activity is altered in patients with long-standing diabetes [26–28]. Although the tissue sensitivity to catecholamine is sometimes increased [29], the release of adrenaline from the adrenal gland is often decreased [27, 30]. These observations are based on the studies using isolated adrenal glands of BB-Wistar rats, a spontaneously diabetic model known to develop both functional [31, 32] and morphological [33] manifestations of autonomic neuropathy. Using this preparation, Wilke and co-workers have stated that both the splanchnic nerve and chromaffin cells are hypofunctional. Further histological degenerative changes have also been reported in cholinergic nerve terminals that innervate these glands [26]. Diminished sympathoadrenal activity has been reported following stress in diabetic patients suffering from autonomic neuropathy [28]. This decrease in the secretion activity of adrenaline can be of critical clinical importance since adrenaline is intimately involved in the maintenance of glucose homeostasis.

A number of adrenergic agonists, including adrenaline and noradrenaline, are reported to produce hyperglycemia in animals through various mechanisms. This hyperglycemia is blocked by α-adrenergic blockers like phentolamine, yohimbine and to some degree by di-hydroergotamine, but α-blockers like phenoxybenzamine and prazosin are ineffective in antagonizing this hyperglycemia induced by α-adrenergic agonists. Based on these results it has been suggested that there are marked differences in the capacity of various α-adrenergic blockers to inhibit α-adrenergic receptors of the pancreatic β-cells. Since phentolamine and yohimibine (α-2 type) are more potent in blocking presynaptic than postsynaptic α-adrenoceptors and because phenoxybenzamine and prazosin (α-1 type) are ineffective, it seems reasonable to suggest the presence of the α-2 type of adrenoceptors on the post-synaptic membrane of pancreatic β cells [34].

4 Effect of adrenalectomy and chemical sympathectomy

Adrenalectomy is reported to have no significant effect on acute (24 h) or maintenance of (7 days) hyperglycemic response in rats produced by intravenous injection of STZ [35]. Doses of 6-OHD which are reported to have a selective effect in destroying sympathetic nerve terminals in the rat [36-37] do not produce a significant change in the hyperglycemic response to intravenous administration of STZ in the rat. Even the hypoglycemic effect of tolbutamide and phenformin is unaltered in these sympathectomized animals when compared to controls [35]. In rhesus monkeys, 6-OHD treatment does not show any glucose intolerance or any effect on insulin release [38].

From the above results it can be concluded that at least in the rat, the sympathetic nervous system does not play any significant role in the diabetogenic effect of STZ and hypoglycemia induced by tolbutamide and phenformin in the rat. Even in the rhesus monkey, sympathectomy produced by 6-OHD does not modify the glucose tolerance test (GTT) and insulin release. The inability of 6-OHD to modify GTT may be related to the sparse adrenergic innervation of β cells in the monkey [39].

5 Effect of various agents on hyperglycemic response of streptozotocin (STZ)

5.1 α- and β-adrenoceptor blocking drugs

Pretreatment of rats with α- and β-adrenoceptor blocking drugs like phentolamine and oxprenolol has been reported to produce no significant change in the hyperglycemic response produced by STZ. Both these treatments do not have any effect on the acute (24 h), or maintenance of, hyperglycemic response (7days) following STZ injection. Furthermore, the hypoglycemic response to an oral hypoglycemic agent (tolbutamide) is unaltered with α- and β-adrenoceptor blocking drugs like phentolamine, phenoxybenzamine and oxprenolol in the rat [35]. Physiological doses of phenoxybenzamine do not produce any alleviation in the blood sugar. The effect of β-adrenergic blocking drugs on the blood sugar response is variable. Born and Spratto [40] have reported a significant effect on the blood glucose response in mice but no effect in rats. It has been emphasized that the species difference exists between rats and mice with respect to the action of β-adrenergic blocking agents on blood glucose response.

Although the phentolamine did not modify the hyperglycemic response to STZ (50 mg/kg, IV) it is reported to potentiate the diabetogenic effect of low doses of STZ (20–25 mg/kg, IV) in the rat [41]. Phentolamine is also reported to decrease the resistance of KK (Kasukaba (K) group of Japan) mice to the diabetogenic action of STZ [42]. This property of potentiating the diabetogenic effect to the threshold doses of STZ is not shared by other α-adrenergic blocking drugs like tolazoline and phenoxybenzamine. This potentiation does not seems to be related to α-adrenergic blockade or to the vasodilatory effect since phenoxybenzamine, which is a more potent α-adrenergic blocking drug and produces a marked vasodilatory effect, has no significant effect even when given 4 h before STZ.

Phentolamine has been reported to stimulate insulin secretion as a result of unopposed endogenous β-receptor stimulation [43, 44]. The potentiating effect of phentolamine cannot be ascribed to insulin release since insulin and tolbutamide (a known insulin releaser) do not modify the STZ response. β-Adrenergic blocking drugs like propranolol and oxprenolol do not potentiate the diabetogenic effect of STZ. In fact, oxprenolol treatment is reported to significantly antagonize the potentiating effect of phentolamine. These results with oxprenolol suggest that the potentiating effect of phentolamine may be due to its having β-adrenergic stimulating properties, which is further supported by the results with the β_2 agonist salbutamol, where the number of animals which became hyperglycemic was significantly higher than the controls [41]. It is also possible that phentolamine in some way alters the permeability of β cells to STZ and thereby potentiates the diabetogenic effect. This effect cannot be ascribed to a membrane-stabilizing action, since propranolol, a known membrane-stabilizing agent, does not show this potentiation [45]. There is hardly any example in the rat where potentiation of STZ has been demonstrated. Most of the earlier studies relate to inhibition of the diabetogenic effect of STZ [46, 47].

A number of pharmacological agents are known to produce hyperglycemia in experimental animals. In the majority of the cases, the adrenal medulla seems to be involved in producing this hyperglycemia, since this hyperglycemic response is abolished by adrenalectomy or adrenal demedullation. Some of these agents are diazoxide, GO 8288, 6-amino-nicotinamide, prostaglandins, angiotensin II, dopamine derivatives, etc.).

5.2 GO 8288 and diazoxide

Both GO 8288 and diazoxide have been reported to produce hyperglycemia in rats which are blocked by adrenalectomy or demedullation [48, 49], suggesting the role of catecholamine release. The ability of hydrocortisone to restore the hyperglycemia partially or completely seems to suggest some role of adrenal cortical hormones in the hyperglycemia produced by these two agents, which is more pertinent in diazoxide-induced hyperglycemia as compared to GO 8288. In the case of GO 8288, the hyperglycemic response is antagonized by glibenclamide and insulin but not with tolbutamide and phenformin, whereas in the case of diazoxide, both glibenclamide and tolbutamide antagonize the hyperglycemic response, but phenformin was ineffective. The ability of glibenclamide to prevent hyperglycemia may be related to stimulation of insulin release in diazoxide- and GO 8288-treated animals. Diazoxide-induced inhibition of insulin release is reported to be antagonized by tolbutamide *in vitro* [50] and this could perhaps explain the ability of tolbutamide to antagonize the diazoxide-induced hyperglycemia. The failure of tolbutamide to antagonize the hyperglycemic effect of GO 8288 significantly could probably be related to its inability to overcome GO 8288-induced inhibition of insulin release [48].

From the above results it seems that the inhibition of insulin release may be more important in case of GO 8288 than diazoxide since (a) GO 8288 does not increase the pre-existing hyperglycemia in diabetic rats and (b) the intensity of hyperglycemia produced by diazoxide is much more when compared to GO 8288, despite the fact that inhibition of insulin release is less marked [49]. It can be concluded that, although there are many similarities between the biological profiles of GO 8288 and diazoxide, there are some differences, e.g., treatment with β-adrenoceptor-blocking drugs like oxprenolol antagonized the diazoxide-induced hyperglycemia but not GO 8288. Again guanethedine antagonized the hyperglycemic effect of GO 8288 but not of diazoxide. Unlike GO 8288, diazoxide further accentuated the hyperglycemic effect in STZ diabetic rats.

5.3 6-amino-nicotinamide (6-AN)

6-AN, an antimetabolite to pyridine nucleotide synthesis [51], is reported to induce delayed hyperglycemia in rats and the peak effect is seen by about 7 h. Initial studies attributed this hyperglycemic response to the inhibition of insulin release [52, 53] and adrenal medullary discharge [54] but the exact mechanism of this delayed hyperglycemia has now been reported [55]. The results showed that 6-AN-induced adrenaline release from the adrenal glands is mainly responsible for the development of hyperglycemia in rats. This observation is based on the following observations: (a) adrenalectomy and adrenal demedullation completely block the hyperglycemic response to 6-AN, (b) 6-AN induced adrenaline release from the adrenals, (c) phentolamine and not propranolol blocks the hyperglycemic response, (d) catecholamine depleters like reserpine (which depletes adrenal catecholamine) and not guanethidine (which does not deplete adrenal catecholamine) inhibit the hyperglycemic response and (e) a decrease in liver glycogen was seen after 6-AN was administered following adrenaline release.

Although phentolamine is reported to increase insulin secretion in rats, this effect is of very short duration [56, 41]. It is therefore reasonable to assume that the antagonism to the hyperglycemic effect of 6-AN is due to the antagonism of catecholamine release by 6-AN and not due to the antagonist effect of elevated insulin concentration, since elevated levels of insulin are not seen up to 7 h following phentolamine administration. Failure to inhibit the hyperglycemic response following administratin of β-adrenergic blockers is not surprising since these drugs even in large doses have been reported to have no effect in adrenaline-induced hyperglycemia [57–59].

Although 6-AN is reported to have no effect on the fasting plasma glucose, it inhibits glucose-induced insulin release (*in vivo* and *in vitro*) [52], which would suggest that the sustained hyperglycemia seen with 6-AN may be due to the combined effect of stimulation of adrenaline release from the adrenals and inhibition of insulin release.

The sustained hyperglycemia reported following administration of 6-AN may also be due to the inhibition of the pentose phosphate shunt (PPS) in the adrenal medulla and pancreas, since administration of 6-AN results in the formation of a 6-amino analogue of NADP which, by inhibiting 6-amino phosphogluconate dehydrogenase, blocks the PPS [60]. The PPS may be involved in catecholamine synthesis in the adrenal medulla [61] or glucose-induced insulin release in the pancreas [52]. This is supported by the fact that simultaneous administration of nicotinic acid or nicotinamide has no effect on blood sugar, but could block the 6-AN-induced hyperglycemia. Furthermore, the hyperglycemic effect of adrenaline could not be blocked by nicotinic acid and nicotinamide.

The delayed hyperglycemic response of 6-AN suggests that the hyperglycemic effect of 6-AN is contingent upon metabolic conversion *in vivo*, probably by being incorporated in pyridine nucleotides in place of nicotinamide, which is supported by the fact that the accumulation of 6-phosphogluconate, which reflects (inhibition of PPS) in the adrenal medulla, is delayed in the rat following 6-AN administration [61].

5.4 Prostaglandins

The effect of prostaglandins (PG) on the central nervous system regulation of blood sugar homeostasis has been reported [62]. Injection of PGD_2, PGE_1, PGE_2 and $PGF_{2\alpha}$ into the third cerebral ventricle produces hyperglycemia in rats. The relative potency of various prostaglandins to produce hyperglycemia is $PGF_{2\alpha} > D_2 > E_1 > E_2$. Besides the glucose, concentration of glucagon, adrenaline and noradrenaline has been reported to increase following injection by $PGF_{2\alpha}$. This hyperglycemic effect of $PGF_{2\alpha}$ is blocked by adrenal demedullation and phentolamine but not by propranolol, indicating the role of the central nervous system in producing hyperglycemia by increasing adrenaline secretion from the adrenal medulla.

5.5 Chlorpromazine

Subcutaneous administration of chlorpromazine produces a dose-dependent increase in plasma glucose in fed mice. Phentolamine, yohimbine, and higher doses of dihydroergotamine completely suppressed the elevation of plasma glucose, whereas phenoxybenzamine and propranolol had no effect. These results suggest that chlorpromazine-induced hyperglycemia is mediated through the stimulation of alpha-adrenoceptors [62, 63].

5.6 Glucagon

Intracerebroventricular (ICV) administration of glucagon in the rat produces more prolonged and pronounced elevation of plasma glucose than with identical intravenous doses. This elevation in plasma glucose following ICV administration is accompanied by insignificant changes in plasma immunoreactive insulin (IRI) and immunoreactive glucagon (IRG). In contrast, intravenous administration of glucagon produces a marked increase in IRI and IRG. The prolonged hyperglycemic effect of glucagon can be explained by the fact that a glucagon-sensitive mechanism exists in the brain, probably in the hypothalamus, and glucagon may play a neurotransmitter or mediator role in the brain. This evidence is supported by the fact that glucagon-induced hyperglycemia is blocked by prior administration of atropine, phentolamine and hexamethonium, but not by propranolol. These findings also suggest the involvement of cholinergic (muscarinic) and adrenergic mechanisms. Involvement of the adrenal medulla in the ICV-administered, glucagon-induced hyperglycemia is small since the bilateral adrenalectomy partially blocked the hyperglycemic response [64].

5.7 Angiotensin II

Intravenous administration of angiotensin II causes a rapid rise of blood sugar, which is enhanced by pre-treatment with guanethidine. Adrenal demedullation does not alter the hyperglycemic response but giving adrenal demedullated animals guanethedine causes a decrease in the hyperglycemic response to angiotensin II. These data indicate that angiotensin II has a direct hyperglycemic effect, in addition to its action on sympathetic nervous system activation and adrenomedullary secretion [65].

5.8 Histamine

Intracerebroventricular administration of histamine is reported to produce hyperglycemia, which is enhanced markedly by metoprine (an inhibitor of HA-n-methyl transferase). Administration of a H_1 receptor antagonist, like mepyramine, chlorpheniramine or promethazine, antagonized the hyperglycemia but H_2 receptor antagonists had no effect. Adrenalectomy blocked the hyperglycemic effect of histamine. Phentolamine but not propranolol blocked the hyperglycemic response by 50%. The same doses of phentolamine and propranolol, when given together, blocked the hyperglycemic response completely, which seems to suggest that the central hyperglycemic response to histamine is produced mainly by an increasing sympathetic outflow followed by an increase in catecholamines from the adrenal medulla [66].

5.9 Dopamine derivatives

A number of synthetic derivatives of dopamine, apomorphine and RDS 127 (2-di-n-propylamino-4,7-dimethoxyindane), di-n-propyldopamine, 2-di-n-propylamino-5,6-dihydroxytetralin (TL 102) and bromocriptine, are reported to produce dose- and time-dependent hyperglycemia in conscious unrestrained rats through activation of dopamine receptors. Amongst all compounds TL 102 was the most potent in producing hyperglycemia. The hyperglycemic response of apomorphine and RDS 127 was blocked by adrenalectomy, demedullation and by pimozide, a dopamine (DA) receptor antagonist. Both apomorphine and RDS-127 caused abnormal glucose intolerance and inhibited the compensatory increase in serum immunoreactive insulin. These effects were again blocked by phentolamine and pimozide. These results seem to suggest that central dopamine receptors modulate sympathetic neuronal activity to the adrenal medulla to other glucoregulatory mechanisms [67, 68].

5.10 Clonidine

Centrally acting α2 adrenoceptor agonists are reported to produce hyperglycemia in the fed rats whereas peripherally acting α2 agonists (DPI) produce hypoglycemia. Clonidine is reported to produce hyperglycemia in a variety of experimental animals like dogs, mice, chicks, rabbits, cats and man [69–71]. The hyperglycemic effect of clonidine can be reversed by phentolamine, yohimbine and rauwolscine (α2 adrenergic antagonist) but not by prazosin or corynanthine (selective α1-antagonist). The hyperglycemic effect seems to be mediated by enhanced gluconeogenesis, as this response is partially blocked by 3-MPA, an inhibitor of gluconeogenesis. This hyperglycemic response is un-altered by the H_2 receptor antagonist, prostaglandins or glucagon release. These results seem to be consistent with the major role of the growth hormone, which is elevated during clonidine treatment and which can stimulate gluconeogenesis and decrease peripheral glucose utilization.

Selective α2 adrenoceptor agonists like UK 14304, clonidine and guanbenz produce hyperglycemia which is accompanied by inhibition of insulin secretion. Hyperglycemia induced by α2 adrenoceptor agonists like UK 14304 is mediated through stimulation of the postsynaptic α2 adrenoceptor located on the pancreatic β cells, leading to inhibition of insulin release. Adrenalectomy, depletion of catecholamines by reserpine and α-MMT fail to modify the hyperglycemic response [72].

6 Stress and hyperglycemia

Stress has been implicated in the development of hyperglycemia by activating pituitary-adrenocortical and sympathoadrenal systems [73]. A number of stressors elicit the elevation of circulating glucocorticoids and catecholamine, resulting in an increase in blood glucose. As mentioned before, it is not very clear whether a stress-induced increase in blood sugar is mediated primarily by hormonal or neural stimulation of the liver. In normal situations, a stressful stimulus causes an increase in blood sugar by activating neural connections from the brain to the adrenal medulla or liver. The contribution of each of the pathways will depend on many factors, e.g., anaesthetized or awake animal, intensity of stimuli, nutritional state of the animal (fasted and fed). The role of adrenal hormones is mediating an increase in blood sugar levels following several stressful stimuli in conscious rats has been reported [74]. These authors used brief foot shock stress, injection of 2-deoxy-D-glucose, exposure to the odor of a predator and electrical stimulation of the hypothalamus. Following these treatments, the blood sugar levels were elevated, which were completely blocked by removal of the adrenal medulla, a procedure that does not damage the hypothalamic noradrenaline system or the multi-synaptic neural pathway from the hypothalamus to the liver, suggesting that the increase in blood sugar following these stressors is mediated by release of adrenaline from the adrenal medulla. Rats depleted of brain noradrenaline potentiated the responses to stressful stimuli as compared to the controls, indicating that the hypothalamic noradrenaline systems are not involved in the elevation of blood sugar.

In the case of diabetics, the hormonal response to stress is reported to be abnormal or less adaptive because of the alterations in the system secondary to the loss of pancreatic β cells [75, 76]. Diabetics have a different response profile when compared to non-diabetics, and different stressors can produce different responses. Altered responses to environmental stress have been reported for STZ diabetic rats [12]. Metabolic stability in diabetics is also known to be affected by stress [73], which can lead to ketoacidosis even when insulin is given routinely [77]. Insulin treatment in these cases can further contribute to the metabolic complication of stress, since lowering of blood sugar following insulin treatment can actually stimulate release of catecholamines and cortical hormones which further contribute to decompensation in the face of stress [78].

A number of recent reports have shown enhanced responses to stress in rats and mice with STZ and spontaneous diabetes. Increases in the levels of glucocorticoids and catecholamines are reported in STZ diabetic rats following intraperitoneal cold water injections [79, 80], whereas in obese C57BL/6 ob/ob mice, a greater elevation of plasma glucose and catecholamines following immobilization and shaking was observed, as compared to the controls [81]. As indicated before, increased activity of the sympathetic nervous system (SNS) has been reported in STZ diabetic rats and this increased activity of the SNS in diabetes suggests mechanisms by which stress would lead to increased metabolic complications in diabetes mellitus [12].

7 Conclusions

The results reported in this review show that the SNS does not play any significant role in STZ-induced hyperglycemia, glucose tolerance and insulin release, at least in the rat and monkey. Furthermore, the hyperglycemic response to oral hyperglycemic agents is unaltered in sympathectomised animals and after treatment with adrenoceptor-blocking drugs like phentolamine, phenoxybenzamine and oxprenolol. Adrenalectomy and chemical sympathectomy also do not show any significant effect on the diabetogenic effect of STZ in the rat. Phentolamine potentiates the diabetogenic effect of threshold doses of STZ, which is probably related to its having β-adrenergic stimulating properties. Adrenal medullary catecholamine release, stimulation of the adrenoceptor, direct action on the SNS increase sympathetic outflow followed by increase in catecholamine release and enhanced gluconeogenesis are some other mechanisms which produce hyperglycemia in experimental animals. Using a combination of these drugs, it is possible to delineate the possible mechanism of action of some of the pharmacological agents which produce hyperglycemia.

References

1 T. Shimazu: Diabetologia *20*, 343 (1981).

2 T. Shimazu, in: A.J. Szabo (ed.): Advances in Metabolic Disorders, Vol. 10 (CNS Regulation of Carbohydrate Metabolism). Academic, New York 1983, 355.

3 T. Shimazu, in: S. Lightman, B. Everitt (eds.): Neuroendocrinology. Blackwell, Oxford UK 1986, 304.

4 G. Smythe, H. Grunstein, J. Bradshaw, M. Nicholson and P. Crompton: Nature (Lond) *38*, 65 (1984).

5 N.J. Christensen: J. Clin. Invest. *51*, 779 (1972).

6 N.J. Christensen: Diabetes *23*, 1 (1974).

7 S. Ferraro, S. Fazio, M. Santomauro, G. Cianfrani, S. Mossetti, G. Turco, E. De Simone, M.G. Gravina, E. Matera et al.: Diab. Res. Clin. Pract. *8*, 91 (1990).

8 A.R. Christlieb: Am. J. Cardiol. *32*, 592 (1973).

9 C.L. Kaul and R.S. Grewal: Pharmacology *21*, 223 (1980).

10 C.L. Kaul: Clin. Exp. Hypertens. *21*, 95 (1999).

11 R.A. Cohen, B. Tesfamarian, R.M. Weisbrod and K.M. Zitnay: Am. J. Physiol. *259*, H55 (1990).

12 L.L. Bellush. and W.N. Henley: Physiol & Behav. *47*, 231 (1990).

13 A.D.B. Harrower: Br. J. Clin. Pract. *31*, 47 (1977).

14 C.L. Kaul and R.S. Grewal: Pharmacol. Res. Commun. *12*, 945 (1980).

15 H. Kawashima, T. Igarashi, Y. Nakagima, Y. Akiyama, K.R. Usuk and S. Ohtake: Naunyn Schmiedbergs. Arch. Pharmacol. *305*, 123 (1978).
16 C.J. Chang, J.S. Wu, F.H. Lu, I.M. Liu, T.C. Chi and J.T. Cheng: J. Auton. Nerv. System *74*, 116 (1998).
17 T. Yoshida, H. Nishioka, Y. Nakamura and M. Kondo: Diabetologia *28*, 692 (1985).
18 A. Giachetti: Diabetes *27*, 969 (1978).
19 N.A. Hillarp and B. Hokfelt: Acta Physiol. Scand. *30*, 55 (1953).
20 R.R. Vollmer: Clin. Exp. Hypertens. *18*, 731 (1996).
21 D.A. Carbonaro, J.R. Mitchell, F.L. Hall and P.R. Vulliet: Brain Res. Bull. *21*, 451 (1988).
22 R.E. Coupland: J. Endocrinol. *17*, 191 (1958).
23 R.R. Vollmer, A. Baruchin, S.S. Kolibal-Pegher, S.P. Corey, E.M. Stricker and B.B. Kaplan: Am. J. Physiol. *263*, R 716 (1992).
24 A. Scheurink and S. Ritter: J. Neurochem. *50*, 1302 (1993).
25 R.R. Vollmer, J.J. Balcita, A.F. Sved and D.J. Edwards: Am. J. Physiol. *273*, R 1758 (1997).
26 R.A. Wilke, D.A. Riley, P.I. Lelkes and C.J. Hillard: Diabetes *42*, 862 (1993).
27 P.E. Cryer: Diabetes *38*, 405 (1989).
28 T. Frost, A. Pfutzner, J. Christine, H. Schmitz, K. Lichtwald, J. Beyer and H. Lehnert: J. Auton. Nerv. System *61*, 31 (1996).
29 J. Hilstead, E. Richter, S. Madsbad, B. Triner, N.J. Christensin, P. Hildebrand, M. Damkjaer and A.H. Galbo: N. Engl. J. Med. *317*, 421 (1987).
30 J. Hilstead: Diabetes *31*, 730 (1982).
31 T.A.J. McEwan and A.A.F. Sima: Diabetes *36*, 251 (1987).
32 M. Paro, M. Prosdocimi and W.X. Zhang: Diabetes *38*, 1023 (1989).
33 S. Yagihashi and A.F.F. Sima: Am. J. Pathol. *121*, 138 (1985).
34 T. Nakadate, T. Nakaki, T. Muraki and R. Kato: J. Pharmacol. Exp. Ther. *215*, 226 (1988).
35 C.L. Kaul, P.K. Talwalkar and R.S. Grewal: Experientia *32*, 1072 (1976).
36 R.S.Grewal and C.L. Kaul: Br. J. Pharmacol. *42*, 497 (1971).
37 H. Thoenen and J.P. Tranzer: Naunyn Schmiedbergs. Arch. Pharmacol. *261*, 271 (1968).
38 C.L. Kaul, P.K. Talwalker and R.S. Grewal: Ind. J. Exp. Biol. *18*, 623 (1980).
39 L. Cegrell: Acta Physiol. Scand. Suppl. *314*, 60 (1968).
40 C.K. Born and G.R. Spratto: Fed. Proc. *30*, 315 (1971).
41 P.K. Talwalker, C.L. Kaul and R.S. Grewal: J. Pharm. Pharmacol. *31*, 598 (1979).
42 H. Iwatsuka, A. Shino and S. Taketomi: Diabetes. *23*, 856 (1974).
43 R.P. Robertson and D. Porte: Diabetes *22*, 1 (1973).
44 S.C. Woods and D. Porte: Physiol. Rev. *54*, 596(1974).
45 A. Langslet: Eur. J. Pharmacol. *13*, 6 (1970).
46 W.E. Dulin and B.M. Wyse: Diabetes *18*, 459 (1969).
47 O.P. Ganda, A.A. Rossini and A.A. Like: Diabetes *25*, 595 (1976).
48 R. Yabo, J. Vitoria, M. Staquet and F. Wolff: Diabetes *14*, 591(1965).
49 C.L. Kaul, P.K. Talwalkar and R.S. Grewal: Arch. Int.Pharmacodyn. *233*, 92 (1978).
50 J.C. Basabe, N.L. Lopez, J.K. Victoria and F.W. Wolff: Diabetes *20*, 457 (1971).
51 L.S. Dietrich, J.M. Friedland and A. Kaplan: J. Biol. Chem. *233*, 964 (1958).
52 H.T.P. Ammon and J. Steinke: Diabetes *21*, 143 (1972).
53 H.P.T. Ammon, T.N. Patil and J. Steinke: Biochem. Biophys. Acta *297*, 352 (1973).
54 G. Schultz, G. Senft, W. Losert and U. Schacht: Arch. Exp. Pathol. Pharmacol. *253*, 345 (1966).
55 C.L. Kaul, P.K. Talwalkar and R.S. Grewal: J. Pharm. Pharmacol. *32*, 701 (1980).

56 B.L. Furman and F.M. Tayo: J. Pharm. Pharmacol. *26*, 512 (1974).
57 V. Claassen and E.L. Noach: Arch. Int. Pharmacodyn. *126*, 332 (1960).
58 K.R. Hornbrook and T.M. Brody: Biochem. Pharmacol. *12*, 1407 (1963).
59 B.W. Lei and R.S. McCutcheon: J. Pharm. Sci. *53*, 503 (1964).
60 H. Herken, K. Lange and H. Kulbe: Biochem. Biophys. Res. Commun. *36*, 93 (1969).
61 S.E. Jansson, J. Gripenberg and M. Harkonen: Acta Physiol. Scand. *99*, 467 (1977).
62 A. Yatomi, A. Iguchi, S. Yanagisawa, H. Matsunaga, I. Niki and N. Sakamoto: Endocrinology *121*, 36 (1987).
63 T. Nakadate, T. Muraki and R. Kato: Jap. J. Pharmacol. *30*, 199 (1980).
64 S. Marubashi, M. Tominaga, T. Katagiri, K. Yamatani and Y. Yawata: Acta Endocrinology *108*, 6 (1985).
65 I. Mihessen-Neto, A.M. Reis, U. Marubayashi and C.C. Coimbra: Neuropeptides *30*, 303 (1996).
66 M. Nishibori, Y. Itoh, R. Oishi and K. Saeki: J. Pharmacol. Exp. Ther. *241*, 582 (1987).
67 S.P. Arneric, S.A. Chow, R.K. Bhatnagar, R.L. Webb, L.J. Fischer and J.P. Long: Neuropharmacol. *23*, 134 (1984).
68 S.P. Arneric, S.A. Chow, J.P. Long and L.J. Fischer: J. Pharmacol. Exp. Ther. *228*, 551 (1984).
69 W. Kobinger, in: G. Onestir and K.E. Kimp (eds.): Hypertension Mechanism and Management. Grune and Stratton, New York 1973, 369.
70 T. Nakadate, T. Nakaki, T. Muraki and R. Katu: J. Pharmacol. *25*, 226 (1980).
71 S.A. Metz, J.B. Halter and R.P. Robertson: Diabetes *27*, 554 (1978).
72 I. Angel, S. Bidet and S.Z. Langer: J. Pharmacol. Exp. Ther. *246*, 1098 (1988).
73 F.W. Kemmer, R. Bisping, H.J. Steingruber, H. Baar, F. Hardtmann, R. Schlaghecke and M. Berger: N. Engl. J. Med. *314*, 1078 (1986).
74 R.J. Bialik, J.W. Smythe, M. Sardelis and D.C. Roberts: Brain Res. *502*, 88 (1989).
75 H. Shammon, R. Hendler and R.S. Sherwin: Diabetes *29*, 284 (1980).
76 A.M. Jacobson, L.I. Rand and S.T. Hauser: Psychosom. Med. *47*, 372 (1985).
77 M.H. Macgillivary, E. Bruck and M.L. Voorhess: Pediatric Res. *15*, 99 (1981).
78 J.E. Gerich and P.J. Camphell: Diab. Metab. Rev. *4*, 93 (1988).
79 J.H. Lee, M. Konarsha and R. McCarty: Physiol.Behav. *40*, 447 (1987).
80 A.F. De Nicola, O. Fridman, E.J. Del Castillo and V.G. Foglia: Horm. Metab. Res. *9*, 69 (1977).
81 R.S. Surwit, M.W. Feinglos, E.G. Livingstone, C.M. Kuhn and J.A. McCubbin: Diabetes *33*, 616 (1984).

Progress in Drug Research, Vol. 57 (E. Jucker, Ed.)

From outer to inner space: Traveling along a scientific career from astrochemistry to drug research

By Jay A. Glasel

Global Scientific Consulting LLC
15 Colton St.
Farmington, CT 06032, USA
<jaglasel@home.com>

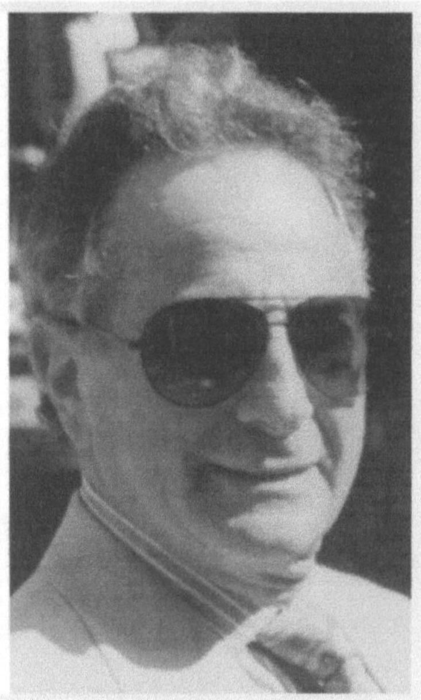

Jay A. Glasel

obtained a B.S. in chemistry and physics from CalTech. His Ph.D. was in chemical physics for work on chemical reactions on comets at the University of Chicago. After postdoctoral appointments at the University of California at La Jolla, Imperial College in London and active duty in the U.S. Air Force, he took up a faculty position in biochemistry at Columbia University where he performed biostructural research on bioactive peptides. After a sabbatical at Oxford University he took up positions as an Associate Professor and later as a Professor of Biochemistry at the University of Connecticut Health Center in Farmington, Connecticut. There, his research interests changed slowly from biostructural work to the biochemistry of opiates and opiate receptors. He pioneered the uses of anti-morphine monoclonal antibodies and anti-opiate receptor anti-idiotypic antibodies in research on the biochemistry of narcotics. In 2000 he founded Global Scientific Consulting, LLC.

Summary

This professional history describes my journey as a research scientist after my early training and experiences in the pre- and early post-World War II United States. My graduate training concentrated on a problem in astrochemistry: phenomena on comets. As my career developed, I felt confident enough in myself as an experimentalist to enter, and make contributions to, several different fields: structural biochemistry (*via* nuclear magnetic resonance spectroscopy), molecular immunology, pharmacology, neurochemistry, and cell biology. One emphasis is on the nature and quality of my scientific training that permitted me to do cross-disciplinary work. A second emphasis is on the technical and intellectual developments in late twentieth-century science and how, along with the changes in American society as it passed through three major wars, they influenced my life and thought.

"What we cannot speak about we must pass over in silence."

The last proposition from
Tractatus Logico-Philosophicus, Ludwig Wittgenstein, 1921

Contents

1	Introduction: so few degrees of separation	185
2	Early days	185
2.1	Beginning education	186
2.2	Scientific beginnings	187
3	CalTech years	188
3.1	Among smart people	188
3.2	CalTech's philosophy – then	189
3.3	Humility, humiliation and teaching caltech style	189
3.3.1	My research beginnings	190
3.3.2	A 1950s CalTech education in summary	191
4	A Ph.D. candidate at the University of Chicago	192
4.1	Starting to become a chemical physicist and teacher	192
4.2	My independent research career's foundation: Harold Urey	193
4.2.1	A research problem in astrochemistry	194
4.2.2	Teaching myself free radical chemistry and low temperature physics	195
4.2.3	First slip-ups, discoveries and encounters with "experts"	197
4.3	Urey leaves, Joe Mayer takes over	200
4.4	Thesis and graduation	200
5	Postdoctoral work with Harold Urey: the new University of California at San Diego	201
5.1	If I can learn nuclear magnetic resonance spectroscopy I have a job at Columbia University	202
6	Postdoctoral research in London learning NMR	203
6.1	Department of Chemistry, Imperial College	203
6.1.1	Making a MUDDLE	203
6.1.2	The Berlin Wall affects my life	205
7	A nuclear research officer, United States Air Force	205
7.1	Military science and life	206
8	Back to academic life as a biochemist	207
8.1	New in biochemistry and NMR	207
8.1.1	Research on water and biomolecular interactions *via* NMR	207
8.1.2	Developing instrumentation: the era of minicomputers arrives	209
8.2	Biomolecular structural work	210
8.2.1	Peptide hormones	210
8.2.2	Fourier-transform spectroscopy arrives: homemade	211
8.2.3	David Rittenberg	212
9	Sabbatical at the University of Oxford	213
9.1	Lanthanide ion chemistry	213
9.1.1	Determining biomolecular structures using NMR and lanthanide ions	214
9.1.2	Families of structures and computer data fitting	215
9.2	Putting it all together: our first lanthanide-derived structural family	216

10	Connecticut years – Part I, 1970–1980	216
10.1	Water relaxation in heterogeneous systems – pre-magnetic resonance imaging	217
10.2	Peptide hormones redux: encountering a central problem in structural drug research	218
10.2.1	A regional NMR facility	219
10.3	Research developments, 1970–1980	220
10.3.1	Instrumentation	220
10.3.2	Starting to branch out from NMR	220
10.3.3	NMR and bioactive peptides	221
10.3.4	Beginnings of opiate work	222
10.3.5	Determination of structural families of flexible molecules from spectral density functions	222
11	Beginning wet biochemistry	225
11.1	Neurohypophyseal proteins: physical and biochemical properties	225
12	Sabbatical at Imperial College: neurochemistry and opiates	226
12.1	Opiate receptors	226
12.1.1	Learning subcellular fractionation	226
12.1.2	Monoclonal antibodies and the germ of an idea about anti-idiotypic antibodies	227
13	Connecticut years – Part II, 1980–2000	228
13.1	Structural work on opiates	228
13.2	Anti-morphine monoclonal antibodies, opiate receptors	229
13.3	Radiation inactivation studies of opiate receptors – knowledge before its time had come	230
13.4	Molecular immunology and opiates	231
13.5	Are binding sites for drugs on antibodies good models for drug-receptor binding?	232
13.6	Learning molecular biological skills	233
13.7	More structural work on opiates	233
14	Sabbatical at the Australian National University	234
14.1	Transferred NOEs	234
15	Research 1990–2000	235
15.1	Using anti-idiotypic antibodies to observe opiate receptors *via* confocal microscopy	235
15.2	Beginning to understand the molecular biology of opiate receptors	237
15.2.1	A good tool for determining drug signaling pathways to the nucleus?	238
15.2.2	Still thinking quantitatively	239
15.2.3	High school algebra pays off	239
15.3	Final work: out of funds but not out of ideas	241
15.3.1	Pleotropic effects of drugs: a rapidly developing field	241
15.3.2	"Not innovative"	243
	References	243

1 Introduction: so few degrees of separation

This narrative describes my career as a research scientist from my beginning work to my present interests concerning the interaction of drugs with gene expression.

Depending on how you look at it, I had the great fortune or the great misfortune to become a scientist just at the time when science was becoming a profession.

After his first viewing of a rocket launch at Cape Canaveral, Harold Urey (1893–1981) told me in wonder "it was as big as a locomotive standing on end!" I think that only an American with one foot in the 19th century and the other in the 20th could have come up with this technological simile. Now I am a scientist with feet bridging two centuries: Dr. Urey was my principal Ph.D. thesis advisor and to me his remark symbolizes how few degrees of separation[1] there are between chemists of my era and origins of quantitative chemistry.

As science has become more specialized during my career, so has what might be called the languages and thought processes used in the different areas of specialization.

Looking back, I believe I can claim this: I speak physical chemistry and biophysical chemistry well, am quite fluent in molecular pharmacology and immunology, speak serviceable biochemistry and molecular biology, and really stumble along in biology. To work in these different areas one must use different languages and think along different lines. The molecular science underlying all biological disciplines is identical, but just as translation between social languages is often difficult, the translation between scientific languages is too. I was privileged to have been given the opportunity to teach myself some of the translations – an option for young scientists that is unfortunately rapidly disappearing because, while self-teaching is personally more satisfying to the individual, it is very inefficient.

Let me start at the beginning.

2 Early days

My cultural background contains two streams of Judaic tradition – Germanic and Russian – that individually have been influential in American culture, business and science. On my father's side, the Glasels came to this country from the Tyrol in the second half of the 19th century. On my mother's side, the heritage was Russian/Hungarian farmers.

2.1 Beginning education

My family resided in New York City and Rye, New York, until I was seven years old. My formal education began on Sunday mornings, when my father taught me to read – pre-kindergarten – using the comic strips in the Sunday papers as a textbook. I also had the good fortune to subsequently attend Rye Grammar School – a very advanced school for its time. For example, it had its own student news broadcasts to classes every morning.

Aged 41 when the United States entered World War II (WWII), my father requested and obtained active duty in the Navy (he was a Chief Warrant Officer in the Naval Reserve). He was immediately transferred to the West Coast and then shipped out to the Pacific theater about the time (June, 1942) of the Battle of Midway. My mother and I followed and the rest of my education until graduate school took place in California (San Diego, Los Angeles, San Francisco). With my father away throughout the war, my mother continued my outside-school education by reading many volumes of Dickens aloud to me.

The psychological impact of WWII on me was enormous. I followed the news very closely and my father wrote me about the men he was with *via* v-mail. Although I was too young to fully understand the sweep of world events, I followed them closely in the newspapers and they became firmly imprinted in my memory. While he was on leave, I remember my father crossing out sunken submarines from a list he had and telling me about crew members he knew on them. Because of these events, I became acutely aware of the precarious nature of life and through the war years, I was never certain that I would see my father again.

In San Diego (where we landed after the war and my father's discharge from the Navy), I continued to be well served by a fully functional public school system. I still remember individual teachers at the junior high school and high school levels. In particular, in high school, I had a science teacher who allowed me to supplement formal classes with after-hours chemistry experiments on my own, working with real chemicals, and trying reactions whose descriptions I dug out of advanced texts.

2.2 Scientific beginnings

As did many young people at the beginning of the nuclear age, I had become interested in nuclear physics and in my case, cosmic rays. I became (I think) one of the first people in San Diego after the war to have a licence from the Atomic Energy Commission (AEC #1828, Aug. 16, 1950) to purchase radioactive materials, and with it, I purchased one ounce of thorium nitrate at a cost of $ 0.83 in August, 1950. I used the nitrate as a test source of ionizing radiation for a continuous cloud chamber I constructed when I was in my junior year in high school. It was an even greater thrill observing cosmic ray tracks with the thorium source removed: it produced a great sense of mystery about the origin of these rays that I knew had traveled enormous distances to leave their calling cards in my little peanut butter jar apparatus.

At about the same time I became interested (I think because of an article I read in *Popular Science* magazine) in field emission microscopy. I wrote to Erwin Müller (1911–1977), who invented the technique that allows the visualization of individual atoms in 1937, at the Kaiser-Wilhelm Institute in Berlin telling him of my plans to build such a microscope. Müller wrote me back a very nice letter in German along with a reprint of his latest work. In the letter he gently told me that "Um gute Resultate zu erreichen, muss man allerdings einige Erfahrungen in der Vakuumtechnik besitzen." ("To get good results, one must have experience in vacuum technique"). I wasn't destined to have such technique for another 8 years.

Looking back now, it is clear to me that my early scientific interests focused on the mystery surrounding things we can't see with our own eyes: for example, cosmic rays and atoms.

When it came time for college, the tuition-free (at that time) University of California at Berkeley seemed to be the answer for a family with our income. The only drawback was the reportedly huge classes – especially in freshman chemistry. However, after a visit to an open house at The California Institute of Technology (CalTech) my father decided on the spot that no matter what the financial sacrifice on his and my mother's part, I had to go to CalTech, where I was accepted a few months later.

3 CalTech years

Matriculating at CalTech was then meant to be (and was) intimidating. Speaking to the assembled incoming freshman before classes started, Dean Foster Strong casually said something like, "look right and left, at the end of the first term one of those classmates will no longer be here". Try saying something like that to modern college freshmen! With these beginning words we were let loose for long days of classes and homework.

The Korean War continued through my beginning undergraduate years, as did the military draft. Knowing I would soon be eligible for the military draft, I joined The Air Force Reserve Officers Training Corps (AFROTC) which recruited actively on the CalTech campus. As described later, joining the AFROTC had definite effects on my career and attitudes.

3.1 Among smart people

Including the students, there were some weighty intellects at CalTech when I was there. Linus Pauling was in his prime, Richard Feynman had recently arrived, and there were many other famous or soon-to-be-famous members of the faculty. But there were also many faculty members whom the rapid advances in the sciences had left completely behind. And, for the first time, I met men my own age (only men – CalTech then was like a Jesuit school for scientists) who were very smart and had scientific abilities far outstripping anything I had.

I still have a CalTech examination book with an essay written for – and corrected personally by – Linus Pauling during freshman chemistry. Pauling was insistent on proficiency in language so he gave a snap essay exam each year for the whole freshman class of 125 students taking the course. Pauling had this much work to do because one of the features of a CalTech education then was that future engineers and scientists took all classes together the first two years. For example, I took engineering drafting (which helped me greatly later when I had to design apparatus in graduate school).

3.2 CalTech's philosophy – then

This idea – that there is fundamental knowledge that engineers and scientists both need to know – is completely out of fashion and all students that I meet now have specialized very early and assume they will join teams of people with interlocking abilities. I don't want to enter into a debate here about the merits of this and other changes in undergraduate scientific education that have taken place since my era. But I do know that, with the preparation I got as an undergraduate, I've been able to keep up with a general understanding of the major developments in all branches of science that have taken place since I left formal training.

3.3 Humility, humiliation and teaching CalTech style

CalTech was both a place for humility and for humiliation. It was and is mainly a graduate school and regularly graduate students deemed not prepared for the CalTech standard were made to attend undergraduate courses (where they would usually slip into seats in the back of the class and attempt to be invisible). In my junior year, James Watson was on campus, just back from England where he had collaborated with Crick in the monumental work that changed biology forever. My undergraduate friends majoring in biology appreciated and understood his work (even if some of the faculty had missed its implications.) One of my friends told me how important Watson's work was going to be and I searched Watson out and got a reprint of one of the two famous *Nature* papers [1] (he said it was his last copy, and I still have it).

Pauling and Feynman were great lecturers who knew the full value of stagecraft in teaching. At that time, Feynman confined his lower-level formal lecturing to what were called "Friday Evening Demonstration Lectures" that were open to students and public alike. Some inkling of Feynman's lecture style can be obtained by reading his *Lectures on Physics* [2] (the books were based on lectures given in 1961–62) or listening to recordings of them, now available on audio cassette [3].

Constantly smiling during his dynamic lectures, Pauling obviously delighted in undergraduate education. Later on I heard it said that Enrico Fermi could lecture on physics in one continuous development of thought starting with Newton's laws and going all the way up to the edge of what is known. Pauling could do the same thing with chemistry and I still use his textbook *General Chemistry* as a reference. I was 17 years old and being exposed to, and challenged by, some of the finest analytical minds of the 20th century.

3.3.1 My research beginnings

Beginning near the end of my sophomore year, and continuing until I graduated, I did some real research. John D. Roberts, a great and forward-looking organic chemist at CalTech, suggested to me that he thought the mechanism of an organic reaction (I forget which) that appeared in all undergraduate organic chemistry textbooks was wrong. He suggested a simple and straightforward experimental way of testing the mechanism. I proved Roberts to be correct and the textbooks wrong. This research left a lasting impression on me of how clearly a great scientist thinks about a problem. The experiment Roberts suggested to me was so simple that for the first time in science I could have kicked myself for not thinking of doing it the same way.

I went on from my research start with Roberts to solve a crystal structure (of a Li-Sn metallic compound) using X-ray diffraction. I worked on this directly with B. Gunnar Bergman (then officially Pauling's student but actually working mainly with David P. Shoemaker, another about-to-be well-known crystallographer).

In my third year at CalTech, I became friendly with another Pauling protégé, Norman Davidson, who proved to have a great influence on my career. Although he later did as I was to do – unilaterally declare himself a molecular biologist – Davidson at the time was doing research on gas phase reactions using shock tubes. However, Davidson suggested I do some research with the then relatively new and primitive electron microscope. I took up his suggestion, and although the research didn't come to anything, I learned a lot about staining samples and, as a side issue that would turn out to be lucky in my future thesis project, learned a lot about high vacuum systems (mainly, in those days, about the plenty of things that could go wrong with them).

Looking back now, my second and third years at CalTech must have been a time when I widened my mental horizons greatly. I read Harold Urey's new book *The Planets, Their Origin and History* when it came out in 1952 even though I had no idea who Urey was or that I was to become his student and, briefly, an astrochemist!

I also read Edmund Berkeley's *Giant Brains* about the development of computers. This was several years before the first commercial stored-program computer (the UNIVAC) appeared on the market. I remember tabulating data from my X-ray diffraction experiments using Hollerith cards and IBM sorters, but all calculations were done by hand on Marchant electro-mechanical calculators. Thus I humbly entered the computer age and have followed it along like a surfer picking up a wave that gets bigger and bigger.

I was also a little unusual as a chemistry major insofar as I took enough courses in physics to officially minor in that subject. This was especially difficult for me because, much as I like physics, I was (and am) a terrible and unnatural mathematician (that is, at a level necessary to do creative physics). That problem of being fluent in another scientific language struck again: I found that I didn't speak mathematical physics well.

When my senior year started, I began looking at graduate schools. CalTech science graduates were in great demand: I even got an unsolicited invitational telegram from a well-known infrared spectroscopist at the University of Minnesota inviting me to enter the chemistry department there. Evidently, to recruit them, student-hungry departments around the country were finding the names of CalTech's about-to-graduate students. And our entire chemistry class totaled 8 students!

For graduate school, I was determined to go to a big city school in the eastern U.S. and under the influence of Norman Davidson, who had graduated from there in 1941, I decided to apply to the University of Chicago's Chemistry Department and was accepted with a teaching assistantship.

3.3.2 A 1950s CalTech education in summary

To summarize a CalTech education at that time: it produced pretty arrogant boy-men with a superb education in the foundation of quantitative science: the integration of mathematics and basic physics, and – if they wanted it – the beginnings of a liberal education. The system also produced the ability to calculate the answers to numerical problems, knowledge of what a mathematical derivation is, knowledge of what a scientific experiment is, knowledge of what a control for an experiment means, and what experimental errors are and where they come from. In my case, it did furnish me with a basic liberal arts education, and allowed me to expand my interests in that direction. It was a superb school.

In June 1955, I graduated from CalTech with "Academic Honors" (granted to the upper 10% of the around 100 remaining original members of the class) with my father and grandfather present. (My mother had died the previous fall.)

4 Ph.D. candidate at the University of Chicago

In the 10 years after WWII ended, the University of Chicago had swept up many scientists who had engaged in nuclear weapons research: Enrico Fermi, Harold Urey, Leo Szilard, Joseph and Maria Mayer to name only a few. It had built its Institute for Nuclear Studies to house this faculty directly across from the grandstand under which was the famous squash court (when I got there, still standing but empty) where Enrico Fermi supervised – with a break for an Italian lunch – the criticality of the first nuclear pile. Fermi had died a year before I arrived, but his personal and scientific influence still pervaded the Institute.

4.1 Starting to become a chemical physicist and teacher

I took the usual variety of graduate chemistry courses (e.g., chemical thermodynamics, quantum chemistry, statistical mechanics, etc.) but also completely overstretched myself with courses in quantum electrodynamics (given by Richard Dalitz, a well-known particle physicist) and of all things, magnetohydrodynamics – given by the then 45-year-old S. Chandrasekhar (1910–1995) in his scientific prime.

Although I had financial support from UC, first as a teaching assistant and then later *via* fellowships, it was still not enough to live on. After taking courses for a year, I discovered I could be awarded a Master of Science degree from UC without any further work and this would enable me to teach freshman chemistry at the University of Illinois at Navy Pier (UINP) at a pretty good salary.

Teaching freshman chemistry was challenging, especially at that University and in that era: UINP was mainly attended by students who couldn't afford to go the main University of Illinois campus downstate, and included many who didn't speak English at home. Chicago was then, and still is, divided into very definite ethnic areas whose inhabitants were mixed only in certain circumstances like getting an education. It was very intriguing to learn to teach effectively at a level different from CalTech or UC.

4.2 My independent research career's foundation: Harold Urey

During this time, I also began looking for someone to direct my eventual thesis work. A visiting scientist working with Harold Urey suggested I talk to Urey about doing a thesis with him. In my interview with Urey as his prospective student, he related to me the mystery of explosions on comets (where does the stored energy come from?) and at the end of the interview he asked me whether I would like to solve this problem. The answer was yes.

I was to be Urey's last student. His previous one before me had been Stanley Miller who had received worldwide scientific and public recognition for his experiments suggesting how life on earth may have begun.

Urey had a wonderful way with any professional or would-be professional scientist he met, students included, that intimidated many of them. He treated everyone absolutely the same: we were all assumed to be on the same scientific level. There are merits and demerits to this way of treating people, but the merits far outweigh the demerits. During my thesis work and thereafter as a postdoctoral worker, and finally as a faculty member, when I would come to him with what often were half-baked scientific ideas, Urey would invariably take them seriously, consider them, and then give me succinct and dead-on *scientific* reasons why they were half-baked. The result was that I never left his presence humiliated, just chastened and with new understanding of what science was all about.

Urey was a great scientist, but a very un-complex man. He has been variously described by different authors as "boorish and thin skinned" [4], "short, intense, enthusiastic" [5], and "a bantam cock of a physical chemist" [6], among others. I think the derogatory descriptions are grossly unfair: he was just a very ordinary man outside of his scientific talents. Urey's secret weapon in social situations was his wife Frieda who made everyone she met, students especially, feel at home and relaxed almost instantly after meeting her.

After I passed the preliminary examinations allowing me to enter thesis research, Urey arranged for me to have space in the old chemistry building (his office and laboratories were a couple of blocks away in the Institute) and gave me account numbers for purchasing equipment and chemicals. I can't remember seeing him in my laboratory for another year.

During that year I was fortunate in attending the almost daily afternoon tea sessions in his mass spectrometry labs at the Institute. After WWII, Urey had gone into geochemistry, using mass spectrometry as a tool, mainly to get away from the secrecy he had been involved with when working on separation of uranium isotopes for the nuclear weapons project. His Chicago laboratory had turned out some outstanding geochemists before I got there (among them Gerald Wasserburg, Harmon Craig and Cesare Emiliani).

4.2.1 A research problem in astrochemistry

Starting my thesis research project was heady stuff. The basic scientific problem was that comets, drawing near to the sun, experience large outbursts with energy production inconsistent with known chemical or photochemical reactions [7]. Just before I started the project, Bertram Donn and Urey [8] had postulated that comets accumulated free radicals in concentrations up to 10% *via* soft photochemical reactions as they moved away from the sun in their orbits. Upon their return to the close proximity to the sun, their idea was that the free radicals reacted with each other, causing the observed outbursts.

My job was to do experiments to prove the Donn-Urey theory of comet explosions correct.

Reactions on comets take place in the high-vacuum, low-temperature environment of deep space. My job was to design methods for studying photolytic reactions under high-vacuum, low-temperature conditions that simulated actual cometary conditions as closely as possible. The problem was that this was somewhat pioneering work. As the introduction to my thesis [9] states:

> "...it was found that the field of low temperature spectroscopy in the regions of interest had not been explored to any great extent. Until

> recently there were two main reasons for this: the apparatus and refrigerants needed were not widely available, and in many cases sufficient data had not been obtained concerning exact assignments of spectral lines in molecules of interest."

My approach to the problem, approved perfunctorily by Dr. Urey, was to place a cryostat, that I would design, containing an internal liquid hydrogen-cooled window in a spectrophotometer in such a manner that the window could be rotated within the cryostat in one direction to receive gases to be condensed on it, in another direction for irradiation of the condensed gases with hard ultraviolet radiation from a hydrogen discharge lamp of my (future) design, and in a third direction to allow spectra from the ultraviolet to near-infrared (near-IR) of the condensed and irradiated material to be acquired. This was a complicated design that required the outer cryostat to have windows at room temperature through which the beam of the spectrometer passed, an inner liquid nitrogen-cooled shield, and finally the inner liquid hydrogen cryostat tipped with the cooled window. The technical problem was that the whole inner assembly had to be rotated in a high vacuum to receive the gases for condensing, irradiation, and to obtain the spectra of the irradiation products. Urey trusted me, without any evidence that I could do the job, to specify and order the spectrophotometer, to design the apparatus, to arrange its construction, and to do the experiments completely on my own.

The first entry in my lab book on Nov. 21, 1957 starts "Beckman DK-1 recording spectrophotometer delivered and installed."

4.2.2 Teaching myself free radical chemistry and low temperature physics

With the spectrophotometer at hand, I set about designing the cryostat, cooled window assembly, high-vacuum system, hydrogen discharge lamp, and the modifications to the spectrophotometer (then a relatively expensive piece of instrumentation), made engineering drawings, specified materials and supervised the fabrication by the superb professional machine shop at the Institute, and built part of it (teaching myself machining) in the student-faculty workshop. I also took a course in glass blowing given by the old world master glassblower in the Chemistry Department and then proceeded to

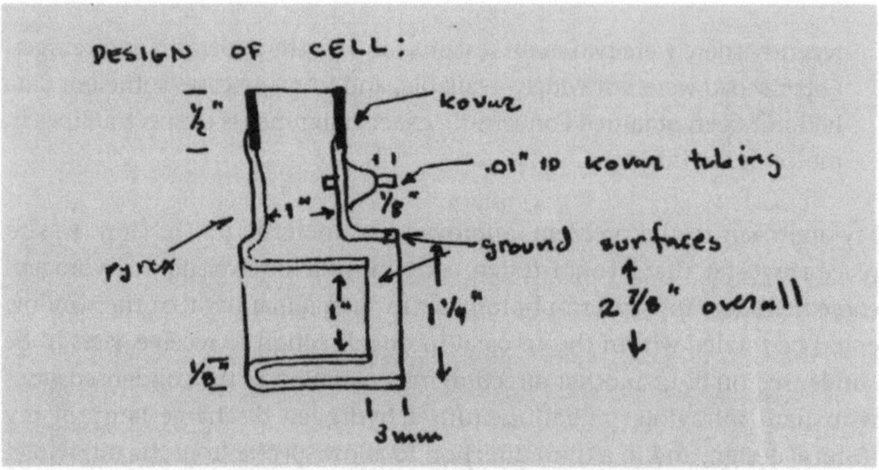

Fig. 1
Liquid-hydrogen-cooled spectrophotometer cuvette designed by the author for viewing putative cometary photolytic products. The windows that were later glued on had to be parallel, so this was a very difficult design to execute for the glassblowers in the Chemistry Department at the University of Chicago. They did a wonderful job.

make the glass manifold for the vacuum system. Figure 1 shows my first window design sketch in my lab notebook.

In my first design the windows were of CaF_2, a substance transparent to light from the far ultraviolet through the near-IR. The use of liquid hydrogen as the coolant was in the interests of technical simplicity and would never be allowed today (hydrogen gas forms an explosive mixture with oxygen in almost all proportions!). The alternative of using liquid helium as the refrigerant would have required much more extensive apparatus and the heating during irradiation of substances on the window would have boiled off much more helium than we could afford. In my design, the liquid hydrogen that boiled off was simply vented into the Hyde Park neighborhood *via* a hose that went through a hole I punched in one of my laboratory's windows. Figure 2 shows a photograph of the completed apparatus, including some of its main features.

Figure 1 shows that light from the monochromator passed through a 3 mm pathway of liquid hydrogen which should have been transparent to light of all the wavelengths I was using. However, almost from the first filling with liquid hydrogen, I found that I got a spectrum in the near-IR without any condensate on the windows of the cuvette.

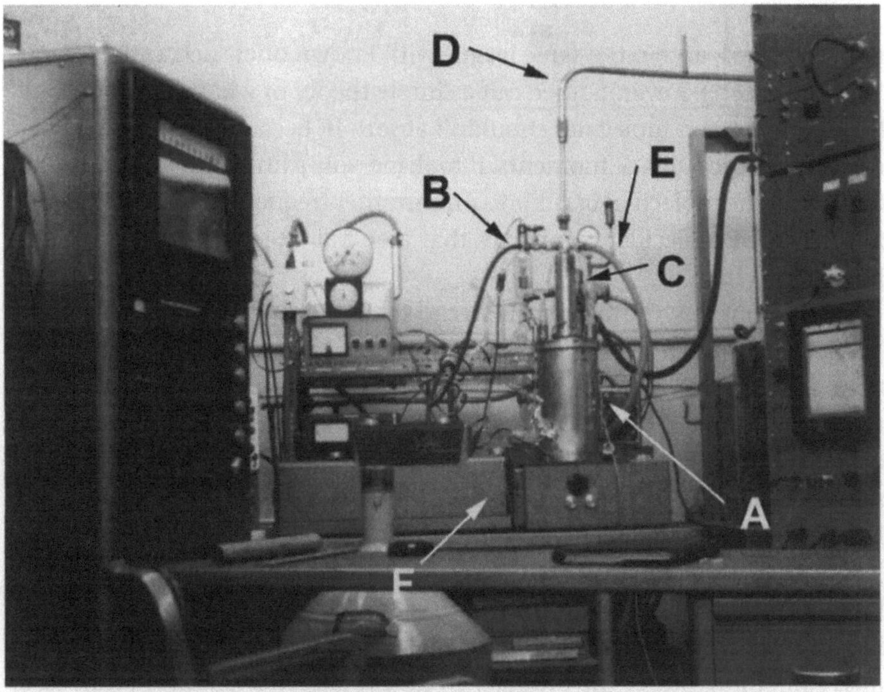

Fig. 2
The author's thesis apparatus. A, the outer cryostat; B, the vacuum gauge; C, the rotating inner cryostat; D, liquid hydrogen fill tube; E, hose to the window for liquid hydrogen boil-off; F, the Beckman DK-1's monochromator. Not visible, the hydrogen discharge lamp for irradiating samples.

4.2.3 First slip-ups, discoveries and encounters with "experts"

This led to the first important non-discovery of my career.I tried cleaning the windows, changing the vacuum pump oil, evaporating liquid hydrogen to see if there was an impurity that left a residue, everything I could think of; but the near-IR spectrum was always still there. Finally, I just concluded the spectrum was due to liquid hydrogen itself.

News of my finding excited quite a few faculty because it violated quantum theoretical spectroscopic "selection rules" pertaining to a symmetrical molecule like hydrogen: hydrogen shouldn't have an absorption spectrum in the near-IR. Willard Stout, a faculty member who was also editor of the *Journal of Chemical Physics* (a journal Urey had founded), told me that it could be "a name effect" (e.g., the "Glasel effect"; the first of many bearing my name, I hoped, and in the same league with known ones such as the famous "Raman Effect"). I even figured out a simple theory of what was happening. Isolated hydrogen molecules shouldn't absorb IR because they have no permanent electrical dipole moments. It took me only a little thinking to see that in a liquid the molecules crash into one another frequently and create short-lived crushed molecular complexes that aren't at all symmetrical and *could* have IR spectra.

As I set out to write a short "Letter to the Editor" about this effect to the *Journal of Chemical Physics* at Stout's invitation, I came across a nasty surprise: there were several papers by a Canadian group that had recently found and reported on the same phenomenon. Alas, no Letter to the Editor, no named effect, and friends and faculty that had encouraged me about the work now said I should have looked for it in the literature *before* getting them excited. Dr. Urey shook his head and said it could happen to anyone.

I learned a lot from this affair. Perversely, I was happy with myself because I now knew I would *never* drop an observation into the mental trash bin just because I didn't understand it. It also gave me confidence that I would never miss something out of the ordinary in an experiment. Finally, I resolved to do literature searches before reporting something I thought was totally new.

I redesigned the window to be a single sheet of synthetic sapphire (which conducts heat better than copper at liquid hydrogen temperatures). When this was built, I began new condensation and irradiation experiments. Outside the problems with high vacuum leaks that gave me constant headaches, I found a new interpretational problem: as I deposited materials on the window, the recorded baseline as a function of wavelength went from flat, to one with big waves, to smaller waves, and finally flat again when there was a lot of material on the window (Fig. 3).

Because of the familiarity of wavy backgrounds to anyone with a passing knowledge of optics – and I had a good course in optics as an undergraduate – it didn't take me too long to figure out that I was observing interference patterns between light striking the vacuum-deposit interface and that striking the sapphire-deposit one. Using these interference patterns, I knew I had a way of measuring the thickness of the deposited layer. This was very exciting to me, because knowing the thickness of the deposited layer was necessary to calculate the concentration of any molecules in the layer and there was no other way I could figure out to know these concentrations.

This was my first true discovery, but alas it became a non-event.

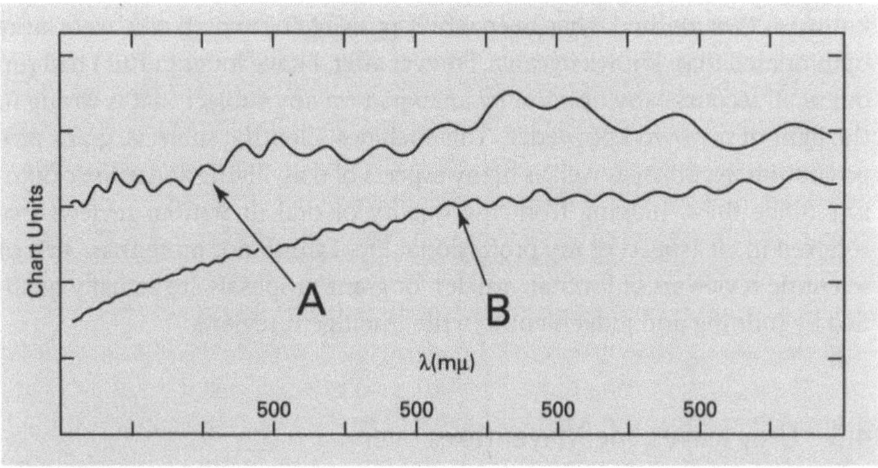

Fig. 3
Near-IR spectra of water deposited on a sapphire window at 20 K in high vacuum. A, 15′ deposition; B, 30′ deposition. Note that the waves become smaller in amplitude and closer together as the deposit becomes thicker.

This time I did do my homework: my method for determining the thickness of layers condensed from vacuum hadn't been reported yet. I submitted a quick paper to *The Review of Scientific Instruments* (where techniques of this type are best reported). It was very quickly rejected: the reviewers sternly offered their decision that the phenomenon of interference fringes had been known since Newton's time and therefore my technique was not new.

I then made a big mistake that I have never repeated in any walk of life: I believed the "experts"(in this case, my paper's scientific reviewers) and I did not fight back by rebutting the experts or arguing with the editor, or by submitting the paper to another journal. I just put the manuscript away and didn't look at it again because, at the time, it seemed like a repeat of the liquid hydrogen spectrum debacle. The problem was that the reviewers were correct in only a minor sense: interference fringes had been known since Newton's time. However, for them not to acknowledge that there were different uses for interference fringe effects, such as I had found, was like saying that the spectrum of colors from a prism had been known since Newton's time and therefore no part of spectroscopy was new.

A few years later someone else published the same use of interference fringes to measure concentrations of deposited reactants and it became known as *their* method. I had been rabbit-punched by experts who were more opinionated than knowledgeable. Forever after, I have fought until I had run out of all recourse any opinion by an expert on any subject that is wrong in the light of my own knowledge. This includes scientific subjects, grant proposal study sections, as well as many aspects of daily living and artistic opinion. Since then, judging from the quality of oral or written reviews I've received in all aspects of my professional life, I think not more than 30% of scientific reviewers of journal, articles, or grant proposals are actually qualified by training and judgement to write intelligent reviews.

4.3 Urey leaves, Joe Mayer takes over

In 1958, without telling many people, including me, Harold Urey was recruited by the new University of California's branch in San Diego (now known as the University of California at San Diego, UCSD) and left the University of Chicago forthwith.

Searching for another faculty member who could take over my thesis research led me to Joseph Mayer (1904–1983). Joe was well known for his theoretical work in statistical mechanics and he and his wife Maria Goeppert Mayer (1906–1972), a nuclear physicist even more famous than Joe, were long-standing friends of Urey's.

I became part of Joe's small group – all theoreticians – and started attending the weekly lunches that the group had with him at local restaurants. Joe was the first scientific intellectual I had ever met (and one of the very few I have since met) and a very sophisticated thinker about many non-scientific things, including larger world issues. We became friends and the more I learned about him as a scientist and a man, the more I admired him.

4.4 Thesis and graduation

In late 1958, I told Joe that I thought I satisfied the requirements for a Ph.D. in chemical physics. Somewhat bemused, Joe said, "I still don't know what you've done, but OK". I hadn't solved the comet problem (to date, nobody has) but I had enough data to submit manuscripts for several papers on low-temperature spectroscopy [10–13].

My thesis project did not succeed in proving the Donn-Urey theory of cometary outbursts to be correct (I reviewed the whole problem at a later date [7]): the maximum concentration of free radicals I could achieve was way below what could lead to the observed energy yields in cometary explosions. I did manage to show experimentally a fact that was confirmed many years later for comets: at low temperatures, the NH radical was one of the most stable [13].

In my thesis research, I learned a good deal about spectroscopy at low temperatures and a lot of spectroscopic theory and experimental methods – almost all self-taught. The most satisfying paper to come out of this research concerned the stabilized nuclear spin states of protons in the hydrogen atoms of H_2O frozen in an argon matrix [10]. It was satisfying because it was a complete story and showed I had mastered basic spectroscopic technique and could deal with a problem that I had recognized and solved on my own.

As a result of my mainly solitary learning experience in graduate school, I left Chicago with a rock-solid conviction that has never left me: I believe there is no scientific experiment of any kind that I can't learn to do quickly and if there are meaningful results to be obtained in the experiment, I will obtain them.Urey insisted that I join him in California after getting my Ph.D. and with his help I was awarded a National Science Foundation Postdoctoral Fellowship in 1959 (at that time only 50 of these were given out yearly). I immediately traveled to the West Coast to begin work.

5 Postdoctoral work with Harold Urey: the new University of California at San Diego

The UCSD campus was so new that there was no room for my instruments (which UC had let me take with me), so Urey arranged for me to have a space in the nearby General Atomic Corp. research building.

I can't say that I had a happy time that year. The quality of the personnel in Urey's laboratory was nowhere near as good as at UC, I was isolated several miles away at General Atomic, the Air Force was trying to make me live up to my CalTech AFROTC obligation of 2 years active duty (which I was now trying to avoid as long as possible), and yes, the beach was distracting. Also, I knew that the comet problem wouldn't be solved without firing an instrument-bearing rocket right into a comet, taking spectroscopic and other data all the while, and that wasn't likely.

Since much of my later career involved me in computer technology and programming, it is significant that during my stay in La Jolla, I began learning FORTRAN II.

For reasons I can't explain I made a sudden decision to change my career and go into biochemistry. And not just biochemistry, but into applying the then new tool of nuclear magnetic resonance (NMR) spectroscopy to biochemistry. I suppose my decision was also based on what little I knew about the structures of molecules involved in biochemical reactions: the few structures known were almost always more complicated or "unusual" to me than the ones I had encountered in my training in chemistry. Since NMR was emerging as the tool for determining structures, I thought it could build a career pioneering the use of NMR in biochemistry.

With Urey's support, I received a second National Science Foundation Postdoctoral Fellowship to go to Great Britain to take up NMR.

5.1 If I can learn nuclear magnetic resonance spectroscopy I have a job at Columbia University

I obtained a position in Lloyd Jackman's laboratory in the Chemistry Department at the Imperial College of Science and Technology in London. I chose Jackman because he was young and becoming well known for his structural-organic chemical work using NMR.

While I waited to leave La Jolla, with propitious timing, Stanley Miller (by then on the UCSD faculty) introduced me to the visiting David Rittenberg (1906–1970), Chairman of the Department of Biochemistry at Columbia University's College of Physicians and Surgeons in New York. Rittenberg had been one of Urey's first graduate students at Columbia in the 1930s.

After he got his Ph.D. with Urey in Chicago, Stanley had taken an Assistant Professorial position in Rittenberg's Department, leaving there after a few years to go to La Jolla. I have always assumed that Stanley had spoken to him beforehand, because Rittenberg offered me a job as an Assistant Professor in his Department almost immediately. When informed that I had an active duty commitment to the Air Force, Rittenberg replied that he would wait the two years. Our agreement was that I would set up a laboratory at Columbia to do NMR spectroscopy applied to biochemical problems. It didn't seem to bother Rittenberg that I had only seen an NMR spectrometer once, and knew nothing about biochemistry.

Although I was still too much into the world of physical sciences to appreciate the honor, Columbia's Biochemistry Department was then one of the most prestigious in the United States. The Department's faculty contained such notables (besides Rittenberg) as Erwin Chargaff (1905–), David Shemin (1911–1991) and David Nachmansohn (1899–1983), while elsewhere at the College of Physicians and Surgeons (P&S) were scientists such as Elvin Kabat (1915–2000). I also didn't know that it had been a long time since there was any turnover in the Department. Stanley Miller had been the last appointment before me.

6 Postdoctoral research in London learning NMR

Fifteen years after the end of WWII, England was still showing the deprivations it had suffered. There were still bomb craters visible in the City of London and coffee was still rationed. After Southern California, London was cold, dark and smelled of coal smoke, and I loved it immediately (and have never stopped).

6.1 Department of Chemistry, Imperial College

I duly reported to Imperial College (IC). It was then a great Victorian pile as far as architecture was concerned, but with a scientific reputation in America as the "MIT" of Great Britain. In fact, I had come at a time of great change in the faculty at IC: Patrick Blackett (1897–1974), Derek Barton (1918–1998) and Ernst Chain (1906–1979) had all recently joined the Departments of Physics, Chemistry, and Biochemistry respectively, making them certainly the equal of any such departments in the world.

6.1.1 Making a MUDDLE

A brilliant spectroscopist, David W. Turner was also on the Chemistry Department faculty doing NMR research, and Lloyd suggested I work closely with him. Previous to my arrival, David had come up with a typical (for him) astute observation: the resonant frequency ratios of some nuclei (in particular, ^{1}H:^{14}N) were very nearly a rational fraction (in this case 13/180).

In those days magnetic field drifts, along with radio frequency drifts, made it difficult to accurately irradiate two nuclei simultaneously (desirable in some important experiments such as spin decoupling). David saw that if the oscillator supplying the resonant radio frequency for ^{1}H were locked to that of ^{14}N by radio frequency division by 180 followed by multiplication by 13, the job of getting the exact resonant frequency for ^{14}N could be transferred to a low-frequency oscillator (much more stable than a radio frequency oscillator). Then the two nuclei could be irradiated simultaneously, regardless of magnetic field drifts, because their resonant frequencies would be accurately locked together. David, with Lloyd's agreement, suggested I make it my job to make this idea practical.

I did two things. First, I purchased Abragam's just-published classic monograph on NMR spectroscopy [14]. Reason: I knew nothing about theoretical or practical NMR. Second, I started researching in the IC library for circuitry for dividing and multiplying radio frequencies, also something I knew nothing about. This was still the vacuum tube era in Great Britain and it was still the postwar era of frugality as far as funding for academic science was concerned (for example, IC's new Varian NMR spectrometer was shut off each evening to conserve electricity; it then required hours of wasted time in the morning to regain magnetic field homogeneity adequate for doing research). While I was able to convince the Prof that we were worthy of an expenditure (not small, given our budget) for an oscilloscope, it fell to me to get most of the electronic components from war surplus stores (then mostly located in the red-light section of Soho).

I was quickly successful in designing and building this radio frequency divider/multiplier (I believe the original is the property of London's Science Museum now; at least I saw it on display there in recent years.) Acronyms began being popular then, so in honor what I perceived to be the English attitude, I promptly named our device MUDDLE (*M*odulated *U*nclear *D*ecoupler and *D*amn *L*ittle *E*lse) and so labeled its front panel in bold lettering. We published a paper describing MUDDLE [15], but never even thought to patent the method. Several years later I was told that the method became the basis of Varian's "gyrospin" feature on their next-generation NMR instruments.

But world events finally overtook my life and four years were to pass before I published another paper in the physical sciences.

6.1.2 The Berlin Wall affects my life

During the night of August 12–13, 1961, the Berlin Wall went up and President Kennedy was faced with how to react to this provocation. As we know, despite his calling for a full war alert for the American military, no shots were fired then and the Wall became a reality for almost the next 30 years.

As a direct consequence of the war alert, six months after the Wall was built, I was called to active duty in the USAF. The reason was that "chemical physics" was not an Air Force personnel qualification descriptor so when I provided information to the USAF personnel office upon my graduation from UC, the nearest thing that seemed to apply was "nuclear chemistry", which seemed near enough to the stable isotopic chemistry most of Urey's laboratory was doing. However, the Air Force now suddenly found a need for nuclear chemists and, on paper, my qualifications fit and I was called to active duty.

I knew nothing about nuclear chemistry – the work I was about to engage in. I found out later that the outfit I was to be assigned to had detected an increase in Russian plutonium production at about the time of the Wall's construction and needed trained nuclear chemists to beef up their analytical capabilities: hence the Air Force's sudden need for me.

My orders sent me to Sacramento, California and my assignment as a First Lieutenant in the "1155th Technical Operations Squadron" of the "1066 Field Activities Group". These were innocuous cover names to shield the mission of the units.

7 A nuclear research officer, United States Air Force

The 1066th bore the responsibility in the United States for detecting and analyzing nuclear explosions – specifically above-ground Russian nuclear tests at that time – for yield, weapon design, etc., along with foreign fissionable materials production. Both testing and production were monitored largely *via* radiochemical and physical examination of airborne debris gathered by U-2 planes assigned to the Group.

7.1 Military science and life

On the basis of my smattering of Fortran II training during my La Jolla postdoctoral appointment, my first non-chemical assignment came when I was instructed to "learn to program" a new IBM 1620/1400 computer combination that arrived in Sacramento one day. Such was the hurry, I taught myself this higher-level programming language without disciplining myself to write flow diagrams for my programs, an unfortunate practice I have never been able to shed. But I got the job done and within a few weeks we could use the computer to help physically reconstruct a weapon from the sets of data available.

I learned a lot, both scientific and personal, during my active duty in the military. After my first year, I was put in charge of a small group whose responsibility was setting up and running a electron microprobe analyzer (a then newly developed apparatus for using secondary electron emissions to do elemental analysis of solid specimens – such as bomb debris). This technique was déjà vu insofar as it involved wrestling with vacuum systems but it also taught me how to teach non-commissioned officers and enlisted men with no scientific training how to do experimental physics. Also, during my off-duty time in the Air Force, I moonlighted by teaching undergraduate "physics for non-physics majors" at Sacramento State College and quantum chemistry at the graduate level for the University of California Extension Program.

I was scheduled to be discharged from active duty in the USAF on February 16, 1964. One day while I waited, I was called into the squadron commander's office and asked if I would accept a regular commission in the Air Force! To be offered this is a singular honor for any reservist in the U.S. military. Even though I was anxious to get out of uniform and back to big-league science and my own ideas for research, I hesitated. Although I finally turned it down, I've often wondered in years since whether or not I made a good decision. I haven't had many honors in my life, but this offer of a commission was certainly a sterling one, and I turned it down. I was discharged from the Air Force, resigned my reserve commission, and traveled to New York to begin my career as an academic scientist.

8 Back to academic life as a biochemist

8.1 New in biochemistry and NMR

While I was still on active duty, I had written my first grant proposal – to set up a laboratory at Columbia equipped with the best NMR instrumentation then available (the 0.141T electromagnet Varian DA-60EL proton high resolution and multi-nuclear wideband instrument), with Rittenberg as a co-investigator. We got the grant, and using my design, a temperature- and humidity-controlled room was built and the instrumentation installed within about six months after I arrived after my discharge.

After the instrument was running satisfactorily, I started an ambitious program to apply proton and multinuclear NMR to problems I thought might be of biochemical interest. My subsequent NMR work at Columbia fell into three categories: the involvement of water structure in biochemical interactions, biomolecular structures (in particular bioactive peptides), and instrumental developments.

8.1.1 Research on water and biomolecular interactions *via* NMR

My work on water structure involved the then new approach of studying the rotational motions of water molecules *via* the NMR relaxation properties of water labeled with the stable isotopes ^{2}H and ^{17}O. My decision to work on this project stemmed from my knowledge of what was happening in chemical physics as well as biochemical research.

The structure of liquids was a hot theoretical and experimental topic in chemical physics at that time and some of this focus was applied to biochemistry. In particular, both Pauling and Stanley Miller had recently published papers hypothesizing that water structure played a role in general anaesthesia [16, 17]. Their basic idea was that anaesthetics altered the structure of water around neurons so as to inhibit transmission of impulses. Furthermore, their arguments implicated anaesthetics that promoted formation of hydrates. The rare gas xenon, a good anaesthetic, is an example of a chemically unreactive species that forms hydrates.

I decided to see if NMR could be applied to the problem of how water molecules interacted with biological structures.

Rittenberg had close connections with many scientists in Israel (he had helped set up the Biochemistry Department in the Weitzmann Institute after the war). He arranged for Yeda Research and Development Co. in Rehovoth, Israel, to present me with a gift of a few milliliters of 10% enriched $H_2{}^{17}O$ – at that time worth thousands of dollars.

I wanted to see whether or not xenon in solution altered water structure as indicated by changes in water molecules' rotational reorientation times – quantities that I knew could be derived from ^{17}O NMR spin-lattice relaxation times.

In thick-bore NMR tubes, I made stoichiometric xenon-$H_2{}^{17}O$ mixtures that formed a waxy solid hydrate below 27 °C and melted to a clear solution above this temperature. The paper that appeared describing this work [18] contained all the equations necessary to interpret ^{17}O relaxation experiments and to quote its conclusion, "in essence, the xenon lowers the effective temperature of the water." I'm not aware of any papers following up this phenomenological explanation for xenon's anaesthetic properties but I followed up with another paper giving a theoretical analysis of the observed relaxation parameters for both $H_2{}^{17}O$ and ^2H_2O [19]. Using $H_2{}^{17}O$ I was also able to report (prior to many subsequent X-ray crystallographic studies showing the same thing) that proteins contained patches of relatively immobile water [20]. I confirmed this observation using ^2H_2O [21].

Even though no competitors were working with $H_2{}^{17}O$, I decided that using it was too expensive and time-consuming for one person to perform numerous measurements with because it needed to be re-purified carefully after work with each solute was completed. I therefore turned to measurements of biomolecular motions in solution using much less expensive ^2H_2O and ^2H-labeled compounds. To do the labeling work, I had to redevelop a proficiency in simple organic synthesis. Fortunately, I enjoyed doing syntheses as a respite from instrumental and theoretical NMR work and was grateful for the thorough training in organic chemistry that came from working with Jack Roberts as an undergraduate.

My Columbia work with ^2H_2O and ^2H-labeled compounds resulted in a series of papers [22–25] dealing with: a correction to the commonly assumed microviscosity value necessary to describe water molecule rotation [26], the interactions of water molecules with biopolymeric conformation [23], the roles of water-solute interactions in denaturing agent and surfactant actions [24], the motions of nucleotide bases in polynucleotides [22], and NMR relaxation times for water in highly heterogeneous systems [25].

In retrospect, the conclusions of the last two papers [22, 25] were somewhat ahead of their time. Working with deuteron-labeled polynucleotides, I showed for the first time that the librational motions of the bases are far more rapid than had previously been assumed. As I stated, "studies of this nature should reveal a large amount of quantitative data on the microscopic motions within macromolecules". Subsequently, much work along these lines has been reported.

The work on heterogenous systems contrasted ^1H and ^2H relaxation in ^1H_2O and ^2H_2O, respectively. The NMR tubes were packed with uniform-diameter glass beads from 0.2 cm down to 0.0015 M in diameter. I showed that as the surface-to-volume ratio increased (the system becoming more heterogeneous), there were very large effects on the water ^1H spin-lattice and spin-spin relaxation times (T_1 and T_2). This paper was followed up by a more quantitative treatment (see below) and I have been told that these papers were later referred to frequently during the development of magnetic resonance imaging (MRI), a technique that was then just beginning its development and which depends partly on the relaxation properties of molecules in a heterogenous system.

8.1.2 Developing instrumentation: the era of minicomputers arrives

Three largely instrumental development papers were part of my Columbia work. Two of them, a "poor man's" technique for measuring spin-lattice relaxation times [27] and a method of improving the DA-60 spectrometer [28], rapidly became obsolete as NMR spectrometers improved. However, a notable instrumentation improvement, done with a Yugoslav postdoctoral worker (the only postdoc I had during my Columbia years) in consultation with workers at Brookhaven [29], was much more interesting: we designed and made a device for the digital production of radio frequency (rf) phase shifts in the rf pulses used for NMR relaxation measurements. It was my first venture into digital technology and the paper is interesting on two counts: (1) it describes our use of some of the first commercially available integrated circuits in combination with the new Digital Equipment Corp. PDP-8/I minicomputer I had been able to obtain; (2) it also describes one of the first uses of computer-generated gated rf pulses for use in NMR – now ubiquitous on all commercial NMR instruments.

8.2 Biomolecular structural work

My first two papers [30, 31] on biomolecular structure (using high-resolution 60 MHz proton NMR) reflect my early belief that three-dimensional conformations of biologically interesting molecules could be approached by NMR methods. Both these papers drew some simple conclusions concerning intramolecular and H-bond stabilization of the molecules involved (biotin and cysteines) and discussed how these might be involved in their function. This NMR approach was new to biochemistry, and both papers continue to be cited sporadically in the literature.

8.2.1 Peptide hormones

These early biomolecular structure papers involved analyzing the NMR spectra of "off-the-shelf" chemicals using standard analytical methods. I saw a dead-end in doing routine work of this sort: work that anyone with an NMR instrument could do. Fortunately, in the late 1960s I began a collaboration with Frank Bovey's laboratory at Bell Telephone Laboratories (specifically with a member of Frank's laboratory, Anne Brewster) and Victor Hruby from the University of Arizona. The focus of our attention was the conformation of oxytocin in solution as determined by NMR using vicinal coupling constants and amide proton exchange rates. At this stage in the development of applications of NMR to bioactive peptides, one often needed a proprietary source of hard-to-get peptides. In this case Victor, who had obtained his Ph.D. under Vincent du Vigneaud (1901–1978), was the source of NMR quantities of oxytocin and some of its derivatives.

The study of peptide conformations *via* NMR was stimulated by a paper [32] from Lyman Craig's laboratory at the Rockefeller Institute (now University) analyzing the conformation of a gramicidin using one of the few superconducting NMR spectrometers available at the time: the 5.2 T instrument at Bell Laboratories. Shortly after this paper was published, another 5.2 T instrument was installed at Rockefeller and both instruments became available to outside investigators.

Although not apparent at the time, our results [33] illustrated a strength and some weaknesses of NMR structural determinations – characteristics that in my opinion persist to the present day. Oxytocin is a biologically important cyclic polypeptide with a prolyl-leucyl-glycinamide "tail" attached to the ring at a cystinyl residue. Several groups were competing to determine the solution conformation of this peptide.

Our contribution was to show that there were two conformations for the hormone: two almost equally populated *cis* and *trans* conformers about the Cysteine-Proline bond. The conformers interchanged very slowly (theoretically the energy barrier interchange was on the order of 20 kcal/mole). The strength of NMR was to show the existence of this isomerization clearly and to explain why X-ray diffraction studies on the same peptide were difficult. The weaknesses of NMR structural methods that this [34, 35] and other groups' studies on peptide hormones showed were that although they *suggested* possible structure-function relationships, they didn't indicate how to experimentally confirm the suggestions.

It was perhaps around this time that I began to have doubts about the utility of the reductionist approach of relating biomolecular structure to solving actual biological problems. If so, I ignored the doubts for another 15 years.

In technology, a quieter revolution was going on: it was the advent of minicomputers employing the first integrated circuits. As mentioned above, I was able to buy one of the first Digital Equipment Corporation PDP-8/Is to come off the production line. The reason I wanted the computer was that it had been clear from my initial research ideas about using NMR in biochemical studies that many materials of interest were only available in small quantities or were insoluble in aqueous media, so signal-to-noise averaging was going to be a vital point.

8.2.2 Fourier-transform spectroscopy arrives: homemade

In the mid 1960s the advent of the Cooley-Tukey algorithm [36] for doing fast Fourier transforms (FFTs) with a computer changed the whole picture of doing NMR and in particular how signal-to-noise averaging would be done in the future. Using the PDP-8/I, we set about using it for relaxation measurements with a digital pulsed NMR modification we designed [29] and for programming the computer to do FFTs. The system worked well, but with only 16 kilobytes of computer memory, it was good only for single resonance relaxation studies and wide-line signal-to-noise averaging (Fig. 4).

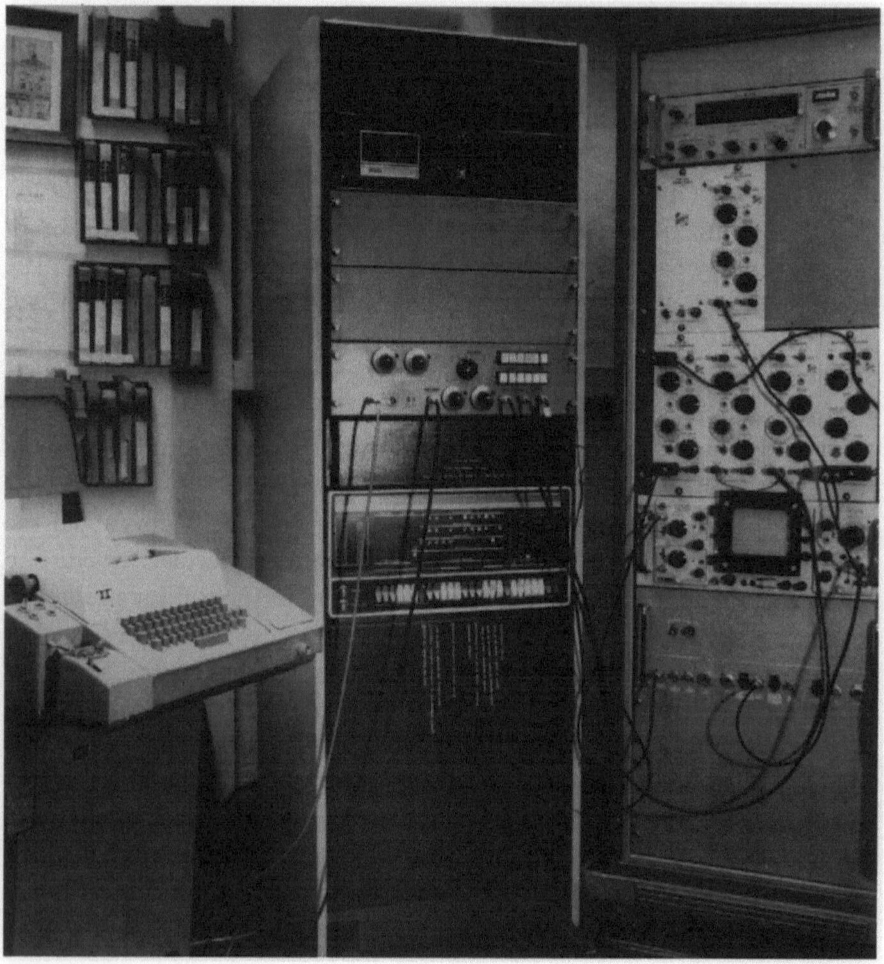

Fig. 4
Our homemade FFT spectrometer circa 1969. Note the punched tape programs to be input *via* the ASR-33 teletype unit. The PDP-8/I used octal arithmetic and the boot program had to be entered by hand using switches.

8.2.3 David Rittenberg

David Rittenberg died of another heart attack at the age of 64 on January 24, 1970. With him gone, I began searching for a job with another biochemistry department. Within a couple of months I had obtained a faculty job as an associate professor in the Biochemistry Department at the first State Medical-Dental School in Connecticut then being constructed (The University of Connecticut Health Center, UCHC). By agreement with the administration at UCHC, I would take a sabbatical in England to allow time for a temporary building to be built at the Connecticut campus to house the NMR equipment I had been given permission to move out of P&S.

9 Sabbatical at the University of Oxford

I had obtained a place in Robert J.P. Williams's laboratory in the Inorganic Chemistry Laboratory at Oxford. Bob Williams was an expert on metallo-enzymes and had published extensively on his imaginative theory of enzyme catalysis. He was also a member of the Oxford Enzyme Group that was very active in structural biochemistry.

The last entry in my laboratory notebook at Columbia was July 26, 1970. It concerned spin-lattice relaxation times for polymers [23]. The first note-book entry at Oxford on September 9, 1970, described measurements using the only NMR instrument conveniently available to Williams at the time, a tiny Varian A-60 spectrometer. The experiments described used the lan-thanide ion Eu (III) as a chemical shift perturbation agent for the NMR spec-trum of ribose-5-phosphate. These measurements, which continued for a week or so, introduced a new method for NMR structural determination.

9.1 Lanthanide ion chemistry

Lanthanide ions have ionic radii that are roughly the same size as many metal ions found in native metalloenzymes. They also have electron paramagnetic properties that are completely different from transition metal ions. Not only do their magnetic moments vary from zero for La (III) and Lu (III), at the beginning and end of the rare-earth element series in the periodic chart (with high values in between), but their electronic states vary so that members of the series, such as Eu(III) and Gd(III), with large paramagnetic moments, affect NMR signals in different ways. For example, Eu(III) causes electron paramagnetic-induced NMR chemical shift perturbations without line broad-ening in molecules where the lanthanide comes into close proximity to the nuclei whose resonances are being measured. On the other hand, Gd(III) causes NMR line broadening but no chemical shifts situated in the same place in the same molecule.

Bob's idea was that these lanthanide ion properties could be used somehow to determine rigid active site structures of metalloenzymes. The idea followed from the recent widespread adoption of lanthanide-containing organic molecules as "shift reagents" to reduce the complexity of second-order NMR spectra. Upon my arrival, Bob Williams suggested that I work with a Ph.D. student of his, Antonio Xavier, on using lanthanide ions in the metalloenzyme work already in progress.

Other than an introduction in an undergraduate course in inorganic chemistry, I had no prior knowledge of the chemistry of the lanthanide ions. However, I did know that one of the current NMR problems being worked on was the functional requirement nucleotides and oligonucleotides had for Mg(II). The structural problem to be solved was what were the conformations of these flexible molecules *in solution* when they interacted with the metal ion. So far NMR work by several other groups had been done using Mn(II) (a transition metal ion with a large electron paramagnetic moment and an ionic radius similar to Mg(II)) as an NMR line-broadening probe. Their published results had so far been very equivocal.

9.1.1 Determining biomolecular structures using NMR and lanthanide ions

My contribution to the ensuing work was simply to suggest that, instead of working on lanthanide-substituted metalloenzymes, we should concentrate on using the lanthanides – which had about the same ionic radii as Mg(II) and Mn(II) – to look at the conformations of flexible nucleotides. Specifically, I suggested that we start out using the shift-inducing properties of Eu(III) on the simple nucleotide, adenosine monophosphate (AMP). It seemed an easy enough thing to do on an A-60 (which anyhow was completely inadequate for any enzyme work) and the reagents were readily available.

The basic experiments consisted of measuring the chemical shifts of the various resonant protons (later ^{13}C was added) as a function of Eu(III) concentrations and forming shift ratios from the various frequency-shifted resonances. Within two weeks after beginning these experiments we had acquired enough data, followed by theoretical analysis, to make it evident that we could obtain conformational information from this type of measurement. We also knew that the derived ion-proton distances were quite accurate, because theory told us that the shift ratios vary as the inverse cubes of the distance between the nuclei and the metal ion.

The method we developed is formally analogous to the present NMR method of obtaining structures of flexible molecules using the nuclear Overhauser effect (NOE). It was clear to us at this time (10–15 years before the start of widespread reporting of NMR-derived structures) that with a limited number of shift ratios there were going to be, in general, many conformations (a "family" of conformations) that differed but which fit the ratios within experimental error. The lanthanide ion structural method we developed has been reviewed [37].

To make the method practical, we needed a way to delineate the families of structures that fit the available data (in the form of shift ratios) for each molecule we worked on.

9.1.2 Families of structures and computer data fitting

A few minutes toying with measuring interatomic distances on a Dreiding model of AMP and calculating shift ratios by hand convinced me that this was no way to do the job – automation was needed. This was long before the day when computer molecular modeling was routine and available to anyone with a minimal desktop computer. Computer molecular modeling was not unknown at Oxford; it was just unknown at the Inorganic Chemistry Laboratory where Bob's laboratory was located. In fact, there was a very good modeling programmer who was part of the Oxford Enzyme Group, C. David Barry.

Working with David Barry was a great pleasure throughout my stay at Oxford. Although not a "wet" chemist or an NMR spectroscopist, he immediately realized the problem we were trying to solve. In effect, as we developed our method, Dave acted as a daily language translator (he spoke computer language), taking our equations and structures and translating them into software that searched out structures that fitted the data. This was accomplished by algorithms that wiggled the molecule (his program was eventually called "Burlesque") through conformation space to find conformational families that fit the data.

9.2 Putting it all together: our first lanthanide-derived structural family

The family we found for AMP, shown in Figure 5, differed from the conformation of AMP in crystals. Our first paper on this method was written in early December 1970, a little over two months after I arrived at Oxford [38]. This was the first paper in a series that extended the method to other molecules, nuclei and solvent systems [39–42].[2]

The least noticed, but to me one of the most important, of these lanthanide papers was one showing that conformations of AMP differed greatly between dimethylsulfoxide and aqueous solutions [41]. This work planted a seed in my mind that conformations of flexible molecules in solution possibly had little relevance to their biologically active conformations: I reasoned that since biomolecules function in so many different environments, if just changing the solvent changes a molecule's conformation, how can we have confidence that any solution conformation predicts the biologically active one?

Despite the development of this new structural method, subsequent advances in determining structures by NMR without perturbation probes that took place several years later seemed to attract more attention around the world. At any rate, very little subsequent lanthanide-perturbation work by any laboratory has been reported, even though it still would be potentially very useful as an adjunct to direct methods to increase conformational accuracy.

10 Connecticut years – Part I, 1970–1980

Shortly after taking up my job at UCHC in 1971, I took out of storage the NMR spectrometer and other equipment I had moved from Columbia. These instruments enabled measurements of proton high-resolution spectra, spin-lattice and spin-spin relaxation times at 60 MHz and broadline and Fourier transform deuteron spectroscopy.

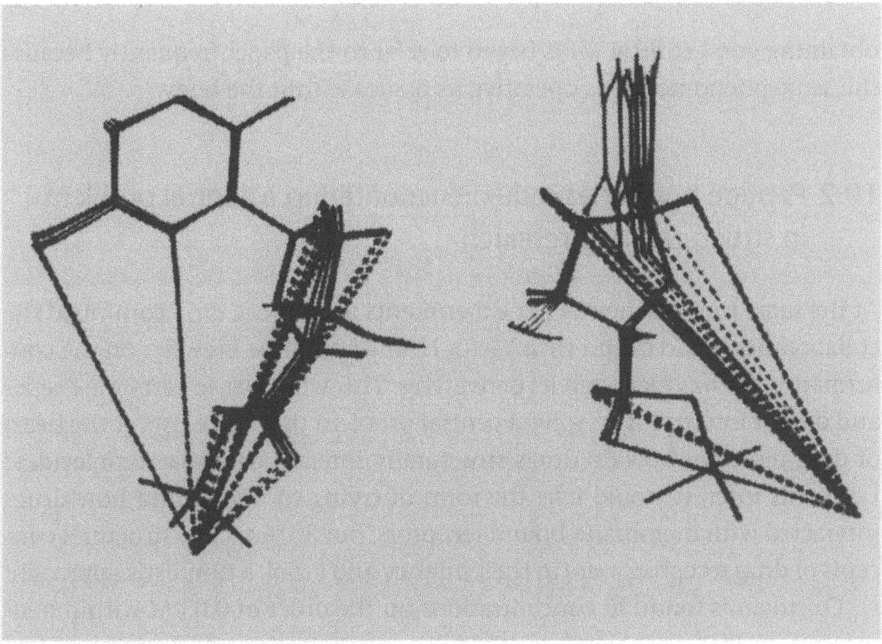

Fig. 5
Orthogonal views of the family of solution conformations for AMP from [38]. Dotted lines indicate metal-ion proton distances for the family that are consistent with the NMR data.

10.1 Water relaxation in heterogeneous systems – pre-magnetic resonance imaging

The first project I started in Connecticut was an extension of the work on water structure begun at Columbia. With a postdoctoral student, Ku Ho Lee, I looked in detail at the spin-lattice relaxation times of deuterons in a series of ^2H_2O-glass microbead systems. The purpose of this work was as we stated in the beginning sentence of the paper that resulted [43], "In spite of its importance, the state of water at foreign surfaces is not well understood". We succeeded in quantitatively analyzing the results in terms of magnetic field inhomogeneity effects at the surfaces of the beads resulting from magnetic susceptibility differences between the beads and bulk water.

While not of seemingly great importance at the time, in the next decade scientists interested in interpreting the roles of spin-lattice relaxation in obtaining good clinical MRIs began to refer to the paper frequently because the same phenomenon is operative in tissues within the body.

10.2 Peptide hormones redux: encountering a central problem in structural drug research

At the same time the new water experiments were going on, I continued the collaboration I had begun with Victor Hruby and Anne Brewster on the conformations of oxytocin and its derivatives. This work was to carry me deeper and deeper into trying to solve a central problem that still exists at the heart of drug research: how do drugs structurally interact with macromolecules? Later this interest would take the form of trying to understand how drugs interacted with membrane-bound receptors, but 30 years ago structural concepts of drug receptors were in their infancy and I took a simplistic approach.

Oxytocin is found in concentrations on the order of 0.03 M within neurosecretory granules, along with similar concentrations of proteins of low molecular weight (approximately 10 kDa) called neurophysins. The role of the neurophysins was unknown but many workers thought that their purpose was to protect oxytocin from enzymatic degradation by binding to the peptide. Fortuitously, we also began a collaboration with Jeffrey McKelvy who was in the Anatomy Department at UCHC, familiar with neurophysin protein chemistry, and interested in NMR techniques.

Since I had one of the few instruments available to do NMR experiments on deuteron-labeled compounds, I proposed that we look at changes in overall rotational and intramolecular motions in deuterated oxytocin and derivatives as they interacted in aqueous solutions with purified neurophysin II.

Our first reported results were on the microdynamical molecular motions of five deuterated derivatives of oxytocin prepared by Victor's laboratory [44]. These experiments showed directly that the "conformation" for flexible molecules can only be regarded as a time-averaged one, whose applicability to biological processes depends on whether or not the motions take place on the same time scale as the physical process being studied. The paper ended with the sentence that summed up our main point: "We believe that these measurements represent the first time that important intramolecular motion has been directly demonstrated in an active hormone." Next, we went on to detailed experiments on the interaction of deuterated oxytocin and derivatives with neurophysin II [45]. This work showed that the Pro-Leu-Gly-NH_2 "tail" of oxytocin was not involved in its interaction with neurophysin II and that there was a rapid exchange between free oxytocin and its neurophysin II bound form.

10.2.1 A regional NMR facility

In 1973 my proposal to the NIH to establish The Southern New England High Resolution NMR Facility was funded for a duration of five years with me as Principal Investigator.

I immediately purchased a 2.35T, JEOL PFT-100 high-resolution Fourier transform spectrometer that incorporated a Texas Instruments 980A computer and had both ^{1}H and ^{13}C probes. To staff the laboratory, I was fortunate to attract Hermann Bleich, a physicist-by-training and NMR-experienced scientist, to run the facility. John Cutnell (on sabbatical leave from the physics faculty at Southern Illinois University) soon joined the laboratory along with Christine Regula as a technician. These five years saw a multiplicity of projects started and my interests switch over rapidly to "wet" biochemistry as I saw our NMR efforts go further and further away from engaging in biological (as opposed to physical biochemical) problems.

In the laboratory during those five years, Hermann, John, Christine and I represented, in our varying interlocking skills, what was to be a dying generation of scientists, "all-arounders". Hermann could switch from designing and building advanced electronic circuits, to NMR theory, then to NMR experiments and back with no effort at all. John could equal Hermann in NMR theory and experiments, along with the ability to do machine and higher-level computer language programming. Christine had the know-how to take a biochemical project that I wanted to carry out from the general idea to performance almost without my help.

In a 1973 talk I gave at the NIH as part of a symposium on recent research methods, I'm pleased that I could see clearly what developments were coming several years later. While Intel had introduced the world's first microprocessor in 1971, the first commercial one, the 8-bit 8080, wasn't available until 1974. In my talk I told an audience of biochemists that "anyone with even a little knowledge of computer technology realizes that inexpensive, advanced microprocessors are very near... one can easily foresee the day when the computer part of the spectrometer will be completely integrated into the experimental part." This came true several years later.

The different research paths I set out on are better explained by category than chronology because most of the time they were all going on in parallel.

10.3 Research developments, 1970–1980

10.3.1 Instrumentation

The PFT-100 was already obsolete when we purchased it because it didn't have quadrature detection (i.e., two-phase sensitive detectors) soon to be used on all commercial spectrometers. Using a design suggested by Alfred Redfield (Hermann Bleich's thesis advisor), Hermann quickly built us a quadrature detector. According to a basic design I suggested, Herman also built water resonance suppression circuitry that worked with an FT spectrometer by selectively saturating the water resonance line before applying the non-selective 90° pulse [46]. During the same period John Cutnell had an idea about how to eliminate annoying phase shifts in FT spin-lattice relaxation measurements that were caused by the invariably imperfect rf pulses that must be used in FT spectroscopy which Herman also built: it proved to be one of the first group of devices built by spectroscopists of that era to use phase alternation to eliminate instrumental artifacts [47].

Later on, when we got interested in rotating-frame spin-lattice relaxation as a way of estimating intramolecular motions in flexible molecules, Herman designed and built a simple modification [48] that allowed these experiments to be done without modifying the software for our spectrometer. This instrumental work was not terrifically innovative, but was in advance of what was then commercially available and so allowed us to do many experiments that only a few other laboratories could do.

10.3.2 Starting to branch out from NMR

As I started becoming a wet protein biochemist, I was able to purchase newly developed equipment: a high-pressure liquid chromatograph (HPLC), the first one at UCHC. While we were using the instrument routinely to characterize peptides using reverse-phase columns, I started wondering about the validity of the then received truth that proteins could only be separated using open column size-exclusion or ion-exchange chromatography. Using the neurophysins as examples, I quickly showed that at least proteins of this molecular mass (about 10 kDa) could be separated by reverse-phase HPLC. I believe the resulting paper [49] was the first report of what has become a standard method of protein separation. The manuscript was originally turned down when a referee stated that "this would never be a practical method of protein separation", thus keeping my opinion of "experts" alive.

10.3.3 NMR and bioactive peptides

By far the major projects we worked on in the period 1973-79 were directed toward learning how NMR relaxation times could contribute to determination of bioactive peptide structures and how these structures interacted with the macromolecules they bound to. We started this work on peptides like oxytocin, vasopressin and tetragastrin, and later branched out to enkephalins. These peptides seemed an ideal way to get at what I believed (and still do) was a major scientific problem to be solved: structurally, wherein lies specificity of binding of bioactive substances to their receptors?

We were doing this work at a time when the possible use of relaxation times and the NOE in determining peptide structures was under increasing investigation by several groups throughout the world.

Our projects differed from other groups insofar as we were focused largely on detailed theoretical analyses of the effects of intramolecular motions on measured relaxation times and NOEs [50–58].

This series of papers established to our satisfaction that in the absence of intramolecular motions in peptides, relaxation times and NOEs could be used to extract main and side-chain torsion angular information. However, we also showed that accurate information of this kind depended upon using dipolar relaxation formalism and that it was deficient where there are intramolecular motions. Since our work showed that *intra*molecular motions *were* important in the peptides we were looking at, the conclusion dawned on me slowly that NMR solution structures of flexible molecules weren't going to contribute much to solving the problem of where their specificity lay.

10.3.4 Beginnings of opiate work

After the existence and identification of the opiate peptides were established in 1975, we were one of three groups to report the first NMR work on one of these, methionine-enkephalin (mENK) [59]. It was satisfying at the time that one of the other contestants made incorrect resonance assignments and the other published their resulting structure in mirror-image stereochemistry.

In subsequent work, we reported on intramolecular motions in mENK, the differences in conformation of mENK in dimethylsulfoxide and water, and the lack of direct interaction of mENK with phospholipid membranes [58, 60, 61] using more and more sophisticated NMR techniques. We also found that lanthanide ions catalyze amide proton exchange in aqueous solutions of peptides [62], an observation we never followed up.

I thought it was not a very satisfactory initial venture into drug-related research: we worked hard but the results showed to my satisfaction that solution conformations of small peptides had *no* implications for their bound conformations on macromolecules, so this body of work actually was another step in my disillusionment with NMR structures of peptides.

However, work which did have important implications for structural determinations of larger, and less flexible, molecules *did* come out of these projects.

10.3.5 Determination of structural families of flexible molecules from spectral density functions

To aid in interpreting the NMR relaxation measurements in structural terms, I began developing a Fortran II source program that included many machine language subroutines for displaying large molecules, determining internuclear distances in them, and printing out ball-and-stick, wire and solid-sphere molecular models of their structures. Most of this was done by a college student, Leonard Spain, under my direction and was done long before computer modeling programs were available for purchase and execution on mini-computers. Our program was in parts called "PEPTID, WOBBLE and WOESS" (Fig. 6), also allowed input of NMR relaxation data and contained some linear programming features that preceded other similar programs by many years.

Since the laboratory was concentrating heavily on the interpretation of ^{1}H and ^{13}C spin-lattice relaxation times and NOEs in peptides, the basic idea of these computer programs was that we could combine these measured NMR parameters with van der Waals filters and vicinal coupling constants to determine self-consistent structures. This idea was already familiar because it was completely analogous to the work that came out of my stay at Oxford 8 years earlier. Just the equations were different.

Jim Visintainer, a new postdoctoral worker, started in on this project along with myself and our programmer. We called the method that developed the SDFM (for spectral density function method) approach to peptide structural analysis. Using one-dimensional NMR, the paper that resulted [63] anticipated the principles and problems of structural determination *via* two- and three-dimensional NMR now in common use.

In the paper, we introduced an NMR "R" value, in analogy to X-ray diffraction models, to estimate the goodness-of-fit of our structures to the NMR data – something later workers in this field didn't get around to doing until the mid-1980s. As we pointed out, the basic problems in determining structures from NMR relaxation or NOE data are the same: determining the spectral density functions $J(h4_i)$; it doesn't make any difference if these appear as a sum (as in spin-lattice relaxation) or a division of sums (as in NOEs) in the equations relating the observables (T_1s or NOEs) to interproton distances. Historically, NMR structure determinations have taken a different course, but I think we were at least among the first groups to put the principles on a firm theoretical and experimental foundation.

Despite our solid NMR work on peptides, it was all getting very boring to me because it seemed farther and farther away from attacking real biological problems. So, with this becoming more important to me, I consciously began teaching myself "wet" biochemistry. The starting point was learning protein chemistry.

When Jeff McKelvy moved away from UCHC in the mid-1970s, he left me with a large quantity of acetone-dried bovine pituitary powder – a rich source of hypophyseal hormones and neurophysins. I decided to teach myself how to isolate and purify neurophysins from this source. Because of some confusions in the literature about the properties of these proteins, it was of interest at the time to characterize them and their interactions with oxytocin at the high concentrations at which they were present in neurosecretory granules.

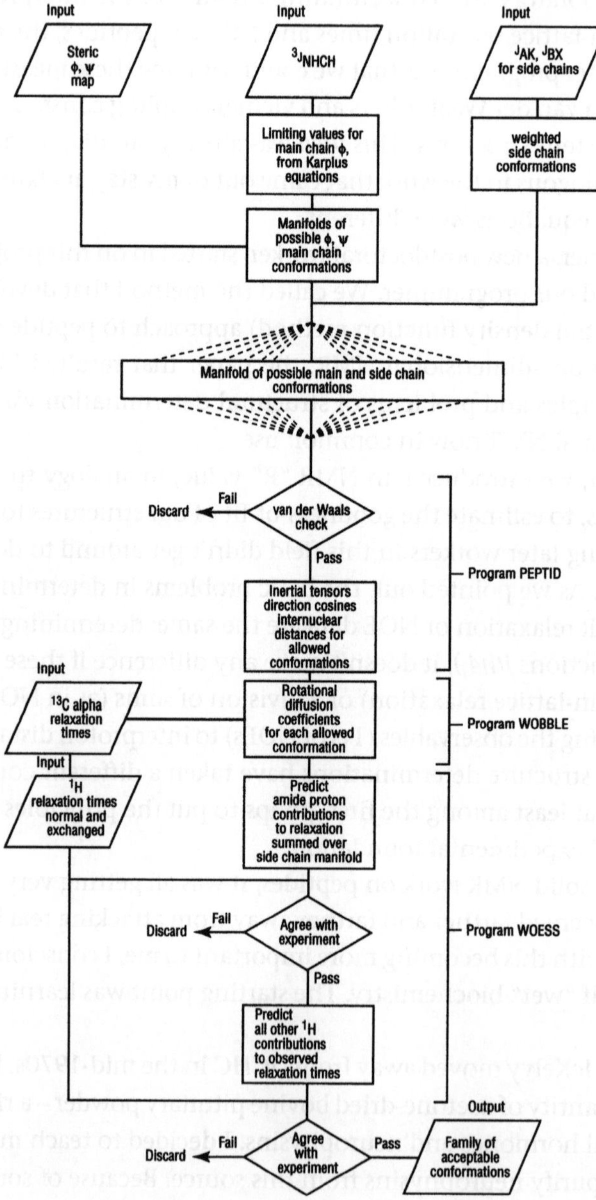

Fig. 6
Flow diagram of the functioning of our 1979 peptide structural determination procedure and programs (given acronyms PEPTID, WOBBLE and WOESS).

11 Beginning wet biochemistry

11.1 Neurohypophyseal proteins: physical and biochemical properties

With Christine Regula's help, I found that protein chemistry was surprisingly easy to pick up: in those days of open column chromatography, all one had to do was master the necessary plumbing! We soon obtained good yields of purified neurophysins.

While we did some work with the neurophysins, using an analytical ultracentrifuge to measure their polymeric associations, similar work was being done by other groups and we never published our results (although I learned a lot about the technique). Instead, we concentrated on determining binding parameters of radiolabeled hormones to the neurophysins (a problem that hadn't been worked on very extensively), choosing equilibrium dialysis as the measurement technique. These experiments went very well and the resulting papers [64, 65] confirmed in my mind my new-found status as a "biochemist."

In one of these papers [65] we dealt with a problem still evident in the literature: common errors in the quantitative analysis of binding data. Many biochemists using Scatchard model analysis of binding were (and are) mathematically incorrect in their analysis of the case of more than one binding site. For example, a later survey paper on analyses of binding experiments that exist in the literature (citing ours as an exception) reported a very large percentage of misinterpretations [66] and I continue to see the same errors made.

As the decade of the 1970s drew to a close we published two papers that typify the way my interests had split. On the one hand I was collaborating in a review of the biochemistry of the hypothalamus with Jeff McKelvy [67] (albeit still concentrating on the physical biochemical aspects), and on the other still trying to use every morsel of NMR information in accurate determinations of solution peptide structures [68].

When a renewal of our "New England NMR Research Resource" grant was not funded in 1979, the staff of the NMR Facility left and I obtained a Fogarty International Fellowship to study the biochemistry of opiate receptors at Imperial College in London.

Jay A. Glasel

12 Sabbatical at Imperial College: neurochemistry and opiates

I chose IC because I had decided to work on the biochemistry of opiates and opiate receptors and Eric Barnard and John Hughes were both in the Biochemistry Department there. Hughes had been a co-discoverer of the enkephalins and Barnard's laboratory was trying to isolate opiate receptors using photoaffinity labeling with derivatized enkephalins.

12.1 Opiate receptors

This was the pre-molecular biology era of "receptology." Isolation and characterization of receptor proteins depended largely on choosing the right starting biological material and the right detergent for solubilization. In correspondence prior to my arrival at IC, Barnard had suggested that I work with his group on their efforts to solubilize affinity-labeled opiate receptors and I initially agreed. My lab notebook in July, 1979, when I started work at IC, is filled with notes on previous attempts by other workers to isolate "the" opiate receptor. To optimize the tissue source of receptors, I began learning a new scientific dialect: subcellular fractionation.

12.1.1 Learning subcellular fractionation

The then accepted premise was that opiate receptors were located in synaptosomes and Barnard's group was using rat brain synaptosomal preparations as starting materials for their receptor isolation work. Reading the literature, and one of Barnard's student's lab notebook, I had found an inconsistency in the assumed synaptosomal location for the majority of opiate receptors.

Harry Bradford's laboratory at IC was noted for work on subcellular fractionation and I began learning how to do this from his people. Within a couple of weeks I had learned to do crude brain dissections to obtain tissues from the caudate nucleus (known to be the anatomical location of maximum opiate ligand binding in the brain) and to make good synaptosomal, microsomal and myelin subcellular fractions, analyze for total membrane-bound proteins in each fraction, and do marker enzyme analyses to characterize the fractions. I was fortunate in having Bradford's group to help me learn these techniques but, in fact, I found that these procedures didn't involve much scientific skill (I later found the same to be true for most molecular biological techniques) – it was more like painting by numbers.

After confirming the purity of my subcellular fractions *via* transmission electron microscopy (calling on my undergraduate research background), I learned how to do filter binding assays using radiolabeled opiate ligands and confirmed what I had suspected: the major location of stereospecific opiate binding was in the microsomal fraction, not the synaptosomal one [69]. Shortly thereafter, the results were confirmed [70].

The importance of these papers was their suggestion that central nervous system (CNS) opiate receptors were not localized to pre- and post-synaptic membranes. To my knowledge, this problem has still not been addressed by neuroanatomists and electrophysiologists.

There were many good scientists in the Biochemistry Department at IC doing new things and talking about new ideas. One of the ideas – the existence of monoclonal antibodies (Mabs) – that were being discussed proved important for my future career.

12.1.2 Monoclonal antibodies and the germ of an idea about anti-idiotypic antibodies

I became friendly with a colleague in the Biochemistry Department who began to fill me in on the, then new, technique for production of Mabs which had first been reported four years previously. Very soon I was writing to Elmer Becker, an immunologist colleague at UCHC, about the feasibility of producing anti-opiate Mabs when I returned home. Elmer had collaborated with us on our NMR structural study of the chemotactic tripeptide [63] and was always interested in new methods. In an April, 1980 letter to him I outlined my sabbatical plans, my views on NMR-determined peptide structures, and ideas I had about how Mabs might be used as receptor structural analogs.

In his answer to this letter, Elmer mentioned another concept that was new to me: anti-idiotypic antibodies (a-Ids) and their properties of binding to idiotypic antibodies (Ids). I had never heard of the concept of immune networks involving Ids and a-Ids and began to learn as much as was known about the concept. As described below, a-Ids were to become an important focus for my research.

I immediately began puzzling about the structural implications of Id-a-Id binding. Antibodies were supposed to have a "cleft" which formed their binding sites. How do two antibodies, each with a binding site in a cleft, bind to each other, I wondered? I still wonder about this question because, after all the subsequent hubbub about a-Ids and their possible uses as therapeutic agents, it is still important but unanswered.

Also, to a lapsed structural biochemist (as I would have referred to myself at the time), the idea that a small organic molecule (a hapten) could be structurally mimicked by a large protein's (the a-Id) binding site was just astounding. I asked myself: wherein lies the structural complementarity between an a-Id's binding site (made up of amino acid residues) and the non-peptide hapten? This seemed to me another fundamental, formidable, and very important structural and biological problem. It has never been solved, or, to my knowledge, been worked on.

After my sabbatical ended, my attempted solution to the problem was to carry me far into molecular immunology and away from where structural NMR was headed.

13 Connecticut years – Part II, 1980–2000

13.1 Structural work on opiates

Upon my return to UCHC my plan was to teach myself molecular immunology while continuing to produce papers on NMR and receptor biochemistry. To this end, I brought over one of Barnard's students, Richard Venn, as a postdoctoral worker to work on the biochemistry.

Only two NMR papers came out of my laboratory during the five years after I returned from IC [71, 72]. They were good papers – we showed that intramolecular motion on a biologically significant time scale existed in morphine, a molecule previously assumed to be rigid – but the quantity was too low to sustain my credibility as an NMR spectroscopist.

13.2 Anti-morphine monoclonal antibodies, opiate receptors

The first thing Venn and I did was to look at the sensitivity of sheep brain opiate receptor-bearing membranes to UV light. As I had suspected from the first days in Barnard's laboratory, these opiate-receptor preparations were extremely sensitive to UV of the same wavelengths that his laboratory and other workers were using for photolabeling [73]. This paper had some influence on ending time-wasting photoaffinity labeling of the opiate receptor because work in that area by others soon halted.

I still had hopes that non-photoaffinity methods could result in a successful opiate-receptor isolation. To do this, I thought we needed to know more about the receptors' properties. Second, to raise opiate-mimicking a-Ids, we needed a starting point. I decided that since polyclonal anti-morphine antibodies had been previously produced, we should use analogous methods to produce anti-morphine Mabs (to be the Ids) which could then be used later to produce morphine-mimicking a-Ids.

Workers in receptology at that time were not attempting to use molecular biological methods to isolate or sequence opiate receptors. Dick Venn and I spent much time, as did other groups, unsuccessfully attempting to solubilize the receptor using conventional detergent methods. To do this we had to set up our own filtration binding assays, which led to an encounter (analogous to the equilibrium dialysis problem mentioned above) with how sloppy some investigators were in performing binding isotherm measurements and analysis. Our critique of this literature contained examples of some of these errors and I'm sure it did little to endear us to many people in the field [74].

Most of the biological assays on agonist and antagonist effects were done using the twitching responses of rodent *vas deferens* or *ileum* tissue preparations. On the other hand, most of the binding assays or attempts to solubilize the receptor used subcellular fractions or membrane preparations from cerebral cortex preparations. Collaborating with Jack Cooper and Jim Reese at Yale, we attempted to meet this logical disconnect directly by performing subcellular fractionation on *ileum* preparations and determining opiate binding parameters on the fractions.

The results succeeded in confusing us completely because they showed that in these rodent autonomic system membrane preparations, the opiate receptor binding was predominantly in the synaptosomal fraction, thus suggesting that the receptors were localized to the pre- and post-synaptic membranes (in contrast to the case in brain) [75]. Since one classical action of opiates (as an anti-diarrhoetic) presumably results from its binding to *ileum* opiate receptors, it is possibly important biologically that CNS receptors are found in the microsomal fraction and *ilium* receptors in the syanaptosomal one. Research on the functions of opiates in the enteric system have lagged far behind the CNS effects and, to this day, few studies have concentrated on the functions of either exogenous or endogenous opiates in the functions of the gastrointestinal system.

13.3 Radiation inactivation studies of opiate receptors – knowledge before its time had come

By now we had published two binding studies and a review of the literature on opiate-receptor binding. The end result was that I had become very disillusioned with binding studies telling much about the molecular properties of the receptor.

We tried another direction: in cooperation with Ellis Kempner, we tried using the radiation inactivation technique he had largely developed by himself [76] to determine a molecular mass of the receptor. When the work was finally published [77], my mathematical analysis of the data predicted that the receptor recognition protein was complexed with other proteins, although my derived mass of the recognition unit (50 kDa) came close to the average receptor protein mass predicted from the receptors' gene sequences (41 kDa) reported 5 years later [78–80], even without taking into account presumed glycosylation of the protein to form the native unit.

The radiation inactivation work was published more than a decade before recent work indicating that, indeed, opiate receptors function as complexes [81]. However, I was still thinking as a physical chemist, and that put me very far apart from the way most other workers in the opiate field regarded progress.I decided to drop the receptor isolation work and, seeking a way out of the research impasse I found myself in, we pushed ahead with re-creating ourselves as molecular immunologists. Part of my reasoning was that nobody else in the opiate field seemed to want to do this type of work.

13.4 Molecular immunology and opiates

Without any previous experience in the area, Venn and I started work to produce anti-morphine Mabs which we then hoped to use to produce morphine-mimicking, anti-receptor, a-Id antibodies.

We soon found that the main requirements to do Mab work were simple manual procedures (sterile technique, freezing and thawing cells, mixing up media accurately, immunizing mice and later performing splenectomies on them) with little intellectual involvement required.

Since both of us were experienced chemists, and polyclonal anti-morphine antibodies had previously been produced by other workers using the hapten, morphine hemisuccinate, conjugated to bovine serum albumin, it was easy for us to make the conjugate. We were able to report the first production of high-affinity anti-morphine Mabs by 1983 [82] and immediately set about characterizing their binding properties.

The cross-binding properties of these Mabs with other opiate agonists were interesting insofar as the antibodies were quite specific for the parts of the morphine molecule that pharmacologists had long associated with opiate potency. But none of the anti-morphine Mabs bound the "universal opiate antagonist," naloxone, significantly. Also, contrary to our expectations, none of our anti-morphine Mabs bound Enks significantly (a fact later independently confirmed with other anti-morphine Mabs produced by a different group) [83].

Taken as a whole, all these results make it very clear that our ideas about the structural features of the interactions resulting in drug binding to proteins are still very cloudy.

For example, after their discovery, structural biochemists had supposed that the opiate peptides and the previously known plant/synthetic opiates had structural similarities; how else could they bind to the same receptor and initiate the same intracellular responses (or in the case of naloxone, block the responses?), it was reasoned. Despite cloning the receptors, and despite innumerable structure-activity-relation (SAR) studies on opiates, I believe the key structural relationships between morphine, opiate peptides and naloxone that result in their all binding to the same receptor with high specificity and affinity remain to this day not only a mystery but a challenge to the applicability of structural chemistry to pharmacology.

At the same time as we were producing our anti-morphine Mabs, there was similar activity in several neuroscience laboratories directed toward producing anti-Enk antibodies. It is illustrative of how much my thinking about the use of these antibodies differed from all the other groups that, when they successfully produced anti-Enk Mabs, not one of them looked at cross-reactivities with plant/synthetic opiates [84, 85]. In fact, to my knowledge the question has been avoided to this day.

With our anti-morphine Mabs in hand we started into, for us, completely unknown territory by attempting to produce the putative morphine-mimicking a-Ids.

13.5 Are binding sites for drugs on antibodies good models for drug-receptor binding?

By 1985 we were able to report the production of polyclonal preparations of morphine-mimetic a-Ids raised by immunization of rabbits with Fab fragments of our anti-morphine Mabs [86–88]. The cross-binding properties of these antibodies were another surprise to me: They blocked both morphine *and* Enk binding to membrane-bound opiate receptors. Here was another paradox: the idiotypic anti-morphine Mabs didn't bind Enks, but the a-Ids mimicked both Enks and morphine. Where did the structural similarities lie? Since at this time there was a great deal of interest by pharmaceutical firms in the development of a-Ids as therapeutic agents, it seemed to me that we had happened onto a structural paradox, the solution of which could lead us to some major insights into the nature of binding-site specificities.Even today, with the push toward "structural biology," our ideas on the origins of antibody binding-site specificity and affinity are largely qualitative and based on very few quantitatively solved structures.

I thought (and still do) that structural studies on a series of Mabs directed against a single hapten form an ideal system for beginning to understand receptor binding specificities and affinities. My reasoning is that this system is, in effect, the result of nature performing site-directed mutagenesis to present us with the best binding sites for each particular hapten. Why guess at trying to produce the same result *via* site-directed mutagenesis when we can have nature's cooperation? Unfortunately, I was unable to obtain funding for a project of this nature and therefore turned further toward molecular biological research.

13.6 Learning molecular biological skills

I taught myself enough molecular biology to enable us to infer sequences of our anti-morphine Mabs from sequencing cDNA we made from the hybridomas producing the Mabs [89], and enough immunology and immunochemistry to contribute papers on new techniques [90–93] and reviews [94] during these years.

13.7 More structural work on opiates

I kept on with NMR work on opiate ligand conformations because I was still hoping to attack the problem that obsessed me: wherein lie specificity and binding affinities of drugs for receptors? With the help of a medical student researcher, and the generosity of Aksel Bothner-By at the NMR laboratory at the University of Pittsburgh we first followed up my paper on Walden inversion in morphine with a more comprehensive treatment of both our 100 MHz and Bothner-By's 600 MHz NMR instruments. In this work [72] we showed that dynamic nitrogen inversion also takes place in the three different opiate agonists and antagonists we examined, and probably takes place in all of the many piperidine ring-containing drugs. These results suggested that a complication in understanding the interactions of agonists and antagonists with receptors is determining which invertomer (or both?) is the biologically active form.

I followed up this NMR work with 500 MHz studies done with the cooperation of Phil Borer, who was working with George Levy at Syracuse University in New York. This combined our anti-morphine antibody work with the NMR studies. My idea was that in the absence of purified soluble receptor, the interactions of ligands with antibodies directed against them might yield information on the specificity/affinity problem that preoccupied me. *Via* transferred NOE measurements, we showed [95] that the bound invertomeric conformations of opiate drugs can be different from their solution conformations, suggesting that the binding can stabilize an invertomeric form that is energetically unfavorable in solution.

The problem with this work was that transferred NOEs can only be used with ligands undergoing rapid exchange between solution and bound forms.

The real biological interest was for the high-affinity binding (and therefore slow exchange) case that could be attacked by the isotope editing technique: work I couldn't get funding for.

I decided to try to attack the problem of bound conformations of drugs by spending a concentrated time at a well-equipped (and well-funded) NMR laboratory.

14 Sabbatical at the Australian National University

In 1988 I took a six-month sabbatical leave with Larry Brown's NMR group at the Australian National University (ANU) in Canberra. Larry's laboratory was well equipped with a new 500 MHz instrument and well staffed with talented people. I had grand plans to finally use the isotope editing scheme to look at two types of binding, the opiate-anti-opiate Mab case and oxytocin-neurophysin binding. This latter was of interest because it was biologically relevant and could be done because some years before Victor Hruby had synthesized some oxytocin peptides specifically labeled with ^{13}C. For the opiate work, I spent several weeks synthesizing morphine specifically labeled with ^{13}C, thus again putting on the hat of an organic chemist. I arrived in Canberra with NMR quantities of all the materials I needed.

14.1 Transferred NOEs

Sadly, I got very little done at ANU. Larry and I just spoke different scientific languages. He didn't see the interest in binding studies, and I didn't understand his lack of interest. I wound up with not much time on the instrument and never got the modifications to the probe necessary to do the isotope editing experiments. I managed to complete the preliminary transferred NOE work from two years earlier in a definitive way [96], but didn't get any data on tightly bound ligands. I didn't know it then, but my NMR days were over.

I decided to go back home and concentrate on using our a-Ids to study the receptors and dropped the idea of using the anti-morphine Mabs as models of receptor binding sites.

15 Research 1990–2000

15.1 Using anti-idiotypic antibodies to observe opiate receptors *via* confocal microscopy

One of the problems with opiate receptors is that they are not very immunogenic. The anti-receptor a-Id approach enabled us to bypass trying to make anti-receptor antibodies by conventional methods. The initial problem I wanted to attack with our a-Ids was the distribution of receptors on cell surfaces. One of the laboratories at UCHC had recently received a new instrument that I knew nothing about – a confocal microscope. Confocal microscopy, which had just come into relatively common use in several laboratories around the world, seemed ideal for the opiate receptor fluorescence labeling experiments I had in mind.

I had the good fortune to be able to employ a Polish national living in the United States, Margaret Ornatowska, M.D. Margaret couldn't practice medicine here, and didn't really want to; she was interested in learning how to do research.

Margaret and I learned how to culture NG-108-15 hybridoma cells (which express large numbers of -subclass opiate receptors) and to biotinylate our a-Ids so that they could be fluorescence labeled with FITC- and Texas Red-conjugated avidin. We were also fortunate in this work to have the cooperation of a computer programmer, Mr. Frank Morgan, who worked in a colleague's laboratory at UCHC. In those early days of confocal microscopy, three-dimensional reconstruction software was not widely available. Frank developed a very useful program to do this reconstruction and made it available to us for one of its first applications (Fig. 7).

Margaret and I published two very thorough papers describing the use of confocal microscopy to study opiate receptor distributions on both asynchronous and synchronized cultures (we had to learn how to do the synchronization) of NG-108-15 cells [97, 98]. Our overall conclusion from this work was that reversibility of anti-Id binding to the receptors by opiate congeners and the stereospecificity of the binding were not connected. That is, we concluded that stereospecific and non-stereospecific receptors co-existed in asynchronous cultures and that in synchronous cultures the percentage of cells displaying stereospecific binding of the anti-Ids was dependent on

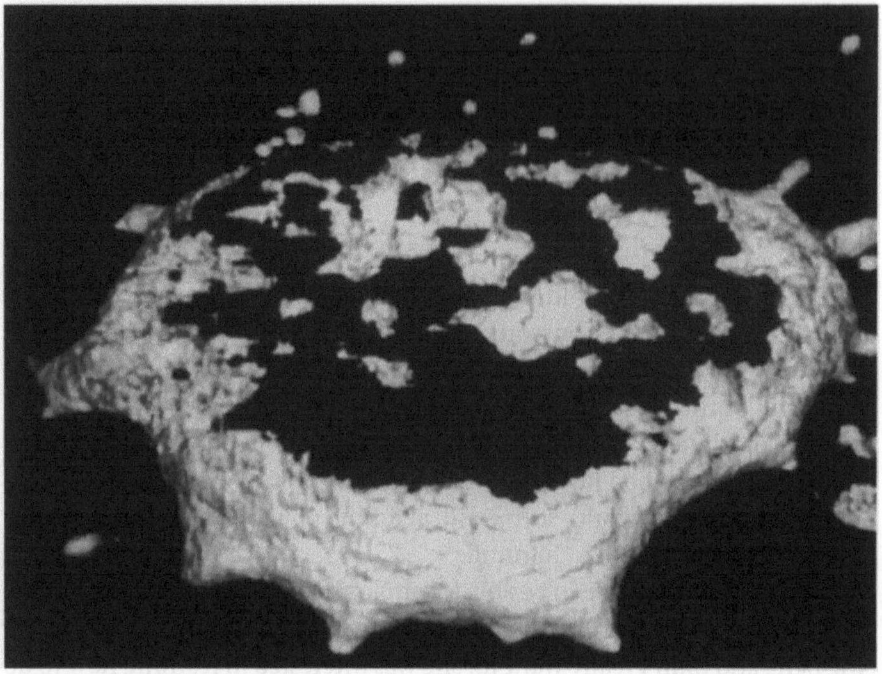

Fig. 7
Confocal fluorescence microscopy of NG108-15 cells. Three-dimensional reconstruction through a middle section of a cell stained with FITC-avidin-a-Id. Note internalization of a-Id binding material. From [97].

cell cycle. This implied that the receptor's binding site(s) mature(s) as the cell grows.

In the confocal microscopic work, in the previous work with radiation inactivation, and in a subsequent paper using non-confocal fluorescence microscopy, I was probably too unimaginative to synthesize the results correctly. Re-reading the papers and the methods, particularly those used to define stereospecificity in the fluorescence work, indicates that what we were really observing were the changes in binding specificities of the receptors as they aggregated into complexes – a conclusion drawn from very new work based on completely different methods than we used [81, 99, 100]. I remain proud of Margaret's and my work with confocal microscopy; it was very new at the time.

In the early 1990s, with a new government in Poland, Margaret returned home, and Dianne Agarwal became my first graduate student.

15.2 Beginning to understand the molecular biology of opiate receptors

Dianne began her thesis work by learning to do cell culture and continuing our fluorescence labeling work. The first mature work she collaborated in was a study of co-localization of δ- and μ-subclass opioid receptors in SK-N-SH cells [101]. Our conclusions were that the results were consistent with a model where μ- and δ-binding sites reside on different subunits of a multimeric complex. In the light of the recent work quoted above [81], this work also seems before its time.

At about this time, opiate receptor research was changed drastically with the cloning and sequencing of the δ-subclass of opiate receptor [78, 79] (followed shortly thereafter by similar work on μ- and κ-receptors). This immediately made obsolete all the solubilization efforts still being made by several groups around the world and opened new avenues of research.

I was determined to try to get a jump on other workers by doing something new in opiate research. In choosing this new direction, I fell back on a habit formed years earlier when I was a full-fledged chemical physicist: I tried to simplify.

From extensive reading about research being done on the effects of drugs, including opiates, on mammalian cells, I had come to the conclusion that there were no good model cell systems; workers in this area got different results depending on what cell lines they were using. This situation resulted in lots of papers, but without much commonality that could be discerned. I believed (and still do) that one of the main problems is the plethora of signals, particularly growth factors, that every cell is bombarded with constantly and which each different cell type responds to differently.

I set Dianne the task of developing a cell system that grew in a *defined* medium and whose growth and proliferation depended on what I hoped would be only a limited number of defined growth factors. Neither Dianne nor I had any real training in mammalian cell culture and biology and in entering this field I was, as usual, depending on attitude and native savvy, not prior training. Dianne rapidly became adept at the manipulations required to culture mammalian cells. Within a year from starting, she had developed a cell line whose origin was the familiar NIH 3T3 fibroblast cell line but which could be cultured in a defined medium containing only insulin as a growth factor. In fact, this cell line (which we named 3T3DA) could be synchronized by withdrawing insulin from the medium. This arrested cell proliferation without killing them and reintroducing insulin started them proliferating in synchronization.

15.2.1 A good tool for determining drug signaling pathways to the nucleus?

With this cell system, I thought we had a very good tool for studying drug effects on cells (once we transfected the cells with receptor-encoding genes), without the confounding effects of multiple exogenous growth signals. This was a typical way of thinking for a physical scientist – proceed from a simple model system to more complex ones – but not for biological scientists; I was unable to get funding for work with our cells.

When I began to have funding difficulties several years before, I had turned to making proposals to pharmaceutical firms for support of the type of work I have been describing in this section. Although I continued to make such proposals, I quickly found that drug firms were even more concerned with fashionable research than academic reviewers. Proposal reviewers from biotechnology and pharmaceutical firms were a bit more polite than those employed by the government, but they universally saw what I proposed as coming up with potential rewards too far in the future for their plans.

Still, using some support from UCHC, small commercial sales of our anti-morphine Mabs, and generous gifts of several receptor-encoding genes from original investigators, Dianne and I plowed on and gathered sufficient data to publish a very complete paper on the mitogenic (as opposed to transforming) effects of drugs on the DA cell line transfected with the receptor-encoding genes and expressing the receptors [102]. In this paper, we showed that proliferation of the DA cell line was down-regulated by chronic morphine treatment, and that the second-messenger signaling by the δ-receptor upon acute morphine treatment was the same as had long been recognized to exist in other cells expressing the same receptor. But we found that the second-messenger signaling pattern changed upon chronic treatment with the drug. We logically surmised that we would have to understand the "downstream" signaling pathways of activated opiate receptor into the nucleus to understand what genes the initial signals were controlling.

I decided that we had to jump ahead directly to finding what genes were affected by chronic morphine treatment. My reasoning was that this is the clinically relevant case. The question was: can chronic treatment with narcotics temporarily or permanently alter the expression of certain proteins that have subsequent effects on cell phenotype? For example, we had found a phenotypic response to withdrawal of DA cells from chronic morphine treatment: they underwent a transient up-regulation of cellular proliferation. I became interested in a quantitative analysis of this up-regulation prior to undertaking work to understand its molecular basis.

15.2.2 Still thinking quantitatively

I found a reference to a computer program (CELLSIM) that analyzed cell proliferation using numerical methods (as opposed to solving differential equations analytically) and was able to obtain a version of the 25-year-old program from its author, Charles Donaghey of the University of Houston. CELLSIM allows a theoretical curve for cell proliferation based on cell cycle variables to be compared with experimental curves. While not mathematically unique (because some variables had to be assumed), the results of the analysis indicated [103] that under chronic morphine treatment, the decrease in proliferation of DA cells was due almost entirely to an increase in the length of time spent in the G1 phase of their cell cycle. On the other hand, we concluded that when withdrawn from chronic morphine treatment, the DA cells undergo an increased rate of proliferation due to a shortening of time spent in G1.

Having published several papers, Dianne had done enough research to write a thesis. She left in 1998 and, continuing to be funded by UCHC with some additions from my own pocket by myself, I continued the work I thought important.

15.2.3 High school algebra pays off

During this period, I published a paper [104] that had nothing to do with the direction I wanted my research to go, took me a half-hour to write, generated controversy and work by other groups, and has proved to be one of the most cited of my biochemical papers. These events convinced me that I really had no place in academic science.

Murray Deutscher, a fellow faculty member at the Health Center, and I were editing a text book on biophysical chemistry methods. He dropped by my office one day and said he thought the chapter on UV spectroscopic methods should contain more practical material and suggested I add an explanation of the popular use by molecular biologists of UV spectroscopy – monitoring the purity of nucleic acid preparations from the ratio of UV absorbances taken at 260 nm and 280 nm. Everybody in molecular biology, including me, used this ratio constantly because it was recommended in all the molecular biology recipe books.

In the library I looked up the original publication that was the origin of the method and was surprised to find that it was developed to determine DNA impurities in *protein* preparations, not the other way around. As it would to anyone trained in high school algebra who examined the problem, it was immediately clear to me that since maximum protein molar extinction coefficients at 280 nm were much smaller than DNA molar extinction coefficients at 260 nm, the A260/A280 was a terrible method for determining purity of DNA preparations. I solved the simple equation for the ratio as a function of the extinction coefficients and showed the ratio's insensitivity by numerical example. I wrote the paper up and it was accepted immediately.

When published it provoked a storm of protest and several subsequent papers attempting to show I couldn't be correct. Even Murray wouldn't believe the results because he told me (as did most of the protesters) that his laboratory's DNA preparations couldn't be as dirty as my results indicated and still be used. Some months later, a scientist who was editing a review on the subject asked me if I was sure of my results and then told me in the next breath that he was going to give a "balanced" account of the pros and cons in the review.

My paper's conclusions, being the result of a simple mathematical relation, couldn't really be refuted and have come to be accepted now. What the protesters didn't think about was that the protein impurities in most DNA preparations are probably complex mixtures that, depending on the subsequent reactions the "purified" DNA was subjected to, sometimes interfere with those experiments and sometimes don't.

I considered the whole incident bizarre and representative of how far away I was from how molecular biologists thought about the world of natural things; group opinion and faith seemed to carry as much weight to workers in this area as (what I call) science. If scientific colleagues didn't believe in the validity of a simple equation – relying on word-of-mouth instead – what hope was there for me who always leaned in exactly the opposite direction.

My further experiences in molecular biological research on opiate receptors drove home this message even more forcibly.

15.3 Final work: out of funds but not out of ideas

In the previous few years Dianne and I had found that DA cells transfected with the δ-opiate receptor gene became active in expressing their (previously not expressed) β_2-adrenergic receptor at high levels. We also found that chronic exposure to procaterol (a specific β_2 agonist) up-regulated proliferation of the cells. Tracing the signaling pathways, we found that separate chronic morphine and chronic procaterol treatments differentially affected the mitogen-activated protein kinase (MAPK) isozymes known to be involved in growth regulation (as it should if one drug up-regulated proliferation and one down-regulated it). We also found that simultaneous chronic treatment with both receptors' agonists had non-additive effects on the levels of these isozymes and on cell proliferation. This meant that the signaling pathways into the nucleus due to simultaneous drug treatments contained a certain amount of "cross-talk." I had been puzzled for a long time over how linear signaling could take place in response to each different drug when the intermediate signaling molecules were identical in many cases.

Our work had, it seemed to me, developed into a clean-cut system to study many phenomena mediated by drug-activated receptors. True, we didn't know why the adrenergic receptor's expression was stimulated by having an opiate receptor introduced into the cell's genome but, however it happened, it gave us a wonderful tool, I thought; we had a cell line that depended on only one media growth factor, expressed two G-protein coupled receptors that could be specifically activated, and responded with different phenotypes to the different agonists and to mixtures of the agonists. These results appeared in another complete paper [105].

15.3.1 Pleotropic effects of drugs: a rapidly developing field

The field of opiate research in the late 1990s had come around strongly to using molecular biological methods. In particular, laboratories interested in studying chronic effects of endogenous and exogenous opiates were concentrating on the effects of drugs on the signaling pathways to the nucleus: something we had started on 4 years previously but could never get funded for.

I decided to try to leap ahead and find out as much as possible what transcripts were differentially regulated by drug treatments. I reasoned that the most important thing was to identify the proteins differentially changed by chronic drug treatments, since some of them would be involved in the phenotypic changes we were observing in cells subjected to the treatments.

Although this problem has become a major focus of modern drug research (prompted by the development of "high-throughput" techniques such as cDNA microarrays), at the time I started the work there was a great deal of controversy over how to observe differential transcription efficiently. For example, the differential display technique was known to discriminate against low-abundance transcripts [106] and to produce many "false positives". However, a newly developed polymerase chain reaction (PCR)-based differential library technique had just been described [107, 108] that appeared to eliminate many of the previous problems.

This new technique proved to be very easy to perform and, within two weeks, I had begun to identify some up-regulated transcripts from DA cells subjected to chronic morphine treatment. Database searching revealed that most of these genes had already been identified and encoded proteins that had been previously related to cell proliferation. In particular, one transcript that was up-regulated as a result of chronic morphine treatment was known to encode a protein that is important in the proliferation of trophoblast giant cells during human embryonic development.

The placenta has been called a "pharmacy" because of its production of a wide diversity of hormones and growth factors, and *via* the literature I found that the trophoblast giant cells not only expressed δ-opiate receptors and opiate peptides, but were subject to damage by exogenous narcotics. To me, it seemed important that even in our model cells, chronic morphine treatment up-regulated a gene that encoded a protein that affected the proliferation of trophoblast giant cells.

I thought that I had been lucky again and jumped into a new and relatively uncrowded area of basic drug research: the effects of narcotic drugs on placental development.

15.3.2 "Not innovative"

Instead, it was a dead end; for the first time in my entire career, a proposal based on the data I had gathered was described by a reviewer as "not innovative." I had been turned down before by reviewers who didn't believe that I could technically do the experiments I proposed, or for not referring to previous grant support in papers (true!) and for various other reasons, but never because I was not innovative. Furthermore, the same proposal was turned down by my colleagues at UCHC when I applied for further support to widen the search for morphine-regulated genes using the newly available cDNA microarrays. The reason given was that I would obtain a lot of data that I wouldn't know how to use.

Faced with very long odds for getting funded to do the things I believed important in my chosen field, and unwilling to try to get funding for work I didn't think important, I decided to offer my generalist experience in science as a consultant.

Science as an intellectual and manual occupation was still wonderful; the practice of academic scientific research became intolerable to me. I had kept the faith as long as I could, and then said goodbye to all that.

Annotations

1 The idea that everyone in the world is connected to everyone else *via* not more than six human contacts. See J. Guare, *Six Degrees of Separation: A Play* and more recently, Duncan J. Watts and Steven H. Strogatz, "Collective Dynamics of 'small-world' Networks", Nature *393*: 440–442 (1998) and references therein.

2 A note on authorship of these and later papers from my laboratory is in order: Bob Williams convinced me that to avoid seniority arguments, authors from each institutional affiliation should be in alphabetical order. At the time this made sense to me so I adopted this method. In reality, for the rest of my career it caused confusion: depending on the name of a co-author my name has been first or last author on subsequent papers with no connotation of who was responsible for the work.

References

1 J.D. Watson and F.H.C. Crick: Nature *171* (1953).

2 R.P. Feynman, R.B. Leighton and M. Sands: The Feynman Lectures on Physics, Addison-Wesley Publishing Co., Inc., Reading, MA 1963.

3 R.P. Feynman: The Feynman Lectures on Physics, The Complete Audio Collection, Perseus Books, Cambridge, MA 2000.
4 N.P. Davis: Lawrence and Oppenheimer, Simon and Schuster, NY 1968.
5 R. Rhodes: The Making of the Atomic Bomb, Simon and Schuster, NY 1986.
6 D.J. Kevles: The Physicists, A.A. Knopf, NY 1978.
7 J.A. Glasel, in: H. Craig, S.L. Miller and G.J. Wasserburg (eds): Isotopic and Cosmic Chemistry, North-Holland Publishing Co., Amsterdam 1964, 530.
8 B. Donn and H.C. Urey: Astrophys. J. *123*, 339 (1956).
9 J.A. Glasel: Absorption Spectroscopy of Molecules and Free Radicals at 20 °K and 77 °K, doctoral thesis, University of Chicago, Chicago 1959.
10 J.A. Glasel: J. Chem. Phys. *33*, 252 (1960).
11 J.A. Glasel: Proc. Natl. Acad. Sci. USA *48*, 491 (1962).
12 J.A. Glasel: J. Chem. Phys. *34*, 1649 (1961).
13 J.A. Glasel: Proc. Natl. Acad. Sci. USA *47*, 174 (1961).
14 A. Abragam: The Principles of Nuclear Magnetism, Oxford University Press, Oxford 1961.
15 J.A. Glasel, L.M. Jackman and D.W. Turner: Proc. Chem. Soc. 426 (1961).
16 L. Pauling: Science *134*, 15 (1961).
17 S.L. Miller: Proc. Natl. Acad. Sci. (USA) *47*, 1515 (1961).
18 J.A. Glasel: Proc. Natl. Acad. Sci. (USA) *55*, 479 (1966).
19 J.A. Glasel: Proc. Natl. Acad. Sci. (USA) *58*, 27 (1967).
20 J.A. Glasel: Nature *218*, 953 (1968).
21 J.A. Glasel: Nature *220*, 1124 (1968).
22 J.A. Glasel, S. Hendler and P.R. Srinivasan: Proc. Natl. Acad. Sci. USA *60*, 1038 (1968).
23 J.A. Glasel: J. Am. Chem. Soc. *92*, 375 (1970).
24 J.A. Glasel: J. Am. Chem. Soc. *92*, 372 (1970).
25 J.A. Glasel: Nature *227*, 704 (1970).
26 J.A. Glasel: J. Am. Chem. Soc. *91*, 4569 (1969).
27 J.A. Glasel: J. Sci. Inst. *1*, 963 (1968).
28 J.A. Glasel: Rev. Sci. Inst. *37*, 1101 (1966).
29 V. Radeka, R.L. Chase, M. Petrinovic and J.A. Glasel: Rev. Sci. Inst. *41*, 1766 (1970).
30 J.A. Glasel: Biochemistry *5*, 1851 (1966).
31 J.A. Glasel: J. Am. Chem. Soc. *87*, 5472 (1965).
32 A. Stern, W.A. Gibbons and L.C. Craig: Proc. Natl. Acad. Sci. USA *61*, 734 (1968).
33 V.J. Hruby, A.I. Brewster and J.A. Glasel: Proc. Natl. Acad. Sci. USA *68*, 450 (1971).
34 A. I. Brewster, J.A. Glasel and V.J. Hruby: Proc. Natl. Acad. Sci. USA *69*, 1470 (1972).
35 A. I. R. Brewster, V.J. Hruby, J.A. Glasel and A.E. Tonelli: Biochemistry *12*, 5294 (1973).
36 J. W. Cooley and J. W. Tukey: Math. Comp. *19*, 297 (1965).
37 S. J. Lippard (eds): Lanthanide Ions as Nuclear Magnetic Resonance Chemical Shift Probes in Biological Systems, John Wiley and Sons, Inc., NY 1973.
38 C.D. Barry, A.C.T. North, J.A. Glasel, R.J.P. Williams and A.V. Xavier: Nature *232*, 236 (1971).
39 B. Birdsall, J. Feeney, J.A. Glasel, R.J.P. Williams and A.V. Xavier: Chem. Comm. 1473 (1971).
40 C.D. Barry, J.A. Glasel, A.C.T. North, R.J.P. Williams and A.V. Xavier: Biochim. Biophys. Acta *262*, 101 (1972).
41 C.D. Barry, J.A. Glasel, A.C.T. North, R.J.P. Williams and A.V. Xavier: Biochem. Biophys. Res. Comm. *47*, 166 (1972).

42 C.D. Barry, J.A. Glasel, R.J.P. Williams and A.V. Xavier: J. Mol. Biol. *84*, 471 (1974).
43 J.A. Glasel and K.H. Lee: J. Am. Chem. Soc. *96*, 970 (1973).
44 J.A. Glasel and J. F. McKelvy: Ann. N.Y. Acad. Sci. *222*, 778 (1973).
45 J.A. Glasel, V.J. Hruby and J.F. McKelvy: J. Mol. Biol. *79*, 555 (1973).
46 H.E. Bleich: J. Magn. Reson. *18*, 401 (1975).
47 J.D. Cutnell, H.E. Bleich and J.A. Glasel: J. Magn. Reson. *21*, 43 (1976).
48 H.E. Bleich and J.A. Glasel: J. Magn. Reson. *35*, 295 (1979).
49 J.A. Glasel: J. Chromat. *145*, 469 (1978).
50 J.D. Cutnell, J.A. Glasel and V.J. Hruby: Org. Magn. Res. *7*, 256 (1975).
51 J.D. Cutnell and J.A. Glasel: Macromolecules *9*, 71 (1976).
52 J.D. Cutnell and J.A. Glasel: J. Am. Chem. Soc. *98*, 7542 (1976).
53 J.D. Cutnell and J.A. Glasel: J. Am. Chem. Soc. *98*, 264 (1976).
54 H.E. Bleich, J.D. Cutnell and J.A. Glasel: Biochemistry *15*, 2455 (1976).
55 J.D. Cutnell and J.A. Glasel: J. Am. Chem. Soc. *99*, 42 (1977).
56 H.E. Bleich and J.A. Glasel: Biopolymers *17*, 2445 (1978).
57 H.E. Bleich, J.A. Glasel, M. Latina and J. Visintainer: Biopolymers *18*, 2849 (1979).
58 H.E. Bleich, A.R. Day, R.J. Freer and J.A. Glasel: Biochem. Biophys. Resch. Comm. *87*, 1146 (1979).
59 H.F. Bleich, J.D. Cutnell, A.R. Day, R.J. Freer, J.A. Glasel and J.F. McKelvy: Proc. Natl. Acad. Sci. USA *73*, 2589 (1976).
60 H.E. Bleich, J.D. Cutnell, A.R. Day, R.J. Freer, J.A. Glasel and J.F. McKelvy: Biochem. Biophys. Res. Comm. *71*, 168 (1976).
61 H.E. Bleich, A.R. Day, R.J. Freer and J.A. Glasel: Biochem. Biophys. Res. Comm. *74*, 592 (1977).
62 H.E. Bleich and J.A. Glasel: J. Am. Chem. Soc. *97*, 6585 (1975).
63 E.L. Becker, H.E. Bleich, A.R. Day, R.J. Freer, J.A. Glasel and J. Visintainer: Biochemistry *18*, 4656 (1979).
64 V.J. Hruby, A.F. Spatola, J.A. Glasel and J.F. McKelvy: Ann. N.Y. Acad. Sci. *248*, 451 (1975).
65 J.A. Glasel, J.F. McKelvy, V.J. Hruby and A.F. Spatola: J. Biol. Chem. *251*, 2929 (1976).
66 J.G. Norby, P. Ottolenghi and J. Jensen: Anal. Biochem. *102*, 318 (1980).
67 J.F. McKelvy, J.A. Glasel and M. Foreman, in: P. J. Morgane and J. Panksepp (eds): Physiology of the Hypothalamus, Marcel Dekker, Inc., New York 1980, 1–81.
68 H.E. Bleich, K.R.K. Easwaran and J.A. Glasel: J. Magn. Reson. *31*, 517 (1978).
69 J.A. Glasel, R.F. Venn and E.A. Barnard: Biochem. Biophys. Resch. Commun. *95*, 263 (1980).
70 B.L. Roth, M.B. Laskowski and C.J. Coscia: J. Biol. Chem. *256*, 10117 (1981).
71 J.A. Glasel: Biochem. Biophys. Resch. Commun. *102*, 703 (1981).
72 J.A. Glasel and H.W. Reiher: Magn. Resn. Chem. *23*, 236 (1985).
73 J.A. Glasel and R.F. Venn: Life Sci. *29*, 221 (1981).
74 J.A. Glasel and R.F. Venn, in: J.L. Barker and J.F. McKelvy (eds.): Current methods in cellular neurobiology, Wiley-Interscience, New York 1984, 185.
75 J.A. Glasel, W.M. Bradbury and R.F. Venn: Life Sci. *34*, 345 (1984).
76 E.S. Kempner and W. Schlegel: Anal. Biochem. *92*, 2 (1979).
77 J.A. Glasel: Biochim. Biophys. Acta *930*, 201 (1987).
78 B.L. Kieffer, K. Befort, C. Gaveriaux-Ruff and C.G. Hirth: Proc. Natl. Acad. Sci. USA *89*, 12048 (1992).

79 C.J. Evans, D.E. Keith Jr., H. Morrison, K. Magendzo and R.H. Edwards: Science *258*, 1952 (1992).
80 J.B. Wang, Y. Imai, C.M. Eppler, P. Gregor, C.E. Spivak and G.R. Uhl: Proc. Natl. Acad. Sci. USA *90*, 10230 (1993).
81 B.A. Jordan, S. Cvejic and L.A. Devi: Neuropsychopharmacol. *23*, S5 (2000).
82 J.A. Glasel, W.M. Bradbury and R.F. Venn: Mol. Immunol. *20*, 1419 (1983).
83 A. Goldstein, R.W. Barrett, I.F. James, L.I. Lowney, C.J. Weitz, L.L. Knipmeyer and H. Rapoport: Proc. Natl. Acad. Sci. USA *82*, 5203 (1985).
84 P.A. Pontarotti, C. le Borgne De Kaouel, M. Verrier and A.A. Cupo: J. Neuroimmunol. 4, 47 (1983).
85 C.A. Jones, D.P. Lane and J. Hughes: Biochem. Biophys. Res. Commun. *113*, 757 (1983).
86 W.E. Myers and J.A. Glasel: Life Sci. *38*, 1783 (1986).
87 J.A. Glasel and L.A. Pelosi: Biochem. Biophys. Res. Commun. *136*, 1177 (1986).
88 J.A. Glasel and W. E. Myers: Life Sci. *36*, 2523 (1985).
89 A. Miller III and J.A. Glasel: J. Mol. Biol. *209*, 763 (1989).
90 J.A. Glasel, W.M. Bradbury and R.F. Venn: J. Immunol. Meth. *63*, 291 (1983).
91 A. Miller III and J.A. Glasel: J. Immunol. Meth. *125*, 35 (1989).
92 J.A. Glasel: Meth. Enzymol. *178*, 222 (1989).
93 M. Ornatowska and J.A. Glasel: Mol. Immunol. *28*, 383 (1991).
94 J.A. Glasel, in: D.S. Linthicum and N.R. Farid (eds): Anti-idiotypes, receptors and molecular mimicry, Springer-Verlag, New York 1988, 135.
95 J.A. Glasel and P.N. Borer: Biochem. Biophys. Res. Commun. *141*, 1267 (1986).
96 J.A. Glasel: J. Mol. Biol. *209*, 747 (1989).
97 M. Ornatowska and J.A. Glasel: J. Chem. Neuroanat. *5*, 95 (1992).
98 M. Ornatowska and J.A. Glasel: Mol. Pharmacol. *40*, 354 (1991).
99 B.A. Jordan and L.A. Devi: Nature *399*, 697 (1999).
100 L.A. Devi: Trends Pharmacol. Sci. *21*, 324 (2000).
101 D. Agarwal and J.A. Glasel: Life Sci. *52*, PL193 (1993).
102 J.A. Glasel and D. Agarwal: J. Cell. Physiol. *171*, 61 (1997).
103 J.A. Glasel and D. Agarwal: Pharmacol. Lett. *61*, PL305 (1997).
104 J.A. Glasel: Biotechniques *18*, 62 (1995).
105 D. Agarwal and J.A. Glasel: Cell Prolif. *32*, 215 (1999).
106 D.J. Bertioli, U.H.A. Schlichter, M.J. Adams, P.R. Burrows, H.-H. Steinbiss and J.F. Antoniw: Nucl. Acid Res. *23*, 4520 (1995).
107 L. Diatchenko, Y.F. Lau, A.P. Campbell, A. Chenchik, F. Moqadam, B. Huang, S. Lukyanov, K. Lukyanov, N. Gurskaya, E.D. Sverdlov and P.D. Siebert: Proc. Natl. Acad. Sci. USA *93*, 6025 (1996).
108 L. Diatchenko, S. Lukyanov, Y.F. Lau and P.D. Siebert: Meth. Enzymol. *303*, 349 (1999).

Index Vol. 57

Abacavir 86
Acetylcholine 35
Aconitine 35
Acyclovir 100
Adenosine deaminase 38
Adenosinetriphosphatase 32
Adenosione 33
Adrenaline 173
Adrenoceptor blockers 166
Adrenoceptors 174
Agenerase 86
AIDS 81
Ajoenes 15, 29, 37, 42
Alkaloids 6
Allicin 25
Alliin 25
Allinase 25
Allium sativum 24
Allium ursinum 37
Allixin 31
Allophatic medicine 5
Allyl sulfides 25
Allylamines 131
Allylmethylsulfide 37
Alpinetin 13, 16
Alpinetinchalcone 13, 16
Alternative therapies 5
Amantadine 96
Amino-nicotinamide 172
Amitriptyline 20
Ampeloside Bfl 33
Ampeloside BS1 33
Amphotericin B 129
Amprenavir 86
Anaphalis adanta DC 7
Angiotensin 174
Allyl mercaptan 39
Aniba gigantifolia 7
Aniba grandiflora 10
Anorexia 6, 43
Anti-arthritic drugs 43
Antibacterial agent 24
Anticancer activity (ginger) 59
Antidepressants 20
Antifungal therapeutics 129
Antifungals 131
Anti-inflammatory activity (ginger) 58
Anti-retroviral drugs 81
Anti-retroviral agent 85
Anti-retroviral treatment 87
Antirhinoviral activity 45
Antithrombotic activity 42
Anxiety 22
Anxiety disorders 22
Apomorphine 175
Apoptosis 42
Arginases 32
Arginine 35
Arrhythmia 35
Arthritic inflammation 59
Arthritis 43
Arylethylene-pyrrones 6
Aspergillus fumigatus 130
Aspirin 42
Atherosclerosis 36
Atherosclerotic process 41

Atorvastatin 127
Azoles 131
Benomyl 125
Benzimidazole 125
Benzodiazepines 6,22
Borneol 55
Bornylcinnamate 14
Brofaromine 20
Bromocriptine 175
Bronchitis 43

Cancer, bladder 37
Cancer, gastric 36
Cancers, colorectal 125
Candida albicans 136
Candida elegans 122
Candida glabrata 136
Candida krusei 131, 136
Candida neoformans 130, 134, 136
Candida parapsilosis 136
Candida species 129, 134
Candidal infection 131
Candidemia 131
Cardiotoxicity 42
Catalases 32
Catecholamine 166
Cepharadione 15
Cerebrosides 31
Chalcones 6, 13
Chest congestion 43
Chicken pox 43, 99
Chlorpromazine 174
Cholera 43
Cholesterol 127
Cholesterol biosynthesis 39
Cholesterol-lowering drugs 127
Cholesterol metabolism 24
Cidofovir 100
Cinnamylidineaceton 14
Cisplatin 58
Clonidine 175
Colchicine 59
Colds 43
Colic 43
Compactin 127
Corynanthine 176
Cough 43
Creatine level 24
Crixivan 86

Cycloalliin 27
Cyclo-oxygenase 37
Cysteine 25
Cytochrome 38
Cytokines 37

Dehydromethysticin 10
Delaviridine 86, 87
Dermatomyositis 24
Desoxyribonucleases 32
Diabetes mellitus 167
Diallylsulfide 25, 37
Diarrhoea 43
Diarylheptanoids 52
Diazoxide 171
Didanosine 86, 93
Dideoxynucleosides 93
Dienketones 6
Diethylnitrosoamine 36
Dihydroergotamine 174
Dihydrokavain 7, 16
Dihydromethysticin 7
Dihydrooroxylin 13,16
Dihydrotectochrysin 13, 16
Diterpenes 55
Dithiins 25
DNA helicase 123
DNA polymerases 80
DNA replication 122
DNA synthesis 59
DNA transcription 122
Dopamine derivatives 175
Dopaminergic neurons 21
Doxorubicin 38, 42
Dropsy 43
Drosophila melanogaster 122
Drugs, mind-altering 5
Dyclonine 144
Dyspepsia 43

Efavirenz 86
Enterovirus 97
Epivir 86
Ergosterol 127, 131, 144
Eruboside B 33
Eschericia coli 137
Esterase 37
Euphoria 6
Eye irritation 23

Famciclovir 104
Fever 43
Fibrillation 35
Fibrosis, cystic 123
Fitness, viral 90
Flatulence 43
Flavanones 6, 13
Flaviviridae family 98
Flavokavain A 16
Flavokavain B 16
Flavonoids 38
Flu 43
Floconazole 131
Flovastatin 127
Foot-and-mouth disease virus 98
Foscarnet 100
Fructans 38
Fructose polymers 38
Fungal infections 129

GABA-A receptors 19
Galanolactone 55
Gallbladder disorders 43
Ganciclovir 100
Garlic 24
Gastrointestinal activities (ginger) 58
Genital disease 99
Gingediols 49
Ginger 43
Ginger oil 44
Gingerdiones 44, 49
Gingerglycolipids 55
Gingerols 44, 48, 58, 59
Gingerproteases 56
Gingesulfonic acid 51, 55
Gingidiols 44
Glibenclamide 171
Glocopyranoside 55
Glutamyl-peptides 27, 38
Glutamyltrans-peptidases 32
Glutathione 42
Gonorrhoea 6
Growth competition 93
Growth hormone 176
Guanidine 98

Hepadnaviruses 98
Hepatitis A virus 97
Hepatitis B 102
Hepatitis C polymerase 98
Hepatitis C virus 81
Hepatocytes 105
Herbal medicine 5
Herpes simplex virus 99
Herpes virus PR inhibitors 102
Herpes viruses 99
Herpesviridae 99
Hexakinases 32
High-throughput methods 148
Hippocampus 21
Histamine 175
HIV infections 81
HIV-1 mutants 81, 83
HIV-1 replication 81
HIV-1 reverse transcriptase 82
Hivid 86
Homeostasis, glucose 164
Homeostasis, sterol 128
Hydrocortisone 171
Hyperacidity 43
Hypercholesterolemia 127
Hyperglycemia 43, 164, 176
Hypertension 43, 167
Hypocholesteremic agent 24
Hypotensive activity 42

Ichthyosis 23
Imipramine 20
Immunodeficiency virus 81
Immunomodulation 37
Immunophilins 144
Immunosuppression 37
Incontinence, nocturnal 6
Indigestion 43
Indinavir 86
Insulin secretion 170
Insulin resistance 167
Interleukin 37
Invertases 32
Invirase 86
Ion channels 19
Isapirone 20
Isoeruboside B 33
Isoproterinol 35

Kaletra 86
Kanakin 8
Kava 6

Kava alkaloids 14
Kavahine 6, 8
Kavains 10, 16
Kavalactones 16, 17
Kavatin 8
Kluyveromyces lactis 122

Labial disease 99
Lactate production 20
Lamivudine 86, 102
Leucorrhoea 6
Leukemia, human 59
Lipases 32
Lipoxygenase 37
Lopinavir 86
Lovastatin 127
Lymphomas 99
Lysozymes 32

Malondialdehyde 42
Medicine, allophatic 5
Medicine, herbal 5
Meiosis 149
Meiotic genes 149
Memantine 17
Memory cells 87
Mesolimbic system 21
Methoxyyangonin 7
Methystic acid 11
Methysticin 16
Mind-altering drugs 5
Mitotic cell cycle 143
Morpholines 131
Multidrug-resistant virus 94
Muscle-relaxing anxiolytic agent 6
Mutagenesis 36
Mycobacterium tuberculosis 59

Nausea 43
Nelfinavir 86
Nevirapine 86, 87
Niacin deficiency 23
Nicotinamide 23
Nicotinic acid 173
Nocodazole 125
Noradrenaline 166, 173
Norvir 86
Nucleoside analogues 100
Nucleotides, pyridine 173

Onion extracts 38
Organoselenium compounds 30
Organosulfides 30
Oseltamivir 96
Osprenolol 170
Oxacepam 22

Paclitaxel 42
Papyrus Ebers 24
Paradol 59
Parasites, intestinal 24
Pathogenesis, viral 81
Pathogenic fungi 129
Pellagroid dermopathy 23
Permease 145
Phenetolamine 170
Phenoxybenzamine 170
Phosphodiesterase 38
Phosphotransferase 100
Pichia pastoris 122
Picornaviridiae family 97
Pimozide 175
Pinostrobinchalcone 13, 16
Pinworms 24
Piper methysticum 7
Pipermethystine 15
Piplatine 15
Pleconaril 97
Pneumocystis carinii 134
Polio virus 97
Polymerase 105
Polyphenoloxidases 32
Prazosin 176
Prednisolone 24
Prostaglandin E2 62
Prostaglandins 173
Protease gene 94
Protease inhibitors 85,94
Protein kinases 151
Proteomics 145
Protoisoeruboside B 33
Psychic disorders 22
Psychoactive anxiolytic agent 6

Rauwolcine 176
Reductases 38
Replication kinetics 93
Replication, viral 80
Rescriptor 86

Reserpine 176
Resistance, antifungal drugs 131
Retrovir 86
Retinitis 99
Reverse transcriptase inhibitors 85, 92
Rheumatism 43
Rhinovirus 97
Ribavirin 81
Rimantadine 96
Ritonavir 86
RNA polymerases 80, 98
RNA viruses 80

Saccharomyces cerevisiae 120
Saccharomyces pombe 124
Saponins 33
Saquinavir 86
Sarcoma 36,99
Sativioside C 33
Scrapie 123
Serotonin 1-A receptor 20
Sesquiphellandrene 45
Shogaols 44, 51, 58
Sigma receptor, human 144
Sodarins 131, 134
Sodium channels 19
Spleen cells 37
Squalene epoxidase 131
Stavudine 86
Sterol homeostasis 128
Sterols 131
Stomatitis, vesicular 81
Streptozotocin 166
Suboptimal therapies 95
Sulcanazole 128
Superoxide-dismutases 32
Sustiva 86
Sympathochromomaffin activity 168

Tachycardia, ventricular 35
Terbinafine 131
Terpenes 44
Tetrahydroyangonin 7
Tetrodotoxin 20
Therapies, alternative 5
Therapies, suboptimal 96
Therapy, antiviral 80
Thiazoles 129
Thioacrolein 30
Thiosulfinates 29, 37
Thrombocyte aggregation 37
Thrombocytes 20
Thynudine kinase 100
Tocopherol 49
Tolbutamide 171
Transfructosidases 32
Triglycerides 39
Tryptophane 33
Tunicamycin 145

Urino-genital tract 6

Vaccines, multi-epitopic 81
Vaccines, multivalent 80
Vaginitis 6
Valacyclovir 100
Valium 6
Varicella zoster virus 99
Vasodilatation 35
Videx 86
Vinyldithiins 29
Viracept 86
Viral replication 80
Viramune 86
Viremia 87
Virions 82
Vomiting 43

Warfarin 42

Yangonin 17
Yarrowia lipolytica 122
Yeast, budding 120
Yohimbine 174

Zalcitabine 86
Zanavir 96
Zerit 86
Ziagen 86
Zidovudine 85, 93
Zingerone 60
Zingeronolol 60
Zingiber officinale Roscoe 43
Zingiberene 45
Zingibiraceae 43

Index of titles
Vol. 1–57 (1959–2001)

Acetylen-Verbindungen als Arzneistoffe, natürliche und synthetische
14, 387 (1970)
Adenosine receptors: Clinical implications and biochemical mechanisms
32, 195 (1988)
Adipose tissue, the role of in the distribution and storage of drugs
28, 273 (1984)
Adrenal cortex, steroidogenic capacity and its regulation
34, 359 (1976)
β-Adrenergic blocking agents
20, 27 (1976)
β-Adrenergic blocking agents, pharmacology and structure-activity
10, 46 (1966)
β-Adrenergic blocking drugs, pharmacology
15, 103 (1971)
Adrenergic receptor research, recent developments
33, 151 (1989)
Adrenoceptors, subclassification and nomenclature
47, 81 (1996)
Adverse reactions of sugar polymers in animals and man
23, 27 (1979)
Aldose reductase inhibitors: Recent developments
40, 99 (1993)
Allergy, pharmacological approach
3, 409 (1961)
Alternative medicine: Herbal drugs and their critical appraisal – Part I
56, 1 (2001)
Alternative medicine: Herbal drugs and their critical appraisal – Part II
57, 1 (2001)
Alternative therapeutic modalities. Alternative medicine
47, 251 (1996)
Alzheimer's disease, implications of immunomodulant therapy
32, 21 (1988)
Alzheimer's disease, neuroimmune axis as a basis of therapy
34, 383 (1990)
Amebic disease, pathogenesis of
18, 225 (1974)
Amidinstruktur in der Arzneistoffforschung
11, 356 (1968)
Amines, biogenic and drug research
28, 9 (1984)
Aminoglycosides and polyamines: Targets and effects in the mammalian organism of two important groups of natural aliphatic polycations
46, 183 (1996)
Amino- und Nitroderivate (aromatische), biologische Oxydation und Reduktion
8, 195 (1965)
Aminonucleosid-Nephrose
7, 341 (1964)
Amoebiasis, chemotherapy
8, 11 (1965)

Amoebiasis, surgical
18, 77 (1974)
Amoebicidal drugs, comparative evaluation
18, 353 (1974)
Anabolic steroids
2, 71 (1960)
Analgesia and addiction
5, 155 (1963)
Analgesics and their antagonists
22, 149 (1978)
Ancyclostomiasis in children, trial of bitoscanate
19, 2 (1975)
Androgenic-anabolic steroids and glucocorticoids, interactions
14, 139 (1970)
Anthelmintic action, mechanisms of
19, 147 (1975)
Anthelminticaforschung, neuere Aspekte
1, 243 (1959)
Anthelmintics, comparative efficacy
19, 166(1975)
Anthelmintics, laboratory methods in the screening of
19, 48 (1975)
Anthelmintics, structure-activity
3, 75 (1961)
Anthelmintics, human and veterinary
17, 110 (1973)
Antianginal drugs, quantitative structure-activity relationships of
56, 121 (2001)
Antiarrhythmic compounds
12, 292 (1968)
Antiarrhythmic drugs, recent advances in electrophysiology of
17, 34 (1973)
Antibacterial agents of the nalidixic acid type
21, 9 (1977)
Antibiotics, structure and biogenesis
2, 591 (1960)
Antibiotic activities, *in vitro* models for the study of
31, 349 (1987)
Antibiotika, krebswirksame
3, 451 (1961)
Antibody titres, relationship to resistance to experimental human infection
19, 542 (1975)
Anticancer agents, metabolism of
17, 320 (1973)
Anticonvulsants, developments in
44, 185 (1995)
Antidepressant agents: Recent developments
46, 243 (1996)
Antidiabetika, orale
30, 281 (1986)
Antifertility substances, development
7, 133 (1964)
Anti-filariasis campaign: Its history and future prospects
18, 259 (1974)
Antifolates, new, in cancer therapy
44, 129 (1995)
Antifungal agents
22, 93 (1978)
Antifungal therapy
37, 183 (1991)
Antifungal therapy
44, 87 (1995)
Antifungal therapy, an everlasting battle
49, 219 (1997)
Antihistamines (H1), developments in
39, 35 (1992)
Antihypertensive agents
4, 295 (1962), *13*, 101 (1969), *20*, 197 (1976)
Antihypertensive agents 1969–1981
25, 9 (1981)
Antihypertensive agents: quantitative structure-activity relationships
53, 53 (1999)
Antihypertensive drugs: Progress in five decades
43, 43 (1994)
Anti-inflammatory agents, nonsteroid
10, 139 (1966)
Anti-inflammatory agents: Development of novel. A pharmacological perspective on leukotrienes and their receptors
46, 115 (1996)

Anti-inflammatory drugs, biochemical and pharmacological properties
8, 321 (1965)
Anti-influenza drugs and neuraminidase inhibitors
56, 195 (2001)
Antikoagulantien, orale
11, 226 (1968)
Antimalarials, 8-aminoquinolines
28, 197 (1984)
Antimetabolites, revolution in pharmacology
2, 613 (1960)
Antimicrobials, penetration of human cells
33, 83 (1989)
Antipsychotic agents
38, 299 (1992)
Antituberculous compounds with special reference to the effect of combined treatment, experimental evaluation of
18, 211 (1974)
Antitumor antibiotics, the chemistry of DNA modification
32, 411 (1988)
Anxiolytic drugs, mechanism of action of
31, 315 (1987)
Apoptosis, the role of, in neurodegenerative diseases
48, 55 (1997)
Appetite suppression, pharmacology of
54, 1 (2000)
Applications of yeast in drug discovery
57, 117 (2001)
Arterial pressure by drugs
26, 353 (1982)
Arzneimittel, neue
1, 531 (1959), *2*, 251 (1960), *3*, 369 (1961), *6*, 347 (1963), *10*, 360 (1966)
Arzneimittel, Wert und Bewertung
10, 90 (1966)
Arzneimittelwirkung, Einfluss der Formgebung
10, 204 (1966)
Arzneimittelwirkung, galenische Formgebung
14, 269 (1970)
Aspirin as an antithrombotic agent
33, 43 (1989)
Asthma, drug treatment of
28, 111(1984)
Asthma, emerging drug targets in the molecular pathogenesis of
47, 165 (1996)
Atherosclerosis, cholesterol and its relation to
1, 127 (1959)
Axoplasmic transport, pharmacology and toxicology
28, 53 (1984)
Ayurveda
26, 55 (1982)
Ayurvedic medicine
15, 11 (1971)

Bacterial cell surface and antimicrobial resistance
32, 149 (1988)
Bacterial resistance to antibiotics: The role of biofilms
37, 91 (1991)
Bacterial vaccines, approaches to the rational design
32, 375 (1988)
Bacteria and phagocytic cells, surface interaction between
32, 137 (1988)
Barbiturates and the GABA receptor complex
34, 261 (1990)
Basic research in the US pharmaceutical industry
15, 204 (1971)
Benzimidazole anthelmintics, chemistry and biological activity
27, 85 (1983)
Benzodiazepine receptor binding studies
45, 67 (1995)
Benzodiazepine story
22, 229 (1978)
Beta blockade in myocardial infarction
30, 71 (1986)
Bewertung eines neuen Antibiotikums
22, 327 (1978)
Biliary excretion of drugs and other xenobiotics
25, 361 (1981)

Biochemical acyl hydroxylations
16, 229 (1972)
Biological activity, stereochemical factors
1, 455 (1959)
Biological response quantification in toxicology, pharmacology and pharmacodynamics
21, 105 (1977)
Biomimicry as a basis for drug discovery
51, 185 (1998)
Bitoscanate, a field trial in India
19, 81 (1975)
Bitoscanate, clinical experience
19, 96 (1975)
Bitoscanate, experience in the treatment of adults
19, 90 (1975)
Brain diseases, immunotherapy for
48, 129 (1997)
Brain, pharmacology of the: The hippocampus, learning and seizures
16, 211 (1972)

Caco-2 cell permeability vs. human gastrointestinal absorption: QSPR analysis
54, 35 (2000)
Caffeine, pharmacology of
31, 273 (1987)
Calcium channel blockers in psychiatry
47, 279 (1996)
Calcium channels: New synthetic ligands for L-type
40, 191 (1993)
Calmodulin: Effects of cell stimuli and drugs on cellular activation
45, 33 (1995)
Calmodulin-mediated enzymatic actions, effects of drugs on
33, 353 (1989)
Cancer, chemopreventive agents, natural products and their derivatives
48, 147 (1997)
Cancer chemotherapy
8, 431 (1965), *20*, 465 (1976), *25*, 275 (1981)
Cancer chemotherapy agents, interaction with the mononuclear phagocyte system
35, 487 (1990)
Cancerostatic drugs
20, 251 (1976)
Cancer therapy, systemic: Four decades of progress and some personal perspectives
34, 76 (1990)
Cannabis, chemistry and pharmacology of
36, 71 (1991)
Carcinogenecity, mutagenecity and cancer preventing activities of flavonoids: A structure-system-activity relationship (SSAR) analysis
42, 133 (1994)
Carcinogenecity testing of drugs
29, 155 (1985)
Carcinogens, molecular geometry and mechanism of action
4, 407 (1962)
Cardiotonic agents: quantitative structure-activity relationships
55, 235 (2000)
Cardiovascular drug interactions, clinical importance of
25, 133 (1981)
Cardiovascular drug interactions
29, 10 (1985)
Cardiovascular system, drug receptors and control of recent advances
36, 117 (1991)
Central dopamine receptors, agents acting on
21, 409 (1977)
Central nervous system drugs, biochemical effects
8, 53 (1965)
Cestode infections, chemotherapy of
24, 217 (1980)
Chemical carcinogens, metabolic activation
26, 143 (1982)
Chemokines as targets for pharmacological intervention
47, 53 (1996)
Chemotherapy of schistosomiasis, recent developments
16, 11 (1972)
Chinese herbal medicine: Immunopharmacological and biochemical bases of
46, 263 (1996)

Chinese traditional medicine, perspective and overview, and contemporary pharmacology
47, 131 (1996)
Chirality and future drug design
41, 191 (1993)
Cholera infection (experimental) and local immunity
19, 471 (1975)
Cholera in Hyderabad, epidemiology of
19, 578 (1975)
Cholera in non-endemic regions
19, 594 (1975)
Cholera, pandemic, and bacteriology
19, 513 (1975)
Cholera pathophysiology and therapeutics, advances
19, 563 (1975)
Cholera, research in India on the control and treatment of
19, 503 (1975)
Cholera toxin induced fluid, effect of drugs on
19, 519 (1975)
Cholera toxoid research in the United States
19, 602 (1975)
Cholera vaccines in volunteers, antibody response to
19, 554 (1975)
Cholera vibrios, interbiotype conversions by actions of mutagens
19, 466 (1975)
Cholesterol, relation to atherosclerosis
1, 127 (1959)
Cholesterol blood levels and other dyslipidemias (Drugs for treatment of patients with high)
43, 9 (1994)
Cholinergic function at the cellular and molecular levels, recent progress in understanding
39, 251 (1992)
Cholinergic mechanism-monoamines relation in certain brain structures
6, 334 (1972)
Cholinergic neurotransmitter system, behavioral correlates of presynaptic events
32, 43 (1988)
Clostridium tetani growth *in vivo*
19, 384 (1975)
Combinatorial chemistry: Polymer supported synthesis of peptide and non-peptide libraries
53, 89 (1999)
Communicable diseases, some often neglected factors in the control and prevention of
18, 277 (1974)
Computer-aided drug design: generation of new lead structures
45, 205 (1995)
Computer-assisted structure – antileukemic activity analysis of purines and their aza and deaza analogs
34, 319 (1990)
Conformation analysis, molecular graphics
30, 91 (1986)
Contraception
21, 293 (1977)
Contraceptive agents, development of
33, 261 (1989)
Convulsant drugs – relationships between structure and function
24, 57 (1980)
Cooperative effects in drug-DNA interactions
31, 193 (1987)
Cyclin-dependent kinase, purine analogs as enzyme inhibitory agents: A survey and QSAR analysis
56, 155 (2001)
Cyclopropane compounds
15, 227 (1971)
Cytokines, clinical application of for immunostimulation and immunosuppression
39, 167 (1992)
Cytokines, the potential role of in cancer therapy
39, 219 (1992)
Cytokines, therapeutic application of for immunostimulation and immunosuppression
47, 211 (1996)

Design and discovery of new drugs by stepping-up and stepping-down approaches
40, 163 (1993)

Developmental biology, application of, to medicine and animal agriculture
54, 191 (2000)
Deworming of preschool community in national nutrition programmes
19, 136 (1975)
Diabetes, experimental, role of adrenal medullary hormone in
57, 163 (2001)
1,2-Diamine functionality, medicinal agents
33, 135 (1989)
Diarrhoea (acute) in children, management
19, 527 (1975)
Diarrhoeal diseases (acute) in children
19, 570 (1975)
Digitalis-like factors (endogenous)
41, 249 (1993)
3,4-Dihydroxyphenylalanine and related compounds
9, 223 (1966)
Dioxopiperazines: Chemistry and biology
35, 249 (1990)
Diphtheria, epidemiological observations in Bombay
19, 423 (1975)
Diphtheria, epidemiology of
19, 336 (1975)
Diphtheria in Bombay
19, 277 (1975)
Diphtheria in Bombay, age profile of
19, 417 (1975)
Diphtheria in Bombay, studies on
19, 241 (1975)
Diphtheria, pertussis and tetanus, clinical study
19, 356 (1975)
Diphtheria, pertussis and tetanus vaccines
19, 229 (1975)
Diphtheria toxin production and iron
19, 283 (1975)
Disease control in Asia and Africa, implementation of
18, 43 (1974)
Disease-modifying antirheumatic drugs, recent developments in
24, 101 (1980)
Diuretics
2, 9 (1960)
DNA technology, significance in medicine
33, 397 (1989)
Dopamine agonists, structure-activity relationships
29, 303 (1985)
Dopamine receptor diversity: Molecular and pharmacological perspectives
48, 173 (1997)
Drug action and assay by microbial kinetics
15, 271 (1971)
Drug action, basic mechanisms
7, 11 (1964)
Drug combination, reduction of drug action
14, 11 (1970)
Drug development, contemporary, art and science of
16, 194 (1972)
Drug discovery, organizing for
32, 329 (1988)
Drug discovery: Past, present and future
50, 9 (1998)
Drug discovery, serendipity and structural research
30, 189 (1986)
Drug latentiation
4, 221 (1962)
Drug-macromolecular interactions, implications for pharmacological activity
14, 59 (1970)
Drug metabolism
13, 136 (1969)
Drug metabolism (microsomal), enhancement and inhibition of
17, 12 (1973)
Drug-metabolizing enzymes, perinatal development of
25, 189 (1981)
Drug potency
15, 123 (1971)
Drug research
10, 11 (1966)
Drug research, fundamental structures in, Part I
20, 385 (1976)
Drug research, fundamental structures in, Part II
22, 27 (1978)
Drug research, interaction of
20, 181 (1976)

Drug research, moral challenges in the organisation and management of
42, 9 (1994)
Drug research and development
20, 159 (1976)
Drug-resistant mutants, viral quasispecies and the problem of
48, 99 (1997)
Drugs in biological cells
20, 261 (1976)
Drugs, biliary excretion and enterohepatic circulation
9, 299 (1966)
Drugs, structures, properties and disposition
29, 67 (1985)

Egg-white, reactivity of in rat and man
13, 340 (1969)
Endocrinology, twenty years of research
12, 137 (1968)
Endothelium-derived hyperpolarizing factor - a critical appraisal
50, 107 (1998)
Endotoxin and the pathogenesis of fever
19, 402 (1975)
Enterobacterial infections, chemotherapy of
12, 370 (1968)
Enzyme inhibitors of the renin-angiotensin system
31, 161 (1987)
Erythropoietin, recent advances in research
41, 293 (1993)
Estrogens, oral contraceptives and breast cancer
25, 159 (1981)
Excitation and depression
26, 225 (1982)
Experimental biologist and medical scientist in the pharmaceutical industry
24, 83 (1980)

Fibrinolysis, mechanisms of and clinical use of thrombolytic agents
39, 197 (1992)
Fifteen years of structural modifications in the field of antifungal monocyclic 1-substituted 1 H-azoles
27, 253 (1983)
Filarial infection, immuno-diagnosis
19, 128 (1975)
Filariasis chemotherapy
9, 191 (1966)
Filariasis in India
18, 173 (1974)
Filariasis, in four villages near Bombay, epidemiological and biochemical studies
18, 269 (1974)
Filariasis, malaria and leprosy, new perspectives in the chemotherapy of
18, 99 (1974)
Fluor, dérivés organiques d'intérêt pharmacologique
3, 9 (1961)
From outer to inner space: Traveling along a scientific career from astrochemistry to drug research
57, 181 (2001)
Fungal metabolites and Chinese herbal medicine as immunostimulants
34, 395 (1990)
Further developments in research on the chemistry and pharmacology of quinuclidine derivatives (synthetic)
27, 9 (1983)

GABA-Drug interactions
31, 223 (1987)
Galenische Formgebung und Arzneimittelwirkung
10, 204 (1966), *14*, 269 (1970)
Ganglienblocker
2, 297 (1960)
Genetic codes: Physicochemical basis of – quantitative analysis
48, 9 (1997)
Genome, from, to drug – optimising the drug discovery process
53, 157 (1999)
Glucocorticoids, anti-inflammatory and immuno-suppressive effects
33, 63 (1989)
Glutamatergic involvement in psychomotor stimulant action
50, 155 (1998)
Glycoproteins, oligosaccharide chains of
34, 163 (1990)

Heilmittel, Entwicklung
10, 33 (1966)
Helminth diseases – challenges and achievements
31, 9 (1987)
Helminthiasis (intestinal), chemotherapy of
19, 158 (1975)
Helminth infections, progress in the experimental chemotherapy of
17, 241 (1973)
Helminthic infections, immunodiagnosis of
19, 119 (1975)
Helminth parasites, treatment and control
30, 473 (1986)
Hepatitis B virus infection: The identification and development of antiviral agents for the treatment of
50, 259 (1998)
Hepatitis C virus infections: recent advances in prevention and treatment of
55, 1 (2000)
Hepatoprotectants, present status of
52, 53 (1999)
Herpesvirus infections, current and potential therapies for the treatment of
56, 77 (2001)
Herbal drugs, alternative medicine
56, 1 (2001); *57*, 1 (2001)
Heterocyclic diversity: The road to biological activity
44, 9 (1995)
High resolution nuclear magnetic resonance spectroscopy of biological samples as an aid to drug development
31, 427 (1987)
High-throughput screening, the application of, to novel drug discovery
51, 245 (1998)
Histamine H_1-receptor agonists, developments
44, 49 (1995)
Histamine H_3-receptor, a targeting for developing new drugs
39, 127 (1992)
Histamine H_3 receptor ligands, the medicinal chemistry and therapeutic potentials
45, 107 (1995)
HIV-Protease inhibitors: Development of, a survey
51, 1 (1998)
Homologous series, pharmacology
7, 305 (1964)
Hookworm anaemia and intestinal malabsorption
19, 108 (1975)
Hookworm disease and trichuriasis, experience with bitoscanate
19, 23 (1975)
Hookworm disease, bitoscanate in the treatment of children with
19, 6 (1975)
Hookworm disease, comparative study of drugs
19, 70 (1975)
Hookworm disease, effect on the structure and function of the small bowel
19, 44 (1975)
Hookworm infection, a comparative study of drugs
19, 86 (1975)
Hookworm infections, chemotherapy of
26, 9 (1982)
Hopanoids, bacterial triterpenoids, and the biosynthesis of isoprenic units in prokaryotes
37, 271 (1991)
Human sleep
22, 355 (1978)
The 5-HT_{1A} receptor and its ligands: structure and function
52, 103 (1999)
Hydatid disease
19, 75 (1975)
Hydrocortisone, effects of structural alteration on the antiinflammatory properties
5, 11 (1963)
5-Hydroxytryptamine and related indolealkylamines
3, 151 (1961)
5-Hydroxytryptamine receptor agonists and antagonists
30, 365 (1986)
5-Hydroxytryptamine $(5\text{-}HT)_4$ receptors and central nervous system function: An update
49, 9 (1997)

Hypertension and brain neurotransmitters
30, 127 (1986)
Hypertension, recent advances in drugs against
29, 215 (1985)
Hypertension: Relating drug therapy to pathogenic mechanisms
32, 175 (1988)
Hypolipidemic agents
13, 217 (1969)

Immune system, the pharmacology of
28, 83 (1984)
Immunization, host factors in the response
19, 263 (1975)
Immunization of a village, a new approach to herd immunity
19, 252 (1975)
Immunization, progress in
19, 274 (1975)
Immunology
20, 573 (1976)
Immunology in drug research
28, 233 (1984)
Immunostimulation with peptidoglycan or its synthetic derivatives
32, 305 (1988)
Immunopharmacology and brain disorders
30, 345 (1986)
Immunosuppressants, recent advances in
52, 1 (1999)
Immunosuppression agents, procedures, speculations and prognosis
16, 67 (1972)
Immunotherapy of leprosy and tuberculosis
33, 415 (1989)
Impact of natural product research on drug discovery
23, 51 (1979)
Impact of state and society on medical research
35, 9 (1990)
Indole compounds
6, 75 (1963)
Indolstruktur, in Medizin und Biologie
2, 227 (1960)
Industrial drug research
20, 143 (1976)
Influenza virus, functional significance of the various components of
18, 253 (1974)
Insulin resistance, impaired glucose tolerance, and non-insulin-dependent diabetes, pathologic mechanisms and treatment: Current status and therapeutic possibilities
51, 33 (1998)
Interferons (Production and action): New insights into molecular mechanisms of gene regulation and expression
43, 239 (1994)
Ion and water transport in renal tubular cells
26, 87 (1982)
Ionenaustauscher, Anwendung in Pharmazie und Medizin
1, 11 (1959)
Isoprenoid biosynthesis via the mevalonate route, a novel target for antibacterial drugs
50, 135 (1998)
Isosterism and bioisosterism in drug design
37, 287 (1991)
Isotope, Anwendung in der pharmazeutischen Forschung
7, 59 (1964)

κ receptor, U-50,488 and the: A personalized account covering the period 1973 to 1990
52, 167 (1999)
κ receptor, U-50,488
53, 1 (1999)
Ketoconazole, a new step in the management of fungal disease
27, 63 (1983)

Leishmaniasis
18, 289 (1974)
Leishmaniasis, present status of
34, 447 (1990)
Leprosy, some neuropathologic and cellular aspects of
18, 53 (1974)
Leprosy in the Indian context, some practical problems of the epidemiology of
18, 25 (1974)
Leprosy, malaria and filariasis, new perspectives on the chemotherapy of
18, 99 (1974)

Leprosy, progress in the chemotherapy: Status, issues and prospects
34, 421 (1990)
Leukotriene antagonists and inhibitors of leukotriene biosynthesis
37, 9 (1991)
Levamisole
20, 347 (1976)
Light and dark as a "drug"
31, 383 (1987)
Lipophilicity and drug activity
23, 97 (1979)
Lokalanästhetika, Konstitution und Wirksamkeit
4, 353 (1962)
Luteinizing hormone regulators: Luteinizing hormone releasing hormone analogs, estrogens, opiates, and estrogen-opiate hybrids
42, 39 (1994)
Luteolytic agents in fertility regulation
40, 9 (1993)
Lysostaphin: Model for a specific enzymatic approach to infectious disease
16, 309 (1972)

Malaria, advances in chemotherapy
30, 221 (1986)
Malaria chemotherapy, repository antimalarial drugs
13, 170 (1969)
Malaria chemotherapy, antibiotics in
26, 167 (1982)
Malaria, eradication in India
18, 245 (1974)
Malaria, filariasis and leprosy, new perspectives on the chemotherapy of
18, 99 (1974)
Mast cell secretion, drug inhibition of
29, 277 (1985)
Mass spectrometry in pharmaceutical research, recent applications of
18, 399 (1974)
Medical practice and medical pharmaceutical research
20, 491 (1976)
Medicinal chemistry, contribution to medicine
12, 11 (1968)
Medicinal chemistry: A support or a driving force in drug research?
34, 343 (1990)
Medicinal research: Retrospectives and perspectives
29, 97 (1985)
Medicinal science
20, 9 (1976)
Membrane drug receptors
20, 323 (1976)
Menses-regulating agents, non steroidal
44, 159 (1995)
Mental illnesses, immunotherapy for
48, 129 (1997)
Mescaline and related compounds
11, 11 (1968)
Metabolism of drugs, enzymatic mechanisms
6, 11 (1963)
Metabolism (oxidative) of drugs and other foreign compounds
17, 488 (1973)
Metronidazol-therapie, trichomonasis
9, 361 (1966)
O-methyltransferase, catechol – characteristics of, and properties of selective COMT inhibitors
39, 291 (1992)
Migraine: Pharmacology
34, 209 (1990)
Monitoring adverse reactions to drugs
21, 231 (1977)
Monoaminoxydase-Hemmer
2, 417 (1960)
Monoamine oxidase, inhibitors of
30, 205 (1986)
Monoamine oxidase inhibitors
38, 171 (1992)
Morphine, the effects of morphine on cell proliferation
55, 33 (2000)
Mycoses, chemotherapy for
33, 317 (1989)

Narcotic antagonists
8, 261 (1965), *20*, 45 (1976)
Natriuretic hormones
34, 231 (1990)

Natriuretic hormones II
45, 245 (1995)
Natural products as anticancer agents
42, 53 (1994)
Necator americanus infection, clinical field trial of bitoscanate
19, 64 (1975)
Nematodes, intestinal, chemotherapy of
16, 157 (1972)
Nematoide infections (intestinal) in Latin America
19, 28 (1975)
Nephrotoxicity (drug) – The significance of cellular mechanisms
41, 51 (1993)
Neuropeptides
38, 149 (1992)
Neuropeptides as native immune modulators
45, 9 (1995)
Neuropeptides in drug research
54, 161 (2000)
Neurotransmitters (Role of) in the central regulation of the cardiovascular system
35, 25 (1990)
Neurotransmitters involved in the central regulation of the cardiovascular system
46, 43 (1996)
Nicotine: An addictive substance or a therapeutic agent?
33, 9 (1989)
Nitroimidazoles as chemotherapeutic agents
27, 163 (1983)
NMDA receptors, regulation of, by ethanol
54, 121 (2000)
NMR spectroscopy in drug discovery: Tools for combinatorial chemistry, natural products, and metabolism research
55, 137 (2000)
Noise analysis and channels at the postsynaptic membrane of skeletal muscle
24, 9 (1980)
NSAIDs, The effects of, and E-prostaglandins on bone: A two signal hypothesis for the maintenance of skeletal bone
39, 351 (1992)
NSAIDs, Effects of, on the kidney
49, 155 (1997)
Nucleosides as drugs, novel and unusual
48, 195 (1997)

Ophthalmic drug preparations, methods for elucidating bioavailability, mechanisms of
25, 421 (1981)
Opiate receptors: Search for new drugs
36, 49 (1991)
Osteoarthritis, glucosamine and chondroitin sulfates in the treatment of: a survey
55, 81 (2000)
Osteoporosis, recent developments in the chemotherapy of
45, 289 (1995)

Parasitic infections in man, recent advances in the treatment of
18, 191 (1974)
Parasitosis (intestinal), analysis of symptoms and signs
19, 10 (1975)
Peptide analogs, bioactive: *In vivo* and *in vitro* production
34, 287 (1990)
Peptide drug delivery into the central nervous system
51, 95 (1998)
Peptide receptor ligand drugs: Progress on nonpeptides
40, 33 (1993)
Peptides (complex), enzymatic generation
48, 27 (1997)
Pertussis agglutinins and complement fixing antibodies in whooping cough
19, 178 (1975)
Pertussis, diphtheria and tetanus, clinical study
19, 356 (1975)
Pertussis, diphtheria and tetanus vaccines
19, 229 (1975)
Pertussis, epidemiology of
19, 257 (1975)
Pertussis vaccine
19, 341 (1975)
Pertussis vaccine composition
19, 347 (1975)
Pharmacology, molecular
20, 101 (1976)

Pharmacology, molecular, basis for drug design
10, 429 (1966)
Phenothiazine und azaphenothiazine
5, 269 (1963)
Phosphodiesterase inhibitors: Biochemistry, pharmacology and therapeutic potential in asthma
40, 9 (1993)
Photochemistry of drugs
11, 48 (1968)
Phosphodiesterase e (PDE4) inhibitors in asthma and chronic obstructive pulmonary disease
53, 193 (1999)
Placeboproblem
1, 279 (1959)
Plasma fibrinogen levels, drug affecting. Implications for new antithrombotic strategies
46, 169 (1996)
Platelets and atherosclerosis
29, 49 (1985)
Podophyllotoxin glucoside – etoposide
33, 169 (1989)
Polyamines, pharmacological properties of, and their depletion by biosynthesis inhibitors
37, 107 (1991)
Polyamines as markers of malignancy
39, 9 (1992)
Polyamines and cerebral ischemia
50, 193 (1998)
Polyamines (the natural) and the immune system
43, 87 (1994)
Potassium channel modulation, recent advances in
49, 93 (1997)
Potassium channel openers: Airway pharmacology and clinical possibilities in asthma
37, 161 (1991)
Progesterone receptor binding of steroidal and nonsteroidal compounds
30, 151 (1986)
Propellants, toxicity of
18, 365 (1974)
Prostacyclin receptors, neuronal
49, 123 (1997)
Prostaglandins
17, 410 (1973)
Prostate cancer and the androgen receptor: Strategies for the development of novel therapeutics
55, 213 (2000)
Protease inhibitors as potential viral agents for the treatment of picornaviral infections
52, 197 (1999)
G Protein coupled receptors as modules of interacting proteins: A family meeting
49, 173 (1997)
Protein kinases in neurogenerative diseases, abnormalities of
51, 133 (1998)
Protozoan and helminth parasites
20, 433 (1976)
Psychopharmaka, Anwendung in der psychosomatischen Medizin
10, 530 (1966)
Psychopharmaka, strukturelle Betrachtungen
9, 129 (1966)
Psychosomatische Medizin, Anwendung von Psychopharmaka
10, 530 (1966)
Psychotomimetic agents
15, 68 (1971)
Pyrimidinones as biodynamic agents
31, 127 (1987)

QSAR, multi-dimensional QSAR in drug research
55, 105 (2000)
Quantum chemical methods to study molecular mechanisms of drug action
34, 9 (1990)
Quaternary ammonium salts, chemical nature and pharmacological actions
2, 135 (1960)
Quaternary ammonium salts – advances in chemistry and pharmacology since 1960
24, 267 (1980)
Quinazoline derivatives
26, 259 (1982)
Quinazolones, biological activity
14, 218 (1970)
Quinazolones, biologically active
43, 143 (1994)

Quinolones
31, 243 (1987)
Quinolone antimicrobials
38, 9 (1992)
Quinuclidine derivatives, chemical structure and pharmacological activity
13, 293 (1969)

Red blood cell membrane, as a model for targets of drug action
17, 59 (1973)
Renin-angiotensin system
26, 207 (1982); *31*, 161 (1987)
Reproduction in women, pharmacological control
12, 47 (1968)
Research, preparing the ground: Importance of data
18, 239 (1974)
Resistance (bacterial) to β-lactam antibiotics: Problems and solutions
41, 95 (1993)
Rheumatherapie, Synopsis
12, 165 (1968)
Ribonucleotide reductase inhibitors as anticancer and antiviral agents
31, 101 (1987)
Risk assessment problems in chemical oncogenesis
31, 257 (1987)
RNA virus evolution and the control of viral disease
33, 93 (1989)

Schistosomiasis, recent progress in the chemotherapy of
18, 15 (1974)
Schwefelverbindungen, therapeutisch verwendbare
4, 9 (1962)
Shock, medical interpretation
14, 196 (1970)
Selenium compounds, synthetic organic, pharmacology of
36, 9 (1991)
Serenics
42, 167 (1994)
Serotonin ($5HT_3$) antagonist series, structural modification patterns from agonists to antagonists and their application to drug-design
41, 313 (1993)
Serotonin, dopamine and norepinephrine transporters in the central nervous system and their inhibitors
54, 59 (2000)
Serotonin in migraine: Theories, animal models and emerging therapies
51, 219 (1998)
Serotonin uptake inhibitors: Uses in clinical therapy and in laboratory research
45, 167 (1995)
Serum electrolyte abnormalities caused by drugs
30, 9 (1986)
Social pharmacology
22, 9 (1978)
Sodium pump inhibition, endogenous: Current status and therapeutic opportunities
46, 9 (1996)
Spectrofluorometry, physicochemical methods in pharmaceutical chemistry
6, 151 (1963)
Stereoselective drug metabolism and its significance in drug research
32, 249 (1988)
Steroids inotropic, in search of ideal
47, 9 (1996)
Stoffwechsel von Arzneimitteln, Ursache von Wirkung, Nebenwirkung und Toxizität
15, 147 (1971)
Strahlenempfindlichkeit von Säugetieren, Beeinflussung durch chemische Substanzen
9, 11 (1966)
Structure-activity relationships
23, 199 (1979)
Substruktur der Proteine, tabellarische Zusammenstellung
16, 364 (1972)
Sulfanilamides and sulfones (antibacterial)-molecular modelling and quantitative structure-activity analysis of
36, 361 (1991)
Sulfonamide research
12, 389 (1968)

Sympathetic nervous system and experimental diabetes: role of adrenal medullary hormones
57, 163 (2001)

T-cell factors, antigen-specific and drug research
32, 9 (1988)
Teratogenesis, chemical
41, 9 (1993)
Teratogenesis, chemical, in humans: Biochemical and molecular mechanisms
49, 25 (1997)
Teratogenic hazards, advances in prescreening
29, 121 (1985)
Terpenoids, biological activity
6, 279 (1963), *13*, 11 (1969)
Tetanus and its prevention
19, 391 (1975)
Tetanus, autonomic dysfunction as a problem in the treatment of
19, 245 (1975)
Tetanus, cephalic
19, 443 (1975)
Tetanus, cholinesterase restoring therapy
19, 329 (1975)
Tetanus, diphtheria and pertussis, clinical study
19, 356 (1975)
Tetanus, general and pathophysiological aspects
19, 314 (1975)
Tetanus in children
19, 209 (1975)
Tetanus in Punjab and the role of muscle relaxants
19, 288 (1975)
Tetanus, mode of death
19, 439 (1975)
Tetanus neonatorum
19, 189 (1975)
Tetanus, pertussis and diphtheria vaccines
19, 229 (1975)
Tetanus, present data on the pathogenesis
19, 301 (1975)
Tetanus, role of beta-adrenergic blocking drug propranolol
19, 361 (1975)
Tetanus, situational clinical trials and therapeutics
19, 367 (1975)
Tetanus, therapeutic measurement
19, 323 (1975)
Tetracyclines
17, 210 (1973)
Tetrahydroisoquinolines and β-carbolines
29, 415 (1985)
Thymoleptika, Biochemie und Pharmakologie
11, 121 (1968)
Toxoplasmosis
18, 205 (1974)
Transfer factor in malignancy
42, 401 (1994)
Transfer factor 1993: New frontiers
42, 309 (1994)
Trichomonasis, Metronidazol-Therapie
9, 361 (1966)
Trichuriasis and hookworm disease in Mexico, experience with bitoscanate
19, 23 (1975)
Troglitazone and emerging glitazones: New avenues for potential therapeutic benefits beyond glycemic control
54, 235 (2000)
Tropical diseases, chemotherapy of
26, 343 (1982)
Tropical medicine, teaching of
18, 35 (1974)
Tuberculosis in rural areas of Maharashtra, profile of
18, 91 (1974)
Tuberkulose, antibakterielle Chemotherapie
7, 193 (1964)
Tumor promoters and antitumor agents
23, 63 (1979)

U-50,488 and the κ receptor
52, 167 (1999); *53*, 1 (1999)

Vaccination (eradication by): The memorial to smallbox could be surrounded by others
41, 151 (1993)
Vaccine escape, viral quasispecies and the problems of
48, 99 (1997)

Vaccines, controlled field trials of
19, 481 (1975)
Vaccines, unsolved problems with
23, 9 (1979)
Vector-borne diseases
35, 365 (1990)
Vibrio cholerae, cell-wall antigens of
19, 612 (1975)
Vibrio cholerae, recent studies on genetic recombination
19, 460 (1975)
Vibrio cholerae, virulence-enhancing effect of ferric ammonium citrate on
19, 564 (1975)
Vibrio parahaemolyticus in Bombay
19, 586 (1975)
Vibrio parahaemolyticus infection in Calcutta
19, 490 (1975)
Viral agents, anti-
22, 267 (1978); *28*, 127 (1984)
Viral agents, anti-, the identification and development of, for the treatment of chronic hepatitis B virus infection
50, 259 (1998)
Virus population dynamics, fitness variations and the control of viral disease: an update
57, 77 (2001)

Wurmkrankheiten, Chemotherapie von
1, 159 (1959)

Yeast, application of in drug research
57, 117 (2001)

Author and paper index Vol. 1–57 (1959–2001)

Pertussis agglutinins and complement fixing antibodies in whooping cough *19*, 178 (1975)	K. C. Agarwal M. Ray N. L. Chitkara
Pharmacology of clinically useful beta-adrenergic blocking drugs *15*, 103 (1971)	R. P. Ahlquist A. M. Karow, Jr. M. W. Riley
Adrenergic beta blocking agents *20*, 27 (1976)	R. P. Ahlquist
Trial of a new anthelmintic (bitoscanate) in ankylostomiasis in children *19*, 2 (1975)	S. H. Ahmed S. Vaishnava
Development of antibacterial agents of the nalidixic acid type *21*, 9 (1977)	R. Albrecht
The mode of action of anti-rheumatic drugs. Anti-inflammatory and immunosuppressive effects of glucocorticoids *33*, 63 (1989)	Anthony C. Allison Simon W. Lee
Biological activity in the quinazolone series *14*, 218 (1970)	A. H. Amin D. R. Mehta S. S. Samarth
Enhancement and inhibition of microsomal drug metabolism *17*, 11 (1973)	M. W. Anders
Reactivity of rat and man to egg-white *13*, 340 (1969)	S. I. Ankier
Enzyme inhibitors of the renin-angiotensin system *31*, 161 (1987)	Michael J. Antonaccio John J. Wright
Narcotic antagonists *8*, 261 (1965)	S. Archer L. S. Harris

Recent developments in the chemotherapy of schistosomiasis *16*, 11 (1972)	S. Archer A. Yarinsky
Recent progress in the chemotherapy of schistosomiasis *18*, 15 (1974) Recent progress in research on narcotic antagonists *20*, 45 (1976)	S. Archer
Molecular geometry and mechanism of action of chemical carcinogens *4*, 407 (1962)	J. C. Arcos
Cell-kinetic and pharmacokinetic aspects in the use and further development of cancerostatic drugs *20*, 521 (1976)	M. von Ardenne
Molecular pharmacology, a basis for drug design *10*, 429 (1966) Reduction of drug action by drug combination *14*, 11 (1970)	E. J. Ariëns
Stereoselectivity and affinity in molecular pharmacology *20*, 101 (1976)	E. J. Ariëns J. F. Rodrigues de Miranda P. A. Lehmann
The pharmacology of caffeine *31*, 273 (1987)	M. J. Arnaud
Recent advances in central 5-hydroxytryptamine receptor agonists and antagonists *30*, 365 (1986)	Lars-Erik Arvidsson Uli Hacksell Richard A. Glennon
Drugs affecting the renin-angiotensin system *26*, 207 (1982)	R. W. Ashworth
Tetanus neonatorum *19*, 189 (1975) Tetanus in children *19*, 209 (1975)	V. B. Athavale P. N. Pai A. Fernandez P. N. Patnekar Y. S. Acharya
Toxicity of propellants *18*, 365 (1974)	D. M. Aviado
Polyamines as markers of malignancy *39*, 9 (1992)	Uriel Bachrach
Neuere Aspekte der chemischen Anthelminticaforschung *1*, 243 (1959)	J. Bally

Problems in preparation, testing and use of diphtheria, pertussis and tetanus vaccines *19*, 229 (1975)	D. D. Banker
Phosphodiesterase 4 (PDE4) inhibitors in asthma and chronic obstructive pulmonary disease *53*, 193 (1973)	Mary S. Barnette
Recent advances in electrophysiology of antiarrhythmic drugs *17*, 33 (1973)	A. L. Bassett A. L. Wit
Chirality and future drug design *41*, 191 (1993)	Sanjay Batra Manju Seth A. P. Bhaduri
Drugs for treatment of patients with high cholesterol blood levels and other dyslipidemias 43, 9 (1994)	Harold E. Bays Carlos A. Dujovne
Stereochemical factors in biological activity *1*, 455 (1959)	A. H. Beckett
Natriuretic hormones II *45*, 245 (1995)	Elaine J. Benaksas E. David Murray, Jr. William J. Wechter
Molecular modelling and quantitative structure-activity analysis of anti-bacterial sulfanilamides and sulfones *36*, 361 (1991)	P. G. De Benedetti
Industrial research in the quest for new medicines *20*, 143 (1976) The experimental biologist and the medical scientist in the pharmaceutical industry *24*, 38 (1980)	B. Berde
Newer diuretics *2*, 9 (1960)	K. H. Beyer, Jr. J. E. Baer
Recent developments in 8-amino-quinoline antimalarials *28*, 197 (1984)	A. P. Bhaduri B. K. Bhat M. Seth
Studies on diphtheria in Bombay *19*, 241 (1975)	M. Bhaindarkar Y. S. Nimbkar
Bitoscanate in children with hookworm disease *19*, 6 (1975)	B. Bhandari L. N. Shrimali
Recent studies on genetic recombination in *Vibriocholerae* *19*, 460 (1975)	K. Bhaskaran

Interbiotype conversion of cholera vibrios by action of mutagens *19*, 466 (1975)	P. Bhattacharya S. Ray
Experience with bitoscanate in hook-worm disease and trichuriasis in Mexico *19*, 23 (1975)	F. Biagi
Analysis of symptoms and signs related with intestinal parasitosis in 5,215 cases *19*, 10 (1975)	F. Biagi R. López J. Viso
Untersuchungen zur Biochemie und Pharmacologie der Thymoleptika *11*, 121 (1968) The role of adipose tissue in the distribution and storage of drugs *28*, 273 (1984)	M. H. Bickel
The β-adrenergic-blocking agents, pharmacology, and structure-activity relationships *10*, 46 (1966)	J. H. Biel B. K. B. Lum
Prostaglandins *17*, 410 (1973)	J. S. Bindra R. Bindra
In vitro models for the study of antibiotic activities *31*, 349 (1987)	J. Blaser S. H. Zinner
The red blood cell membrane as a model for targets of drug action *17*, 59 (1973)	L. Bolis
Epidemiology and public health. Importance of intestinal nematode infections in Latin America *19*, 28 (1975)	D. Botero
Clinical importance of cardiovascular drug interactions *25*, 133 (1981) Serum electrolyte abnormalities caused by drugs *30*, 9 (1986)	D. Craig Brater
Update of cardiovascular drug interactions *29*, 9 (1985)	D. Craig Brater Michael R. Vasko
Some practical problems of the epidemiology of leprosy in the Indian context *18*, 25 (1974)	S. G. Browne
Brain neurotransmitters and the development and maintenance of experimental hypertension *30*, 127 (1986)	Jerry J. Buccafusco Henry E. Brezenoff
Die Ionenaustauscher und ihre Anwendung in der Pharmazie und Medizin *1*, 11 (1959)	J. Büchi

Wert und Bewertung der Arzneimittel *10*, 90 (1966)	J. Büchi
Cyclopropane compounds of biological interest *15*, 227 (1971) The state of medicinal science *20*, 9 (1976) Isosterism and bioisosterism in drug design *37*, 287 (1991)	A. Burger
Human and veterinary anthelmintics (1965–1971) *17*, 108 (1973)	R. B. Burrows
The antibody basis of local immunity to experimental cholera infection in the rabbit ileal loop *19*, 471 (1975)	W. Burrows J. Kaur
Les dérivés organiques du fluor d'intérêt pharmacologique *3*, 9 (1961)	N. P. Buu-Hoï
Teaching tropical medicine *18*, 35 (1974)	K. M. Cahill
Anabolic steroids *2*, 71 (1960)	B. Camerino G. Sala
Immunosuppression agents, procedures, speculations and prognosis *16*, 67 (1972)	G. W. Camiener W. J. Wechter
Dopamine agonists: Structure-activity relationships *29*, 303 (1985)	Joseph G. Cannon
Therapeutic applications of cytokines for immunostimulation and immuno- suppression: An update *47*, 211 (1996)	Gaetano Cardi Thomas L. Ciardelli Marc S. Ernstoff
Analgesics and their antagonists: Recent developments *22*, 149 (1978)	A. F. Casy
Chemical nature and pharmacological actions of quaternary ammonium salts *2*, 135 (1960)	C. J. Cavallito A. P. Gray
Contributions of medicinal chemistry to medicine – from 1935 *12*, 11 (1968) Changing influences on goals and incentives in drug research and development *20*, 159 (1976) Quaternary ammonium salts – advances in chemistry and pharmacology since 1960 *24*, 267 (1980)	C. J. Cavallito

Über Vorkommen und Bedeutung der Indolstruktur in der Medizin und Biologie *2*, 227 (1960)	A. Cerletti
The new generation of monoamine oxidase inhibitors *38*, 171 (1992)	Andrea M. Cesura Alfred Pletscher
Cholesterol and its relation to atherosclerosis *1*, 127 (1959)	K. K. Chen Tsung-Min Lin
Effect of hookworm disease on the structure and function of small bowel *19*, 44 (1975)	H. K. Chuttani R. C. Misra
Recent developments in antidepressant agents *46*, 183 (1996)	James Claghorn Michael D. Lesem
Generation of new-lead structures in computer-aided drug design *45*, 205 (1995)	Nissim Claude Cohen Vincenzo Tschinke
The psychomimetic agents *15*, 68 (1971)	S. Cohen
The identification and development of antiviral agents for the treatment of hepatitis B virus infection *50*, 259 (1998)	Joseph M. Colacino Kirk A. Staschke
Implementation of disease control in Asia and Africa *18*, 43 (1974)	M. J. Colbourne
Structure-activity relationships in certain anthelmintics *3*, 75 (1961)	J. C. Craig M. E. Tate
Contribution of Haffkine to the concept and practice of controlled field trials of vaccines *19*, 481 (1975)	B. Cvjetanovic
Antifungal agents *22*, 93 (1978)	P. F. D'Arcy E. M. Scott
Carcinogenecity, mutagenecity and cancer preventing activities of flavanoids: A structure-system-activity relationship (SSAR) analysis *42*, 133 (1994)	A. Das J. H. Wang E. J. Lien
Some neuropathologic and cellular aspects of leprosy 18, 53 (1974)	D. K. Dastur Y. Ramamohan A. S. Dabholkar
Autonomic dysfunction as a problem in the treatment of tetanus *19*, 245 (1975)	F. D. Dastur G. J. Bhat K. G. Nair

Studies on *Vibrio parahaemolyticus* infection in Calcutta as compared to cholera infection *19*, 490 (1975)	B. C. Deb
Biochemical effects of drugs acting on the central nervous system *8*, 53 (1965)	L. Decsi
Some reflections on the chemotherapy of tropical diseases: Past, present and future *26*, 343 (1982)	E. W. J. de Maar
Drug research – whence and whither *10*, 11 (1966)	R. G. Denkewalter M. Tishler
Immunization of a village, a new approach to herd immunity *19*, 252 (1975)	N. S. Deodhar
Profiles of tuberculosis in rural areas of Maharashtra *18*, 91 (1974)	M. D. Deshmukh K. G. Kulkarni S. S. Virdi B. B. Yodh
The interface between drug research, marketing, management, and social, political and regulatory forces *20*, 181 (1976) Medicinal research: Retrospectives and perspectives *29*, 97 (1985) Serendipity and structured research in drug discovery *30*, 189 (1986) Medicinal chemistry: A support or a driving force in drug research? *34*, 343 (1990) Heterocyclic diversity: The road to biological activity *44*, 9 (1995)	G. deStevens
Hypolipidemic agents *13*, 217 (1969)	G. deStevens W. L. Bencze R. Hess
Antihypertensive agents *20*, 197 (1976)	G. deStevens M. Wilhelm
RNA virus evolution and the control of viral disease *33*, 93 (1989)	Esteban Domingo

Viral quasispecies and the problem of vaccine-escape and drug-resistant mutants *48*, 99 (1997)	Esteban Domingo Luis Menéndez-Arias Miguel E. Quiñones-Mateu Africa Holguín Mónica Gutiérrez-Rivas Miguel A. Martínez Josep Quer Isabel S. Novella John J. Holland
Virus population dynamics, fitness variations and the control of viral disease: an update *57*, 77 (2001)	Esteban Domingo Antonio Mas Eloisa Yuste Nonia Pariente Saleta Sierra Mónica Gutiérrez-Rivas Luis Menéndez-Arias
Transport and accumulation in biological cell systems interacting with drugs *20*, 261 (1976)	W. Dorst A. F. Bottse G. M. Willems
The pharmacology of the immune system: Clinical and experimental perspectives *28*, 83 (1984)	Jürgen Drews
An overview of studies on estrogens, oral contraceptives and breast cancer *25*, 159 (1981)	V. A. Drill
Aminonucleosid-nephrose *7*, 341 (1964)	U. C. Dubach
Impact of researches in India on the control and treatment of cholera *19*, 503 (1975)	N. K. Dutta
The perinatal development of drug-metabolizing enzymes: What factors trigger their onset? *25*, 189 (1981)	G. J. Dutton J. E. A. Leakey
Laboratory methods in the screening of anthelmintics *19*, 48 (1975)	D. Düwel
Recent developments in the chemotherapy of osteoporosis *45*, 289 (1995)	Indra Dwivedy Suprabhat Ray
Present status of luteolytic agents in fertility regulation *40*, 239 (1993)	Indra Dwivedy Suprabhat Ray Arvinder Grover
Progress in immunization *19*, 274 (1975)	G. Edsall

Host factors in the response to immunization *19*, 263 (1975)	G. Edsall M. A. Belsey R. Le Blanc L. Levine
Recent advances in potassium channel modulation *49*, 93 (1997) Endothelium-derived hyperpolarizing factor – a critical appraisal *50*, 107 (1998)	Gillian Edwards Arthur H. Weston
5-Hydroxytryptamine (5-HT)$_4$ receptors and central nervous system function: An update *49*, 9 (1997)	Richard M. Eglen
Drug-macromolecular interactions: Implications for pharmacological activity *14*, 59 (1970)	S. Ehrenpreis
Betrachtungen zur Entwicklung von Heilmitteln *10*, 33 (1966)	G. Ehrhart
Progress in malaria chemotherapy, Part I. Repository antimalarial drugs *13*, 170 (1969) New perspectives on the chemotherapy of malaria, filariasis and leprosy *18*, 99 (1974)	E. F. Elslager
Recent research in the field of 5-hydroxytryptamine and related indolealkylamines *3*, 151 (1961)	V. Erspamer
Recent advances in erythropoietin research *41*, 293 (1993)	James W. Fisher
The chemistry of DNA modification by antitumor antibiotics *32*, 411 (1988)	Jed. F. Fisher Paul A. Aristoff
Toward peptide receptor ligand drugs: Progress on nonpeptides *40*, 33 (1993)	Roger M. Freidinger
Transfer factor 1993: New frontiers *42*, 309 (1994)	H. Hugh Fudenberg Giancarlo Pizza
Drugs affecting serotonin neurons *35*, 85 (1990) Serotonin uptake inhibitors: Uses in clinical therapy and laboratory research *45*, 167 (1995)	Ray W. Fuller
Bacteriology at the periphery of the cholera pandemic *19*, 513 (1975)	A. L. Furniss

Emerging drug targets in the molecular pathogenesis of asthma *47*, 165 (1996)	Jeanne Fürst Jucker Gary P. Anderson
Iron and diphteria toxin production *19*, 283 (1975)	S. V. Gadre S. S. Rao
Effect of drugs on cholera toxin induced fluid in adult rabbit ileal loop *19*, 519 (1975)	B. B. Gaitonde P. H. Marker N. R. Rao
Drug action and assay by microbial kinetics *15*, 519 (1971)	E. R. Garrett
The pharmacokinetic basis of biological response quantification in toxicology, pharmacology and pharmacodynamics *21*, 105 (1977)	E. R. Garrett
The chemotherapy of enterobacterial infections *12*, 370 (1968)	L. P. Garrod
The use of neutrophils, macrophages and organ cultures to assess the penetration of human cells by antimicrobials *33*, 83 (1989)	Zell A. McGee Gary L. Gorby Wanda S. Updike
Progress in the chemotherapy of leprosy: Status, issues and prospects *34*, 421 (1990)	Robert H. Gelber
Metabolism of drugs and other foreign compounds by enzymatic mechanisms *6*, 11 (1963)	J. R. Gillette
The effects of morphine on cell proliferation *55*, 33 (2000) From outer to inner space: Traveling along a scientific career from astro-chemistry to drug research *57*, 181 (2001)	Jay A. Glasel
Orale Antidiabetika *30*, 281 (1986)	Heiner Glombik Rudi Weyer
Calmodulin: Effects of cell stimuli and drugs on cellular activation *45*, 33 (1995)	Margaret E. Gnegy
The art and science of contemporary drug development *16*, 194 (1972)	A. J. Gordon S. G. Gilgore
Basic mechanisms of drug action *7*, 11 (1964) Isolation and characterization of membrane drug receptors *20*, 323 (1976)	D. R. H. Gourley

Zusammenhänge zwischen Konstitution und Wirksamkeit bei Lokalanästhetica *4*, 353 (1962)	H. Grasshof
Recent advances in benzodiazepine receptor (BZR) binding studies *45*, 67 (1995) Quantitative structure-activity relationships of antihypertensive agents *53*, 53 (1999) Quantitative structure-activity relationships of cardiotonic agents *55*, 235 (2000) Quantitative structure-activity relationships of antianginal drugs *56*, 121 (2001)	Satya P. Gupta
Das Placeboproblem *1*, 279 (1959)	H. Haas H. Fink G. Härtefelder
The role of apoptosis in neurodegenerative diseases *48*, 55 (1997)	Iradj Hajimohamadreza J. Mark Treherne
Appetite suppression, pharmacology of *54*, 1 (2000)	Jason C. G. Halford John E. Blundell
Approaches to the rational design of bacterial vaccines *32*, 377 (1988)	Peter Hambleton Stephen D. Prior Andrew Robinson
Clinical field trial of bitoscanate in *Necator americanus* infection, South Thailand *19*, 64 (1975)	T. Harinasuta D. Bunnag
Pharmacological control of reproduction in women *12*, 47 (1968) Contraception – retrospect and prospect *21*, 293 (1977)	M. J. K. Harper
Drug latentiation *4*, 221 (1962)	N. J. Harper
Dopamine receptor diversity: Molecular and pharmacological perspectives *48*, 173 (1997)	Deborah S. Hartman Olivier Civelli
Chemotherapy of filariasis *9*, 191 (1966) Filariasis in India *18*, 173 (1974)	F. Hawking
Production and action of interferons: New insights into molecular mechanisms of gene regulation and expression *43*, 239 (1994)	Mark P. Hayes Kathryn C. Zoon

Recent studies in the field of indole compounds *6*, 75 (1963)	R. V. Heinzelmann J. Szmuszkovicz
Neuere Entwicklungen auf dem Gebiete therapeutisch verwendbarer organischer Schwefelverbindungen *4*, 9 (1962)	H. Herbst
Subclassification and nomenclature of α_1- and α_2-adrenoceptors *47*, 81 (1996)	J. Paul Hieble Robert R. Ruffolo
The management of acute diarrhea in children: An overview *19*, 527 (1975)	N. Hirschhorn
The tetracyclines *17*, 210 (1973)	J. J. Hlavka J. H. Booth
Chemotherapy for systemic mycoses *33*, 317 (1989) Antifungal therapy *44*, 87 (1995)	Paul D. Hoeprich
Endogenous sodium pump inhibition: Current status and therapeutic opportunities *46*, 9 (1996)	Norman K. Hollenberg Steven W. Graves
Calcium channel blockers in psychiatry *47*, 279 (1996)	Leo E. Hollister Enrique S. Garza-Trevino
The use of quantum chemical methods to study molecular mechanisms of drug action *34*, 9 (1990)	H.-D. Höltje M. Hense S. Marrer E. Maurhofer
Troglitazone and emerging glitazones: New avenues for potential therapeutic benefits beyond glycemic control *54*, 235 (2000)	Hiroyoshi Horikoshi Toshihiko Hashimoto Toshihiko Fujiwara
Relationship of induced antibody titres to resistance to experimental human infection *19*, 542 (1975)	R. B. Hornick R. A. Cash J. P. Libonati
Recent applications of mass spectrometry in pharmaceutical research *18*, 399 (1974)	G. Horváth
Risk assessment problems in chemical oncogenesis *31*, 257 (1987)	G. H. Hottendorf
Bacterial resistence to antibiotics: The role of biofilms *37*, 91 (1991)	Brian D. Hoyle J. William Costerton
Recent developments in disease-modifying antirheumatic-drugs *24*, 101 (1980)	I. M. Hunneyball

The pharmacology of homologous series *7*, 305 (1964)	H. R. Ing
Progress in the experimental chemotherapy of helminth infections. Part. 1. Trematode and cestode diseases *17*, 241 (1973)	P. J. Islip
Pharmacology of the brain: The hippocampus, learning and seizures *16*, 211 (1972)	I. Izquierdo A. G. Nasello
Cholinergic mechanism – monoamines relation in certain brain structures *16*, 334 (1972)	J. A. Izquierdo
The development of antifertility substances *7*, 133 (1964)	H. Jackson
Development of novel anti-inflammatory agents: A pharmacological perspective on leukotrienes and their receptors *46*, 115 (1996)	William T. Jackson Jerome H. Fleisch
Agents acting on central dopamine receptors *21*, 409 (1977)	P. C. Jain N. Kumar
Recent advances in the treatment of parasitic infections in man *18*, 191 (1974) The levamisole story *20*, 347 (1976)	P. A. J. Janssen
Recent developments in cancer chemotherapy *25*, 275 (1981)	K. Jewers
Search for pharmaceutically interesting quinazoline derivatives: Efforts and results (1969–1980) *26*, 259 (1982)	S. Johne
Serotonin in migraine: Theories, animal models and emerging therapies *51*, 219 (1998)	Kirk W. Johnson Lee A. Phebus Marlene L. Cohen
A review of advances in prescribing for teratogenic hazards *29*, 121 (1985)	E. Marshall Johnson
A comparative of bitoscanate, bephenium hydroxynaphthoate and tetrachlorethylene in hookworm infection *19*, 70 (1975)	S. Johnson
Polyamines and cerebral ischemia *50*, 193 (1998)	T. David Johnson
Tetanus in Punjab with particular reference to the role of muscle relaxants in its management *19*, 288 (1975)	S. S. Jolly J. Singh S. M. Singh

Virulence-enhancing effect of ferric ammonium citrate on *Vibrio cholerae* *19*, 546 (1975)	I. Joó
Alternative medicine: Herbal drugs and their critical appraisal – Part I *56*, 1 (2001)	Balawant S. Joshi Pushkar N. Kaul
Chemical teratogenesis *41*, 9 (1993) Chemical teratogenesis in humans: Biochemical and molecular mechanisms *49*, 25 (1997)	Mont R. Juchau
Sympathetic nervous system and experimental diabetes: role of adrenal medullary hormones *57*, 163 (2001)	Chaman Lal Kaul Poduri Ramarao
Drug molecules of marine origin *35*, 521 (1990) Alternative therapeutic modalities. Alternative medicine *47*, 251 (1996) Drug discovery: Past, present and future *50*, 9 (1998)	Pushkar N. Kaul
Alternative medicine: Herbal drugs and their critical appraisal *57*, 1 (2001)	Pushkar N. Kaul Balawant S. Joshi
Toxoplasmosis *18*, 205 (1974)	B. H. Kean
NMR spectroscopy in drug discovery: Tools for combinatorial chemistry, natural products, and metabolism research *55*, 137 (2000)	Paul A. Keifer
The application of high-throughput screening to novel lead discovery *51*, 245 (1998)	Barry A. Kenny Mark Bushfield David J. Parry-Smith Simon Fogarty Mark Treherne
Tabellarische Zusammenstellung über die Substruktur der Proteine *16*, 364 (1972)	R. Kleine
Bioactive peptide analogs: *In vivo* and *in vitro* production *34*, 287 (1990) Enzymatic generation of complex peptides *48*, 27 (1997)	Horst Kleinkauf Hans von Doehren
Opiate receptors: Search for new drugs *36*, 49 (1991) Luteinizing hormone regulators: Luteinizing hormone releasing hormone analogs, estrogens, opiates and estrogen-opiate hybrids *42*, 39 (1994)	Vera M. Kolb

Novel and unusual nucleosides as drugs *48*, 195 (1997) Biomimicry as a basis for drug disovery *51*, 185 (1998)	Vera M. Kolb
Experimental evaluation of antituber-culous compounds, with special reference to the effect of combined treatment *18*, 211 (1974)	F. Kradolfer
The oxidative metabolism of drugs and other foreign compounds *17*, 488 (1973)	F. Kratz
Die Amidinstruktur in der Arzneistofforschung *11*, 356 (1968)	A. Kreutzberger
Present data on the pathogenesis of tetanus *19*, 301 (1975) Tetanus: general and pathophysiological aspects: Achievement, failures, perspectives of elaboration of the problem *19*, 314 (1975)	G. N. Kryzhanovsky
Lipophilicity and drug activity *23*, 97 (1979)	H. Kubinyi
Klinisch-pharmakologische Kriterien in der Bewertung eines neuen Antibiotikums. Grundlagen und methodische Gesichtspunkte *23*, 327 (1978)	H. P. Kuemmerle
Regulation of NMDA receptors by ethanol *54*, 121 (2000)	Meena Kumari Maharaj K. Ticku
Recent advances in immunosuppressants *52*, 1 (1999)	Bijoy Kundu Sanjay K. Khare
Combinatorial chemistry: Polymer supported synthesis of peptide and nonpeptide libraries *53*, 89 (1999)	Bijoy Kundu Sanjay K. Khare Shiva K. Rastogi
Adrenergic receptor research: Recent developments *33*, 151 (1989)	George Kunos
Über neue Arzneimittel *1*, 531 (1959), *2*, 251 (1960), *3*, 369 (1961), *6*, 347 (1963), *10*, 360 (1966)	W. Kunz
Die Anwendung von Psychopharmaka in der psychosomatischen Medizin *10*, 530 (1966)	F. Labhardt
The bacterial cell surface and antimicrobial resistance *32*, 149 (1988)	Peter A. Lambert
Therapeutic measurement in tetanus *19*, 323 (1975)	D. R. Laurence

Purine analogs as CDK enzyme inhibitory agents: A survey and QSAR analysis *56*, 155 (2001)	Allen D. Lee Shijun Ren Eric J. Lien
Clinical application of cytokines and immunostimulation and immunosuppression *39*, 167 (1992)	Betty Lee Thomas L. Ciardelli
Physicochemical methods in pharmaceutical chemistry I. Spectrofluorometry *6*, 151 (1963)	H. G. Leemann K. Stich Margrit Thomas
Biochemical acyl hydroxylations 16, 229 (1972)	W. Lenk
Cholinesterase restoring therapy in tetanus *19*, 329 (1975)	G. Leonardi K. G. Nair F. D. Dastur
Perspective and overview of Chinese traditional medicine and contemporary pharmacology *47*, 131 (1996)	E. Leong Way Yong Qing-Liu Chieh-Fu Chen
The histamine H_3-receptor: A targeting for new drugs *39*, 127 (1992)	R. Leurs H. Timmerman
The medicinal chemistry and therapeutic potentials of the histamine H_3 receptor *45*, 107 (1995)	R. Leurs R.C. Vollinga H. Timmerman
Biliary excretion of drugs and other xenobiotics *25*, 361 (1981)	W. G. Levine
Structures, properties and disposition of drugs *29*, 67 (1985) Ribonucleotide reductase inhibitors as anti-cancer and antiviral agents *31*, 101 (1987) Fungal metabolites and Chinese herbal medicine as immunostimulants *34*, 395 (1990) Design and discovery of new drugs by stepping-up and stepping-down approaches *40*, 163 (1993)	Eric J. Lien
Immunopharmacological and biochemical bases of Chinese herbal medicine *46*, 263 (1996)	Eric J. Lien Arima Das Linda J. Lien
Physicochemical basis of the universal genetic codes – quantitative analysis *48*, 9 (1997)	Eric J. Lien Arima Das Partha Nandy Shijun Ren

In search of ideal antihypertensive drugs: Progress in five decades *43*, 43 (1994)	Eric J. Lien Hua Gao Linda L. Lien
Interactions between androgenic-anabolic steroids and glucocorticoids *14*, 139 (1970)	O. Linet
Drug inhibition of mast cell secretion *29*, 277 (1985)	R. Ludowyke D. Lagunoff
Applications of yeast in drug discovery *57*, 11 (2001)	Doreen Ma
Reactivity of bentonite flocculation, indirect haemagglutination and Casoni tests in hydatid disease 19, 75 (1975)	R. C. Mahajan N. L. Chitkara
Characteristics of catechol O-methyltransferase (COMT) and properties of selective COMT inhibitors *39*, 291 (1992)	P.T. Männistö I. Ulmanen K. Lundström J. Taskinen J. Tenhunen C. Tilgmann S. Kaakkola
Interaction of cancer chemotherapy agents with the mononuclear phagocyte system *35*, 487 (1990)	Alberto Mantovani
Mechanisms of fibrinolysis and clinical use of thrombolytic agents *39*, 197 (1992)	Maurizio Margaglione Elvira Grandone Giovanni Di Minno
Drugs affecting plasma fibrinogen levels. Implications for new anti-thrombotic strategies *46*, 169 (1996)	M. Margaglione E. Grandone F. P. Mancini G. Di Minno
Epidemiology of diphtheria *19*, 336 (1975)	L. G. Marquis
Biological activity of the terpenoids and their derivatives *6*, 279 (1963)	M. Martin-Smith T. Khatoon
Biological activity of the terpenoids and their derivatives - recent advances *13*, 11 (1969)	M. Martin-Smith W. E. Sneader
Antihypertensive agents 1962–1968 *13*, 101 (1969) Fundamental structures in drug research - Part I *20*, 385 (1976) Fundamental structures in drug research - Part II *22*, 27 (1978)	A. Marxer O. Schier

Antihypertensive agents 1969–1980 *25*, 9 (1981)	A. Marxer O. Schier
Relationships between the chemical structure and pharmacological activity in a series of synthetic quinuclidine derivatives *13*, 293 (1969)	M. D. Mashkovsky L. N. Yakhontov
Further developments in research on the chemistry and pharmacology of synthetic quinuclidine derivatives *27*, 9 (1983)	M. D. Mashkovsky L. N. Yakhontov M. E. Kaminka E. E. Mikhlina S. Ordzhonikidze
Role of neutrotransmitters in the central regulation of the cardiovascular system *35*, 25 (1990) Neurotransmitters involved in the central regulation of the cardiovascular system *46*, 43 (1996)	Robert B. McCall
On the understanding of drug potency 13, 123 (1971) The chemotherapy of intestinal nematodes *16*, 157 (1972)	J. W. McFarland
Non-steroidal menses-regulating agents: The present status *44*, 159 (1995)	P.K. Mehrotra Sanjay Batra A.P. Bhaduri
Zur Beeinflussung der Strahlen-empfindlichkeit von Säugetieren durch chemische Substanzen *9*, 11 (1966)	H.-J. Melching C. Streffer
Analgesia and addiction *5*, 155 (1963)	L. B. Mellett L. A. Woods
Comparative drug metabolism *13*, 136 (1969)	L. B. Mellett
Prostate cancer and the androgen receptor: Strategies for the development of novel therapeutics *55*, 213 (2000)	Laurane G. Mendelsohn
The oral antiarrhythmic drugs *35*, 151 (1990)	Lisa Mendes Scott L. Beau John S. Wilson Philip J. Podrid
Mechanism of action of anxiolytic drugs *31*, 315 (1987)	T. Mennini S. Caccia S. Garattini
Pathogenesis of amebic disease *18*, 225 (1974) Protozoan and helminth parasites – a review of current treatment *20*, 433 (1976)	M. J. Miller

Medicinal agents incorporating the 1,2-diamine functionality *33,* 135 (1989)	Erik T. Michalson Jacob Szmuszkovicz
Fluorinated quinolones-new quinolone antimicrobials *38,* 9 (1992)	S. Mitsuhashi (Editor) T. Kojima, N. Nakanishi, T. Fujimoto, S. Goto, S. Miyusaki, T. Uematsu, M. Nakashima, Y. Asahina, T. Ishisaki, S. Susue, K. Hirai, K. Sato, K. Hoshino, J. Shimada, S. Hori
Synopsis der Rheumatherapie *12,* 165 (1968)	W. Moll
On the chemotherapy of cancer *8,* 431 (1965) The relationship of the metabolism of anticancer agents to their activity *17,* 320 (1973) The current status of cancer chemotherapy *20,* 465 (1976)	J. A. Montgomery
Present status of Leishmaniasis *34,* 447 (1990)	Anita Mukherjee Manju Seth A. P. Bhaduri
The significance of DNA technology in medicine *33,* 397 (1989)	Hansjakob Müller
Der Einfluß der Formgebung auf die Wirkung eines Arzneimittels *10,* 204 (1966) Galenische Formgebung und Arzneimittelwirkung. Neue Erkenntnisse und Feststellungen *14,* 269 (1970)	K. Münzel
Effects of NSAIDs on the kidney *49,* 155 (1997)	M. D. Murray D. Craig Brater
A field trial with bitoscanate in India *19,* 81 (1975)	G. S. Mutalik R. B. Gulati A. K. Iqbal
Comparative study of bitoscanate, bephenium hydroxynaphthoate and tetrachlorethylene in hookworm disease *19,* 86 (1975)	G. S. Mutalik R. B. Gulati
Ganglienblocker *2,* 297 (1960)	K. Nádor
Nitroimidazoles as chemotherapeutic agents *27,* 162 (1983)	M. D. Nair K. Nagarajan
Recent advances in cholera pathophysiology and therapeutics *19,* 563 (1975)	D. R. Nalin

Preparing the ground for research: Importance of data *18*, 239 (1974)	A. N. D. Nanavati
Computer-assisted structure – antileukemic activity analysis of purines and their aza and deaza analogs *34*, 319 (1990)	V. L. Narayanan Mohamed Nasr Kenneth D. Paull
Mechanism of drugs action on ion and water transport in renal tubular cells *26*, 87 (1982)	Yu. V. Natochin
Progesterone receptor binding of steroidal and nonsteroidal compounds *30*, 151 (1986)	Neelima M. Seth A. P. Bhaduri
Recent advances in drugs against hypertension *29*, 215 (1985)	Neelima B. K. Bhat A. P. Bhaduri
High resolution nuclear magnetic resonance spectroscopy of biological samples as an aid to drug development *31*, 427 (1987)	J. K. Nicholson Ian D. Wilson
Antibody response to two cholera vaccines in volunteers *19*, 554 (1975)	Y. S. Nimbkar R. S. Karbhari S. Cherian N. G. Chanderkar R. P. Bhamaria P. S. Ranadive B. B. Gaitonde
Surface interaction between bacteria and phagocytic cells *32*, 137 (1988)	L. Öhman G. Maluszynska K. E. Magnusson O. Stendahl
Die Chemotherapie der Wurmkrankheiten *1*, 159 (1959)	H.-A. Oelkers
Structural modifications patterns from agonists to antagonists and their application to drug design – A new serotonin($5HT_3$)antagonist series *41*, 313 (1993)	Hiroshi Ohtaka Toshio Fujita
Serenics *42*, 167 (1994)	Berend Olivier Jan Mos Maikel Raghoeba Paul de Koning Marianne Mak

The 5-HT_{1A} receptor and its ligands: structure and function *52*, 103 (1999) Serotonin, dopamine and norepinephrine transporters in the central nervous system and their inhibitors *54*, 59 (2000)	Berend Olivier Willem Soudijn Ineke van Wijngaarden
GABA-Drug interactions *31*, 223 (1987)	Richard W. Olsen
Drug research and human sleep *22*, 355 (1978)	I. Oswald
Effects of drugs on calmodulin-mediated enzymatic actions *33*, 353 (1989)	Judit Ovádi
An extensive community outbreak of acute diarrhoeal diseases in children *19*, 570 (1975)	S. C. Pal C. Koteswar Rao
Drug and its action according to Ayurveda *26*, 55 (1982)	Madhabendra Nath Pal
Oligosaccharide chains of glycoproteins *32*, 163 (1990)	Y. T. Pan Alan D. Elbein
Pharmacology of synthetic organic selenium compounds *36*, 9 (1991)	Michael J. Parnham Erich Graf
Moral challenges in the organisation and management of drug research *42*, 9 (1994)	Michael J. Parnham
3,4-Dihydroxyphenylalanine and related compounds *9*, 223 (1966)	A. R. Patel A. Burger
Mescaline and related compounds *11*, 11 (1968)	A. R. Patel
Experience with bitoscanate in adults *19*, 90 (1975)	A. H. Patricia U. Prabakar Rao R. Subramaniam N. Madanagopalan
The impact of state and society on medical research *35*, 9 (1990)	C. R. Pfaltz
Transfer factor in malignancy *42*, 401 (1994)	Giancarlo Pizza Caterina De Vinci H. Hugh Fudenberg
Monoaminoxydase-Hemmer *2*, 417 (1960)	A. Pletscher K. F. Gey P. Zeller
Antifungal therapy: Are we winning? *37*, 183 (1991)	A. Polak P. G. Hartman

Antifungal therapy, an everlasting battle *49*, 219 (1997)	A. Polak
Neuropeptides in drug research *54*, 161 (2000)	David Poyner Helen Cox Mark Bushfield J. Mark Treherne Melissa K. Demetrikopoulos
What makes a good pertussis vaccine? *19*, 341 (1975) Vaccine composition in relation to antigenic variation of the microbe: Is pertussis unique? *19*, 347 (1975) Some unsolved problems with vaccines *23*, 9 (1979) Eradication by vaccination: The memorial to smallpox could be surrounded by others *41*, 151 (1993)	N. W. Preston
Peptide drug delivery into the central nervous system *51*, 95 (1998)	Laszlo Prokai
Antibiotics in the chemotherapy of malaria *26*, 167 (1982)	S. K. Puri G. P. Dutta
Potassium channel openers: Airway pharmacology and clinical possibilities in asthma *37*, 161 (1991)	David Raeburn Jan-Anders Karlsson
Isozyme-selective cyclic nucleotide phosphodiesterase inhibitors: Biochemistry, pharmacology and therapeutic potential in asthma *40*, 9 (1993)	David Raeburn John E. Souness Adrian Tomkinson Jan-Anders Karlsson
Clinical study of diphtheria, tetanus and pertussis *19*, 356 (1975)	V. B. Raju V. R. Parvathi
Epidemiology of cholera in Hyderabad *19*, 578 (1975)	K. Rajyalakshmi P. V. Ramana Rao
Present status of hepatoprotectants *52*, 53 (1999)	Vishnu Ji Ram Atul Goel
Adenosine receptors: Clinical implications and biochemical mechanisms *32*, 195 (1988)	Vickram Ramkumar George Pierson Gary L. Stiles
New synthetic ligands for L-type voltage-gated calcium channels *40*, 191 (1993)	David Rampe David J. Triggle
Problems of malaria eradication in India *18*, 245 (1974)	V. N. Rao
Pharmacology of migraine *34*, 209 (1990)	Neil H. Raskin

The photochemistry of drugs and related substances *11*, 48 (1968)	S. T. Reid
Natural products and their derivatives as cancer chemopreventive agents *48*, 147 (1997) Development of HIV protease inhibitors: A survey *51*, 1 (1998) Caco-2 cell permeability vs. gastrointestinal absorption: QSPR analysis *54*, 35 (2000)	Shijun Ren Eric J. Lien
Orale Antikoagulantien *11*, 226 (1968)	E. Renk W. G. Stoll
In search of ideal inotropic steroids: Recent progress *47*, 9 (1996)	Kurt R.H. Repke Kathleen J. Sweadner Jürgen Weiland Rudolf Megges Rudolf Schön
Glucosamine and chondroitine sulfates in the treatment of osteoarthritis: a survey *55*, 105 (2000)	Gerlie C. de los Reyes Robert T. Koda Eric J. Lien
Mechanism-based inhibitors of monoamine oxidase *30*, 205 (1986)	Lauren E. Richards Alfred Burger
Anti-influenza drugs and neuraminidase inhibitors *56*, 195 (2001)	Noel A. Roberts
Glutamatergic involvement in psychomotor stimulant action *50*, 155 (1998)	Robin W. Rockhold
The hopanoids, bacterial triterpenoids, and the biosynthesis of isoprenic units in prokaryote *37*, 271 (1991)	Michel Rohmer Philippe Bisseret Bertrand Sutter
Isoprenoids biosynthesis via the mevalonate-independent route, a novel target for antibacterial drugs? *50*, 135 (1998)	Michel Rohmer
Tetrahydroisoquinolines and β-carbolines: Putative natural substances in plants and animals *29*, 415 (1985)	H. Rommelspacher R. Susilo
Functional significance of the various components of the influenza virus *18*, 253 (1974)	R. Rott

Drug receptors and control of the cardiovascular system: Recent advances *36*, 117 (1991)	Robert R. Ruffolo Jr J. Paul Hieble David P. Brooks Giora Z. Feuerstein Andrew J. Nichols
Behavioral correlates of presynaptic events in the cholinergic neurotransmitter system *32*, 43 (1988)	Roger W. Russell
Epidemiology of pertussis *19*, 257 (1975)	J. A. Sa
Surgical amoebiasis *18*, 77 (1974)	A. E. de Sa
Role of beta-adrenergic blocking drug propranolol in severe tetanus *19*, 361 (1975)	G. S. Sainani K. L. Jain V. R. D. Deshpande A. B. Balsara S. A. Iyer
Studies on *Vibrio parahaemolyticus* in Bombay *19*, 586 (1975)	F. L. Saldanha A. K. Patil M. V. Sant
Leukotriene antagonists and inhibitors of leukotriene biosynthesis as potential therapeutic agents *37*, 9 (1991)	John A. Salmon Lawrence G. Garland
Pharmacology and toxicology of axoplasmic transport *28*, 53 (1984)	Fred Samson Ralph L. Smith J. Alejandro Donoso
Clinical experience with bitoscanate *19*, 96 (1975)	M. R. Samuel
Tetanus: Situational clinical trials and therapeutics *19*, 367 (1975)	R. K. M. Sanders M. L. Peacock B. Martyn B. D. Shende
Epidemiological studies on cholera in non-endemic regions with special reference to the problem of carrier state during epidemic and non-epidemic period *19*, 594 (1975)	M. V. Sant W. N. Gatlewar S. K. Bhindey
Epidemiological and biochemical studies in filariasis in four villages near Bombay *18*, 269 (1974)	M. V. Sant W. N. Gatlewar T. U. K. Menon
Hookworm anaemia and intestinal malabsorption associated with hookworm infestation *19*, 108 (1975)	A. K. Saraya B. N. Tandon

The effects of structural alteration on the anti-inflammatory properties of hydrocortisone *5*, 11 (1963)	L. H. Sarett A. A. Patchett S. Steelman
The impact of natural product research on drug discovery *23*, 51 (1979)	L. H. Sarett
Aldose reductase inhibitors: Recent developments *40*, 99 (1993)	Reinhard Sarges Peter J. Oates
Anti-filariasis campaign: Its history and future prospects *18*, 259 (1974)	M. Sasa
Barbiturates and the $GABA_A$ receptor complex *34*, 261 (1990)	Paul A. Saunders I. K. Ho
Platelets and atherosclerosis *29*, 49 (1985)	Robert N. Saunders
Immuno-diagnosis of helminthic infections *19*, 119 (1975)	T. Sawada K. Sato K. Takei
Immuno-diagnosis in filarial infection *19*, 128 (1975)	T. Sawada K. Sato K. Takei M. M. Goil
Quantitative structure-activity relationships *23*, 199 (1979)	Anil K. Saxena S. Ram
Advances in chemotherapy of malaria *30*, 221 (1986) Developments in antihistamines (H_1) *39*, 35 (1992) Developments in anticonvulsants *44*, 185 (1995)	Anil K. Saxena Mridula Saxena
Pyrimidinones as biodynamic agents *31*, 127 (1987)	Anil K. Saxena Shradha Sinha
Phenothiazine und Azaphenothiazine als Arzneimittel *5*, 269 (1963)	E. Schenker H. Herbst
Antihypertensive agents *4*, 295 (1962)	E. Schlittler J. Druey
Endogenous digitalis-like factors *41*, 249 (1993)	Wilhelm Schoner
Die Anwendung radioaktiver Isotope in der pharmazeutischen Forschung *7*, 59 (1964)	K. E. Schulte

Natürliche und synthetische Acetylen-Verbindungen als Arzneistoffe *14*, 387 (1970)	K. E. Schulte G. Rücker
The role of cytokines in macrophage activation *35*, 105 (1990) The potential role of cytokines in cancer therapy *39*, 219 (1992) Newer antifolates in cancer therapy *44*, 129 (1995)	Richard M. Schultz
Central control of aterial pressure by drugs *26*, 353 (1982)	A. Scriabine D. G. Taylor E. Hong
Pharmacological properties of the natural polyamines and their depletion by biosynthesis inhibitors as a therapeutic approach *37*, 107 (1991)	Nikolaus Seiler
The natural polyamines and the immune system *43*, 87 (1994)	Nikolaus Seiler C. L. Atanassov
Aminoglycosides and polyamines: Targets and effects in the mammalian organism of two important groups of natural aliphatic polycations *46*, 183 (1996)	N. Seiler A. Hardy J. P. Moulinoux
Chemistry and pharmacology of cannabis *36*, 71 (1991)	Renu Seth Shradha Sinha
The structure and biogenesis of certain antibiotics *2*, 591 (1960)	W. A. Sexton
Quinolones *31*, 243 (1987)	P. M. Shah
Role of periodic deworming of pre-school community in national nutrition programmes *19*, 136 (1975)	P. M. Shah A. E. Junnarkar R. D. Khare
Advances in the treatment and control of tissue-dwelling helminth parasites *30*, 473 (1986) The benzimidazole anthelmitics chemistry and biological activity *27*, 85 (1983) Treatment of helminth diseases, challenges and achievements *31*, 9 (1987) Vector-borne diseases *35*, 365 (1990)	Satyavan Sharma

Chemotherapy of cestode infections *24,* 217 (1980)	Satyavan Sharma S. K. Dubey R. N. Iyer
Chemotherapy of hookworm infections *26,* 9 (1982)	Satyavan Sharma Elizabeth S. Charles
Ayurvedic medicine – past and present *15,* 11 (1971)	Shiv Sharma
Mechanisms of anthelmintic action *19,* 147 (1975)	U. K. Sheth
Aspirin as an antithrombotic agent *33,* 43 (1989)	Melvin J. Silver Giovanni Di Minno
Immunopharmacological approach to the study of chronic brain disorders *30,* 345 (1986) Implications of immunomodulant therapy in Alzheimer's disease *32,* 21 (1988)	Vijendra K. Singh H. Hugh Fudenberg
Neuroimmune axis as a basis of therapy in Alzheimer's disease *34,* 383 (1990) Immunoregulatory role of neuropeptides *38,* 149 (1992) Neuropeptides as native immune modulators *45,* 9 (1995) Immunotherapy for brain diseases and mental illnesses *48,* 129 (1997)	Vijendra K. Singh
Natural products as anticancer agents *42,* 53 (1994)	Shradha Sinha Sudha Jain
Biologically active quinazolones *43,* 143 (1994)	Shradha Sinha Mukta Srivastava
Some often neglected factors in the control and prevention of communicable diseases *18,* 277 (1974)	C. E. G. Smith
Tetanus and its prevention *19,* 391 (1975)	J. W. G. Smith
Growth of *Clostridium tetani in vivo* *19,* 384 (1975)	J. W. G. Smith A. G. MacIver
The biliary excretion and enterohepatic circulation of drugs and other organic compounds *9,* 299 (1966)	R. L. Smith
Applications of developmental biology to medicine and animal agriculture *54,* 191 (2000)	Rosamund C. Smith Simon J. Rhodes

Noninvasive pharmacodynamic and bioelectric methods for elucidating the bioavailability mechanisms of ophthalmic drug preparations *25*, 421 (1981)	V. F. Smolen
On the relation between chemical structure and function in certain tumor promoters and anti-tumor agents *23*, 63 (1979) Relationships between structure and function of convulsant drugs *24*, 57 (1980)	J. R. Smythies
Gram-negative bacterial endotoxin and the pathogenesis of fever *19*, 402 (1975)	E. S. Snell
Benzodiazepine augmentation of the treatment of disruptive psychotic behavior *35*, 139 (1990)	David A. Solomon Edison Miyawaki Carl Salzman
Chemokines as targets for pharmacological intervention *47*, 53 (1996)	Silvano Sozzani Paola Allavena Paul Proost Jo Van Damme Alberto Mantovani
From genome to drug – optimising the drug discovery process *53*, 157 (1999)	Paul Spence
Emerging concepts towards the development of contraceptive agents *33*, 267 (1989)	Ranjan P. Srivastava A. P. Bhaduri
Strukturelle Betrachtungen der Psychopharmaka: Versuch einer Korrelation von chemischer Konstitution und klinischer Wirkung *9*, 129 (1966)	K. Stach W. Pöldinger
From podophyllotoxin glucoside to etoposide *33*, 169 (1989)	H. Stähelin A. von Wartburg
Chemotherapy of intestinal helminthiasis *19*, 158 (1975)	O. D. Standen
Immunotherapy for leprosy and tuberculosis *33*, 415 (1989)	J. L. Stanford
The leishmaniasis *18*, 289 (1974)	E. A. Steck
The benzodiazepine story *22*, 229 (1978)	L. H. Sternbach

Immunostimulation with peptidoglycan or its synthetic derivatives *32,* 305 (1988)	Duncan E. S. Stewart-Tull
Hypertension: Relating drug therapy to pathogenic mechanisms *32,* 175 (1988)	David H. P. Streeten Gunnar H. Anderson Jr
Progress in sulfonamide research *12,* 389 (1968) Problems of medical practice and of medical-pharmaceutical research *20,* 491 (1976)	Th. Struller
Bacterial resistance to β-lactam antibiotics: Problems and solutions *41,* 95 (1993)	R. Sutherland
Antiviral agents 22, 267 (1978) Antiviral agents 1978–1983 *28,* 127 (1984)	D. L. Swallow
Ketoconazole, a new step in the management of fungal disease *27,* 63 (1983)	J. Symoens G. Cauwenbergh
Antiarrhythmic compounds *12,* 292 (1968)	L. Szekeres J. G. Papp
U-50,488 and the κ receptor: a personalized account covering the period 1973–1990 *52,* 167 (1999) U-50,488 fand the κ receptor. Part II: 1991–1998 *53,* 1 (1999)	Jacob Szmuszkovicz
Practically applicable results of twenty years of research in endocrinology *12,* 137 (1968)	M. Tausk
Stereoselective drug metabolism and its significance in drug research *32,* 249 (1988)	Bernard Testa Joachim M. Mayer
Age profile of diphtheria in Bombay *19,* 412 (1975)	N. S. Tibrewala R. D. Potdar S. B. Talathi M. A. Ramnathkar A. D. Katdare
On conformation analysis, molecular graphics, fentanyl and its derivatives *30,* 91 (1986)	J. P. Tollenaere H. Moereels M. van Loon
Antibakterielle Chemotherapie der Tuberkulose *7,* 193 (1964)	F. Trendelenburg
Alternative approaches to the discovery of novel antipsychotic agents *38,* 299 (1992)	M. D. Tricklebank L. J. Bristow P. H. Hutson

Insulin resistance, impaired glucose tolerance and non-insulin-dependent diabetes, pathologic mechanisms and treatment: Current status and therapeutic possibilities *51*, 33 (1998)	Nicholas C. Turner John C. Clapham
Diphtheria *19*, 423 (1975)	P. M. Udani M. M. Kumbhat U. S. Bhat M. S. Nadkarni S. K. Bhave S. G. Ezuthachan B. Kamath
Biologische Oxydation und Reduktion am Stickstoff aromatischer Amino- und Nitroderivate und ihre Folgen für den Organismus *8*, 195 (1965) Stoffwechsel von Arzneimitteln als Ursache von Wirkungen, Nebenwirkungen und Toxizität *15*, 147 (1971)	H. Uehleke
Mode of death in tetanus *19*, 439 (1975)	H. Vaishnava C. Bhawal Y. P. Munjal
Comparative evaluation of amoebicidal drugs *18*, 353 (1974) Comparative efficacy of newer anthelmintics *19*, 166 (1975)	B. J. Vakil N. J. Dalal
Cephalic tetanus *19*, 443 (1975)	B. J. Vakil B. S. Singhal S. S. Pandya P. F. Irami
G protein coupled receptors as modules of interacting proteins: A family meeting *49*, 173 (1997)	Olivier Valdenaire Philippe Vernier
Multi-dimensional QSAR in drug research *55*, 105 (2000)	Angelo Vedani Max Dobler
The effect and usefulness of early intravenous beta blockade in acute myocardial infarction *30*, 71 (1986)	Anders Vedin Claes Wilhelmsson
Methods of monitoring adverse reactions to drugs *21*, 231 (1977) Aspects of social pharmacology *22*, 9 (1978)	J. Venulet

The current status of cholera toxoid research in the United States *19*, 602 (1975)	W. F. Verwey J. C. Guckian J. Craig N. Pierce J. Peterson H. Williams Jr
Current and potential therapies for the treatment of herpesvirus infections *56*, 77 (2001)	Elcira C. Villarreal
Systemic cancer therapy: Four decades of progress and some personal perspectives *34*, 76 (1990)	Charles L. Vogel
Abnormalities of protein kinases in neurodegenerative diseases *51*, 133 (1998)	Ravenska T. E. Wagey Charles Krieger
The problem of diphtheria as seen in Bombay *19*, 452 (1975)	M. M. Wagle R. R. Sanzgiri Y. K. Amdekar
Drug nephrotoxicity – The significance of cellular mechanisms *41*, 51 (1993)	Robert J. Walker J. Paul Fawcett
Protease inhibitors as potential antiviral agents for the treatment of picornaviral infections *52*, 197 (1999)	Q. May Wang
Recent advances in prevention and treatment of hepatitis C virus infection *55*, 1 (2000)	Q. May Wang Beverly A. Heinz
Nicotine: An addictive substance or a therapeutic agent? *33*, 9 (1989)	David M. Warburton
Cell-wall antigens of *Vibrio cholerae* and their implication in cholera immunity *19*, 612 (1975)	Y. Watanabe R. Ganguly
Steroidogenic capacity in the adrenal cortex and its regulation *34*, 359 (1990)	Michael R. Watermann Evan R. Simpson
Antigen-specific T-cell factors and drug research *32*, 9 (1988)	David R. Webb
Where is immunology taking us? *20*, 573 (1976) Immunology in drug research *28*, 233 (1984)	W. J. Wechter Barbara E. Loughman
Natriuretic hormones *34*, 231 (1990)	W. J. Wechter Elaine J. Benaksas

The effects of NSAIDs and E-prostaglandins on bone: A two signal hypothesis for the maintenance of skeletal bone *39*, 351 (1992)	William J. Wechter
Metabolic activation of chemical carcinogens *26*, 143 (1982)	E. K. Weisburger
A pharmacological approach to allergy *3*, 409 (1961) Adverse reactions of sugar polymers in animals and man *23*, 27 (1979) Biogenic amines and drug research *28*, 9 (1984)	G. B. West
A new approach to the medical interpretation of shock *14*, 196 (1970)	G. B. West, M. S. Starr
Recent progress in understanding cholinergic function at the cellular and molecular levels *39*, 251 (1992)	V. P. Whittaker
Some biochemical and pharmacological properties of antiinflammatory drugs *8*, 321 (1965)	M. W. Whitehouse
Wirksamkeit und Nebenwirkungen von Metronidazol in der Therapie der Trichomonasis *9*, 361 (1966)	K. Wiesner, H. Fink
Carcinogenicity testing of drugs *29*, 155 (1985)	G. M. Williams, J. H. Weisburger
Organizing for drug discovery *32*, 329 (1988)	Michael Williams, Gary L. Neil
Drug treatment of asthma *28*, 111 (1984)	Archie F. Wilson
Cooperative effects in drug-DNA interactions *31*, 193 (1987)	W. David Wilson
Nonsteroid antiinflammatory agents *10*, 139 (1966)	C. A. Winter
A review of the continuum of drug-induced states of excitation and depression *26*, 225 (1982)	W. D. Winters
Basic research in the US pharmaceutical industry *15*, 204 (1971)	O. Wintersteiner
Light and dark as a "drug" *31*, 383 (1987)	Anna Wirz-Justice
Neuronal prostacyclin receptors *49*, 123 (1997)	Helen Wise

Dioxopiperazines: Chemistry and biology *35*, 249 (1990)	Donald T. Witiak Yong Wey
The chemotherapy of amoebiasis *8*, 11 (1965)	G. Woolfe
Antimetabolites and their revolution in pharmacology *2*, 613 (1960)	D. W. Woolley
Noise analysis and channels and the postsynaptic membrane of skeletal muscle *24*, 9 (1980)	D. Wray
Krebswirksame Antibiotika aus Actinomyceten *3*, 451 (1961)	Kh. Zepf
Developments in histamine H_1-receptor agonists *44*, 49 (1995)	V. Zingel C. Leschke W. Schunack
Fifteen years of structural modifications in the field of antifungal monocyclic 1-substituted 1 H-azoles *27*, 253 (1983)	L. Zirngibl
Lysostaphin: Model for a specific enzymatic approach to infectious disease *16*, 309 (1972)	W. A. Zygmunt P. A. Tavormina

Backlist

Vol. 1–47 available

Vol. 48, 1997, 288 pp. ISBN 3-7643-5671-5

Eric J. Lien, Arima Das, Partha Nandy and Shijun Ren: Physicochemical basis of the universal genetic codes – quantitative analysis

Horst Kleinkauf and Hans von Döhren: Enzymatic generation of complex peptides

Iradj Hajimohamadreza and J. Mark Treherne: The role of apoptosis in neurodegenerative diseases

Esteban Domingo, Luis Menéndez-Arias, Miguel E. Quiñones-Mateu, Africa Holguín, Mónica Gutiérrez-Rivas, Miguel A. Martínez, Josep Quer, Isabel S. Novella and John J. Holland: Viral quasispecies and the problem of vaccine-escape and drug-resistant mutants

Vijendra K. Singh: Immunotherapy for brain diseases and mental illnesses

Shijun Ren and Eric J. Lien: Natural products and their derivatives as cancer chemopreventive agents

Deborah S. Hartman and Olivier Civelli: Dopamine receptor diversity: Molecular and pharmacological perspectives

Vera M. Kolb: Novel and unusual nucleosides as drugs

Vol. 49, 1997, 373 pp. ISBN 3-7643-5672-3

Richard M. Eglen: 5-Hydroxytryptamine (5-HT)4 receptors and central nervous system function: An update

Mont R. Juchau: Chemical teratogenesis in humans: Biochemical and molecular mechanisms

Gillian Edwards and Arthur H. Weston: Recent advances in potassium channel modulation

Helen Wise: Neuronal prostacyclin receptors

M.D. Murray and D. Craig Brater: Effects of NSAIDs on the kidney

Olivier Valdenaire and Philippe Vernier: G protein coupled receptors as modules of interacting proteins: A family meeting

Annemarie Polak: Antifungal therapy, an everlasting battle

Vol. 50, 1998, 373 pp. ISBN 3-7643-5821-1

P.N. Kaul: Drug discovery: Past, present and future

G. Edwards and A.H. Weston: Endothelium-derived hyperpolarizing factor – a critical appraisal

M. Rohmer: Isoprenoid biosynthesis via the mevalonate-independent route, a novel target for antibacterial drugs

R.W. Rockhold: Glutamatergic involvement in psychomotor stimulant action

T.D. Johnson: Polyamines and cerebral ischemia

J.M. Colacino and K.A. Staschke: The identification and development of antiviral agents for the treatment of chronic hepatitis B virus infection

Vol. 51, 1998, 330 pp. ISBN 3-7643-5822-X

Shijun Ren and Eric J. Lien: Development of HIV protease inhibitors: A survey

Nicholas C. Turner and John C. Clapham: Insulin resistance, impaired glucose tolerance and non-insulin-dependent diabetes, pathologic mechanisms and treatment: Current status and therapeutic possibilities

P.N. Kaul: Drug discovery: Past, present and future

G. Edwards and A.H. Weston: Endothelium-derived hyperpolarizing factor – a critical appraisal

M. Rohmer: Isoprenoid biosynthesis via the mevalonate-independent route, a novel target for antibacterial drugs

R.W. Rockhold: Glutamatergic involvement in psychomotor stimulant action

T.D. Johnson: Polyamines and cerebral ischemia

J.M. Colacino and K.A. Staschke: The identification and development of antiviral agents for the treatment of chronic hepatitis B virus infection

Vol. 52, 1999, 280 pp. ISBN 3-7643-5979-X

Bijoy Kundu and Sanjay K. Khare: Recenc advances in immunosuppressants

Vishnu J. Ram and Atul Goel: Present status of hepatoprotectants

Berend Olivier, Willem Soudijn and Ineke van Wijngarden: The $5HT_{1A}$ receptor and its ligands: structure and function
Jacob Szmuszkovicz: U-50,488 and the κ receptor: A personalized account covering the period of 1973–1990
Q. May Wang: Protease inhibitors as potential antiviral agents for the treatment of picornaviral infections

Vol. 53, 1999, 290 pp. ISBN 3-7643-6028-3
Jacob Szmuszkovicz: U-50,488 and the κ receptor: Part II: 1991–1998
Satya P. Gupta: Quantitative structure-activity relationships of antihypertensive agents
Bijoy Kundu, Sanjay K. Khare and Shiva K. Rastogi: Combinatorial chemistry: Polymer supported synthesis of peptide and nonpeptide libraries
Paul Spence: From genome to drug – optimising the drug discovery process
Mary S. Barnette: Phosphodiesterase 4 (PDE4) inhibitors in asthma and chronic obstructive pulmonary disease (COPD)

Vol. 54, 2000, 320 pp. ISBN 3-7643-6113-1
Shijun Ren and Eric J. Lien: Caco-2 cell permeability vs human gastrointestinal absorption: QSPR analysis
Jason C.G. Halford and John E. Blundell: Pharmacology of appetite suppression
Berend Olivier, Willem Soudijn and Ineke van Wijngaarden: Serotonin, dopamine and norepinephrine transporters in the central nervous system and their inhibitors
David Poyner, Helen Cox, Mark Bushfield, J. Mark Treherne and Melissa K. Demetrikopoulos: Neuropeptides in drug research
Meena Kumari and Maharaj K. Ticku: Regulation of NMDA receptors by ethanol
Hiroyoshi Horikoshi, Toshihiko Hashimoto and Toshihiko Fujiwara: Troglitazone and emerging glitazones: New avenues for potential therapeutic benefits beyond glycemic control
Rosamund C. Smith and Simon J. Rhodes: Applications of developmental biology to medicine and animal agriculture

Vol. 55, 2000, 344 pp. ISBN 3-7643-6193-X
Q. May Wang and Beverly A. Heinz: Recent advances in prevention and treatment of hepatitis C virus infections
Jay A. Glasel: The effects of morphine on cell proliferation
Gerlie C. de los Reyes, Robert T. Koda and Eric J. Lien: Glucosamine and chondroitin sulfates in the treatment of osteoarthritis: a survey
Angelo Vedani and Max Dobler: Multi-dimensional QSAR in drug research
Paul A. Keifer: NMR spectroscopy in drug discovery: Tools for combinatorial chemistry, natural products, and metabolism research
Laurane G. Mendelsohn: Prostate cancer and the androgen receptor: Strategies for the development of novel therapeutics
Satya P. Gupta: Quantitative structure-activity relationships of cardiotonic agents

Vol. 56, 2001, 300 pp. ISBN 3-7643-6265-0
Balawant S. Joshi and Pushkar N. Kaul: Alternative medicine: Herbal drugs and their critical appraisal – Part I
Elcira C. Villarreal: Current and potential therapies for the treatment of herpesvirus infections
Satya P. Gupta: Quantitiative structure-activity relationships of antianginal drugs
Allen D. Lee, Shijun Ren and Eric J. Lien: Purine analogs as CDK enzyme inhibitory agents: A survey and QSAR analysis
Noel A. Roberts: Anti-influenza drugs and neuraminidase inhibitors

MIX
Papier aus verantwortungsvollen Quellen
Paper from responsible sources
FSC® C105338

If you have any concerns about our products,
you can contact us on
ProductSafety@springernature.com

In case Publisher is established outside the EU,
the EU authorized representative is:
Springer Nature Customer Service Center GmbH
Europaplatz 3, 69115 Heidelberg, Germany

Printed by Libri Plureos GmbH
in Hamburg, Germany